Clinical Applications of Hypnosis

Developments in Clinical Psychology

Glenn R. Caddy, series editor
Nova University

MMPI-168 Codebook, by Ken R. Vincent, Iliana Castillo, Robert I. Hauser, H. James Stuart, Javier A. Zapata, Cal K. Cohn, and Gregory O'Shanick, 1984

Integrated Clinical and Fiscal Management in Mental Health: A Guidebook, by Fred Newman and James Sorensen, 1985

The Professional Practice of Psychology, edited by Georgiana Shick Tryon, 1986

Clinical Applications of Hypnosis, edited by Frank A. DePiano and Herman C. Salzberg, 1986

In Preparation:

The Behavioral Management of the Cardiac Patient, by D. G. Byrne

Advances in the Treatment of Addictive Behaviors, edited by Ted D. Nirenberg

Language and Psychopathology, by Stephen Schwartz

Clinical Applications of Hypnosis

edited by

Frank A. DePiano
Nova University
Ft. Lauderdale, Florida

Herman C. Salzberg
University of South Carolina, Columbia

Ablex Publishing Corporation
Norwood, New Jersey 07648

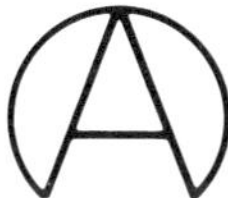

Printed in the United States of America.

Library of Congress Cataloging-in-Publication Data
Main entry under title:

Clinical applications of hypnosis.

(Developments in clinical psychology)
Includes bibliographies and index.
1. Hypnosis–Therapeutic use. I. DePiano, Frank A.
II. Salzberg, Herman C., 1931– . [DNLM: 1. Hypnosis.
WM 415 C6405]
RC495.C49 1985 615.8'512 85-13492
ISBN 0-89391-297-2

Ablex Publishing Corporation
355 Chestnut Street
Norwood, New Jersey 07648

Contents

Introduction

Hypnosis in an Historical Perspective

H. C. Salzberg and F. A. DePiano

It seems fitting to begin with a discussion of how hypnosis was used in the past in order to give us some perspective on how it is used today. Hypnosis once viewed as something mystical, supernatural, and fantastic has become a field of careful scientific inquiry.

Hypnosis, or various forms of suggestion, have been used as a device to treat many disorders since earliest recorded history. The Roman historian, Plutarch, related how Pyrrhus of Epicus would cure cases of colic by touching the sufferer with his big toe (Wolfe and Rosenthal, 1948). Bernheim (1947) wrote about the magnetic stone which the ancient Egyptians used in the preparation of their prophylactic amulets which cured gout, headaches, toothaches, and hysteria.

Rhodes (1915) gave an account of a man of the Christian Science faith who observing blood spurting from the mouth of his daughter who had fallen from a third story window, exclaimed, "There is one law–God's law–under which man remains perfect." The bleeding was said to have immediately stopped. Although temporarily paralyzed, the girl reportedly regained the use of her limbs through her own and her father's faith. Rhodes documents how the power of suggestion worked on some of the Malay inhabitants of Borneo. The cook of a coasting steamer had his baby brought to him when the ship was in port. He was known to be intensely devoted to and proud of the child. While he was cradling the baby in his arms on the deck of the steamer, one of the Malay crew came along with a load of wood which he pretended to nurse in his arms like a baby. He then began to toss the wood in the air catching it again as it fell, getting the man with the child in his arms to imitate him. The man did so, and then the sailor opened his arms and let the wood fall on the deck, the miserable father did likewise with the baby who fell heavily on the deck and never regained consciousness.

Craige (1934) reported an incident in which a Haitian man, after being shot at and missed, was so firmly convinced that he had been mortally wounded that he died. Another old habitant of Haiti announced that a "bocor" had put a "wanga" on him, and that he would die in three days at sunset. He did die, and on schedule. Apparently, the cause was purely psychic as no symptoms of poisoning were found. Baudouin (1921) has cited a report by Artault of a pregnant woman who met a man with a severe malformation of one of the nails on his hand. The woman became obsessed with this deformity. She became terrified lest her child be born with a similar deformity. Unfortunately, her child was born with a similar malformation of one of his fingernails. The above unsubstantiated reports serve to demonstrate how strong an influence suggestion can have on individuals, particularly those who are predisposed to be influenced because of their strong prior beliefs.

The relationship between hypnosis and psychotherapy began with the work of Anton Mesmer in the eighteenth century. An account of his rise and fall can be found in Chapter 7.

It was James Braid, an English surgeon trained in Mesmerism, who finally gave a reasonable scientific explanation of why Mesmer's method produced positive results. Braid dismissed the idea of magnetic fluid and renamed the procedure "hypnotism." He advanced the hypothesis that hypnotism and hypersuggestivity are brought about by having the patient fix his attention on some object. The method of induction he used involved having the patient fix his gaze on the glass stopper of a water bottle.

Jean Martin Charcot, an eminent French neurologist, was the first person to undertake scientific experiments using hypnosis. His studies were the first to deal with the hypothesis that forgotten memories could be retrieved under hypnosis.

Pierre Janet, Charcot's pupil and successor, investigated the use of hypnosis and hypnotic recall to create a sense of emotional catharsis in patients. Joseph Breuer and Sigmund Freud were also investigating the cathartic uses of hypnosis at the same time. Janet hypothesized that traumatic memories played a major role in producing hysterical symptoms and neurotic behavior. He advocated the use of hypnosis to uncover these forgotten memories and to encourage discharge of the affect which accompanied them. This was strikingly similar to the conclusions of Breuer and Freud who were also using hypnosis as the basis of their therapy (See Chapter 7 for an elaborate account of Freud's work with hypnosis).

More recently, Wilson (1951) reported on a prisoner who was capable of extraordinary hypnotic feats. He was said to be able to achieve a state of suspended animation, and come out of it at will, as illustrated when he awakened just in time to avoid having an autopsy performed on him. This prisoner was apparently able to hypnotize a guard who surrendered his belt without being aware of it. In a state of deathlike suspension, the prisoner was able to raise red welts on his skin which approximated the forms of the twelve signs of the zodiac. Wilson invited a neurologist to observe this Indian yogi perform all of these behaviors. The most unusual event reported was of this prisoner telling Wilson and the neurologist that none of the patients in the epileptic ward of the prison would have any seizures for 24 hours. After this period they would all have a seizure at a specific time of day, predicted the yogi. According to Wilson, this unexplained event occurred on schedule.

Another series of similar feats were described by Brunton (1935), a newspaper reporter who was alert for trickery. He related his observations of a yogi in Egypt who seemingly could stop his heart, pulse, and breathing for several hours. He also described seeing a yogi push skewers through his cheek without any apparent pain or bleeding. Brunton also wrote about a professor of chemistry at the University of Calcutta who observed a yogi lick a few drops of poisonous acid, and then stuff glowing charcoal into his mouth and keep it there until it stopped glowing. Later, a group of scientists gathered to watch him lick sulphuric acid, strong carbolic acid, and potassium cyanide. He was reported to have taken enough potassium cyanide to kill a man within three minutes, yet he remained apparently unharmed. He then proceeded to eat ground glass. When his stomach was later pumped, the poison was found. The glass was excreted the following day. Sir C. V. Raman, Nobel Prize winner, was present at the time, and described the performance as a challenge to modern science. The yogi had apparently counteracted the effects of the poison by going into a trance state. At a later time the same yogi attempted a similar feat, but was distracted by some unexpected visitors and did not achieve a trance. He died with tragic swiftness (Brunton, 1935).

Kuda Bux (Flesch, 1953) is reported to have driven a bicycle around town blindfolded. He also walked across red hot coals in his bare feet as attested to by a large number of medical men who set up rigid controls against trickery. There was no blistering or scarring found on his feet afterward. However, a medical student who tried to repeat Bux's feat immediately afterward received severe blistering.

Hypnosis has been used for surgery, instead of anesthetics, for over a century. Esdaile, an English surgeon who practiced in India in the middle of the last century, having learned of mesmerism, performed thousands of minor operations, some 300 major operations including 19 amputations. His specialty was removing the giant scrotal tumors which were common in India at the time. The usual mortality rate for this operation was 50 percent. In 161 of these cases Esdaile had only a 5 percent mortality rate and none of his patients died immediately following the operation (Marks, 1947).

Sampimon and Woodruff (1946), two Australian physicians, were held captive by the Japanese in a prison camp during World War II. They performed many operations on their fellow capitves using hypnosis, since anesthetics were unavailable. They found some advantages to using hypnotic anesthesia such as the elimination of nervousness, full cooperation by the patient, eradication of many postoperative complications like nausea and postoperative pain, less bleeding, and more rapid healing of wounds.

Bramwell (1921) wrote of one of Braid's subjects, a young working girl who did not know the grammar of her own language very well and was completely ignorant about music, but, while hypnotized, was able to accompany Jenny Lind in several songs in different languages, and also in a long and difficult chromatic exercise which was specially improvised to test her. Bramwell also wrote of a case reported by Prince in which his subject, under hypnosis, was able to recall events of which he possessed no knowledge while in a normal conscious state. These recalled events had occurred during the delerium of fever.

Before concluding this section of interesting but rather incredible reports, a personal observation should be mentioned. Gerald Pascal, Salzberg's supervisor and instructor in hypnosis, administered an hypnotic suggestion to a volunteer research subject who reported having boils on her buttocks for three months. Pascal suggested that her boils would heal in two days. The locations of these boils had been observed and mapped out on a drawing by Pascal's female secretary before he hypnotized the subject. When the subject returned two days later, the secretary again observed and drew the subject's buttocks. The boils had almost completely healed.

Except for one or two, all of the above reports are what we may call pseudoscientific. Most are unexplainable from a scientific standpoint. Undoubtedly, many are exaggerations or unexplained coincidences. Some, however, have stimulated further research and opened the door to scientific discoveries later

Interestingly, in addition to Freud, several noted individuals have spent a portion of their professional careers studying and working with hypnosis. Clark Hull, a major learning theorist, wrote extensively about hypnosis. Hans Eysenck, a well known contemporary British psychologist, did some experiments in hypnosis early in his career over 40 years ago. Ernest Hilgard, on the other hand, was an established expert in learning theory before he and his wife Josephine embarked on their extensive research in hypnosis in 1957. In fact, Bowers (1976) has observed that the field of hypnosis is experiencing something resembling a renaissance recently. He attributes this to a loosening of the hold that classical behaviorism has had on American psychology, and a renewal of interest in cognition and subjective experience. This dates from the humanism of the 1960s and early 1970s when young people, disillusioned while the United States was engaged in the Vietnam War, dropped out of society to embrace drugs, Eastern religions, and meditation.

This book attempts to recapture some of the excitement sparked by the refocusing of energy by practitioners and scientists into the study of hypnosis. In Part I, Fundamental Issues in Hypnosis, Chapter 1 describes specific induction techniques along with some commonly used tests of susceptibility. The interested clinician will be able to use this chapter to get very detailed procedural steps for the hypnotic induction process such as how to do the Postural Sway Test, Pendulum Test, Handclasping Test, all of which are tests for susceptibility.

Hand Levitation, Visual Fixation, and Scene Visualization, which are hypnotic induction techniques, are also described. In addition, research on methods of hypnotic induction is discussed and an induction technique used by Pascal and Salzberg is described in detail.

Chapter 2 covers the many experimental designs issues involved in doing hypnosis research. Subject variables such as age, sex, personality characteristics, attitudes and beliefs, level of susceptibility and experimenter variables, subject-experimenter interactions, and situational variables are also discussed. A number of carefully worked out designs are described such as the Own Control Design, Interaction Design, Co-variance Design, and Independent Group Design. Research in hypnosis is rigorous in its methodology, and holds to a standard not met or exceeded by many other scientific fields of inquiry.

Part II, Behavior Modification, begins with Chapter 3, a very scholarly review of the literature on hypnosis and pain control. In addition to informing us about the phenomenon of pain, the chapter covers how hypnosis is used in dentistry, surgery, obstetrics, and terminal cancer and burn patients. Some of the experimental pain research is also covered.

Chapter 4 discusses hypnosis in the treatment of smoking in a scholarly exposition of the research that has been conducted in this area. In addition to discussing the many methodological pitfalls inherent in this kind of research, several treatment approaches are described.

Hypnosis and weight management is the subject of Chapter 5, geared more toward the practitioner than the researcher in this area. It offers some excellent practical suggestions for the implementation of treatment with overweight individuals using hypnosis.

Chapter 6 is a carefully done evaluation of the literature on hypnosis and phobias. In this area behavior therapists have been extensively involved as well as other clinicians who use hypnosis. Because so much of the research has involved behavior therapists, several theoretical issues are brought to light and discussed. Again, methodological aspects are examined.

Part III, Psychodynamic Interventions, moves away somewhat from painstaking methodological research, particularly in Chapter 7 on catharsis and uncovering therapies. Here, some of the more novel and creative uses of hypnosis are discussed. Chapter 8 discusses psychosomatic disorders; it serves as a supplement and update of the DePiano and Salzberg (1979) review article which appeared in Psychological Bulletin. The chapter also presents some surprises.

Part IV, Hypnosis and Enhanced Performances, begins with Chapter 9 on enhanced athletic and physical performance which primarily discusses the laboratory research that has been done in the last decade or so. Some anecdotal material on the clinical application of hypnosis in the sports arena is also presented.

Chapter 10 covers the enhancement of cognitive capacity. It is written in an upbeat style and suggests some potential areas of clinical application.

Chapter 11 is an up-to-date look at the forensic uses of hypnosis. It is written by a lawyer-psychologist who is able to evaluate the work done in this area from both vantage points.

Part V, Conclusion, begins with Chapter 12's discussion of the ethical use of hypnosis. The author questions who should provide the service, what kind of training is necessary, and what kinds of limitations and ground rules should apply to practitioners in their use of hypnosis. Finally, in Chapter 13, we present our views as to how hypnosis could and should be used in the future.

REFERENCES

Baudouin, C. (1921). *Suggestion and autosuggestion.* New York: Dodd, Mead.
Bernheim, H. (1947). *Suggestive therapeutics.* New York: London Book Co.
Bowers, K. S. (1976). *Hypnosis for the seriously curious.* New York: Norton.
Bramwell, J. M. (1921). *Hypnotism.* London: William Rider & Son.
Brunton, P. (1935). *A search in secret India.* New York: Dutton.
Craige, J. H. (1934). *Cannibal cousins.* New York: Minton, Balch.
DePiano, F., & Salzberg, H. (1979). Clinical applications of hypnosis to three psychosomatic disorders. *Psychological Bulletin, 86,* (6), 1223-1235.
Flesch, R. (Ed.). (1953). *Best articles.* New York: Hermitage.
Marks, R. W. (1947). *The story of hypnotism.* New York: Prentice Hall.
Rhodes, G. (1915). *Mind Cures.* Boston: Lure.
Sampimon, R. L. H. & Woodruff, M. F. A. (1946). Observations concerning the use of hypnosis as a substitute for anesthesia. *Medical Journal of Australia, 33,* 292-298.
Wilson, D. P. (1951). *My six convicts.* New York: Rhinehart.
Wolfe, B. & Rosenthal, R. (1948). *Hypnotism comes of age.* New York: Bobbs-Merrill.

PART I

FUNDAMENTAL ISSUES IN HYPNOSIS

Chapter 1

Trance Induction: Methods and Research

David S. Siegel, Ph.D.
Anxiety Disorders Institute
Atlanta, Georgia

It is well known that trance induction and its utilization as a curative aid has an ancient history. There are references made to "sleep temples" in the early civilizations of Greece and Egypt where patients were hypnotized or talked to during their sleep and given suggestions for relief of their symptoms. The Druids, the Celtic priesthood, are supposed to have been experts in its use. In primitive cultures, trance induction has commonly been accomplished through the use of rhythm: drums, chanting, dancing, and so on (Cheek & Le Cron, 1968).

Descriptions of ancient or primitive modes of trance induction, accounts of Mesmer's dramatic use of iron rods for magnetic alteration of the "universal fluids" in which man and all the planets were supposedly immersed, as well as the authoritarian style of many stage hypnotists are responsible for the common lay belief that hypnosis is something very unusual and is more other-directed than inner-directed–that what the hypnotist does is more important than what the subject does. Although some psychoanalytically oriented clinicians (Gill & Brenman, 1959) view hypnotic induction as a transferential process in which the subject submits to the authority and safety of a parental figure, others, such as Erickson (Haley, 1967; Erickson & Rossi, 1979; Erickson, 1980) and Kroger & Felzer (1976) emphasize that the process is less operator-directed than subject-centered. Rather than a means of seizing the subject's attention to "put him under," Erickson considered methods of induction as ways of fixing and focusing the subject's attention upon inner experimental learnings and capacities which are the raw material for hypnotic responsiveness. He criticized (Haley, 1967) what he viewed to be too much emphasis on external factors, such as the rigid use of standardized formulae (there is no method or technique that always works with everyone or even the same person on different occasions), and the use of apparatus (crystal balls, lights, etc.). He found through numerous experiments that visual or auditory imagery produced better induction results than having subjects actually watch pendulums or listen to metronomes (Erickson, 1980).

Hypnosis is a common feature of everyday life although it is not always labeled as such (Cheek & Le Cron, 1968). At one time or another, everyone has daydreamed and therefore has experienced a hypnotic-like state. Concentration and absorption in reading, working, watching a film, or listening to an interesting talk are all common examples of states in which sensory awareness may be restricted and attention amplified. A state of shock or sudden emotion can also produce a hypnotic-like state. Most people have also had other kinds of experiences, such as coming to the end of a page while reading and realizing that the eyes did their job, but the mind's eye was focused internally elsewhere. Another example is the experience of looking for something and having the somewhat annoying sense that it is right in front of one's nose—and having this confirmed later after having left and come back (perhaps with another person). This sort of experience makes the notion of negative hallucination seem less mysterious and unusual. These and other examples of everyday experience may be useful clinically in preparing clients for hypnotic induction.

Wolberg (1948) has given a description of the general steps to be followed when a subject or client is to be hypnotized for the first time. His general procedure is comparable to the steps similarly outlined by Ulett & Peterson (1965). Wolberg's procedure is to:

1. Encourage motivation and desire for hypnosis.
2. Remove misconceptions, fears, and resistances.
3. Give the subject a suggestibility test to demonstrate that he or she can follow suggestions.
4. Encourage relaxation via a preparatory talk.
5. Induce the trance.
6. Deepen the trance.
7. Awaken the subject.
8. Discuss the subject's reaction.

Many of these steps are not necessarily mutually exclusive and can be done simultaneously.

In preparing a subject for hypnosis, it is important to discuss and allay various misconceptions. It is important to ask whether the person has ever seen someone else hypnotized, perhaps by a stage hypnotist and elicit what his or her reactions were. Other common sources of fear and resistance are:

1. That to be hypnotized is a sign of low intelligence or mental weakness.
2. That the process will somehow weaken the subject.

3. That they will be forced to reveal embarrassing things about themselves.
4. That they will be forced to do embarrassing things or commit antisocial acts.
5. That they will be under control of the hypnotist.
6. That they may be unable to awaken from trance.

Particularly resistant subjects may be helped by letting them watch an induction of an experienced subject (Ulett & Peterson, 1965). Subjects should be encouraged to relax, to not try too hard to follow directions but to just allow the process to happen.

After misconceptions and fears have been allayed as much as possible, the subject can be given one of a number of suggestibility tests while still in the waking state. These can help to put the person in the proper response set. Ulett & Peterson describe a number of suggestibility tests:

1. *Postural Sway Test.* The subject is asked to stand with feet together and back turned away from the operator. He (or she) is told to close the eyes and relax. The subject is told that he will begin to feel as if the operator were pulling him backward, that he will find himself swaying backward and forward and that he will begin to fall backward. Reassurance should be given that he will be caught, the operator placing his or her hands firmly behind the subject's shoulder blades. Susceptible subjects typically do not step back as they fall backwards. During the swaying, slight body movements are reinforced by the operator: "Swaying, swaying . . . swaying back . . . now forward . . . falling, falling, falling . . .".

2. *Pendulum Test.* This test capitalizes on the unconscious control of motor movements. A bobbin suspended from a chain is held by the subject with thumb and forefinger above the surface of a table, the subject's elbow resting on the table with the forearm angled upward. The subject, in response to suggestions, visualizes the bobbin swinging around and around in an ever widening circle . . . first in one direction then the other, then in a straight line.

3. *Handclasping Test.* The subject is asked to clasp the hands by interlocking the fingers, and then to tighten the clasp. Suggestions are given that the fingers are being glued together in one piece and that when told to, the subject will be unable to take them apart. "The more you try, the more you cannot do so. Now stop trying. Now they are free again and you can open them."

4. *Eye Catalepsy Test.* The procedure is virtually identical to the handclasp test, only suggestions are given that the eyes are glued, welded, or locked together.

5. *Pencil Dropping Test.* The subject, seated in a chair with eyes closed, is asked to hold a pencil between the thumb and forefinger. Then suggestions are given that "the fingers are coming apart . . . wider . . . wider. The pencil is looser . . . looser. It will soon drop. It is dropping."

6. *Arm Rigidity Test.* The subject is given suggestions that one arm has become "like a steel bar, reaching higher and higher. It won't bend. You cannot pull it down. Any effort in that direction will just make it more rigid and higher."

METHODS OF HYPNOTIC INDUCTION

There are various ways of inducing hypnosis. One general way of describing an induction is according to whether it is delivered in a positive, commanding way employing direct suggestions, or in a permissive manner using indirect suggestions (Barber, 1978). Examples of direct suggestions are statements like the following: "You are going to relax now . . . Notice that with every breath you become more and more heavy . . . Now imagine that a soft wave of relaxation is spreading over your whole body." Any of these sentences can be responded to with a negation: "No I am not/cannot relax now," and so on. Indirect suggestions can communicate the same ideas but are delivered in such a way that, no matter whether the subject is attempting to resist or wants to go along, there is no way to logically reject the suggestions. For example: "I wonder, as you continue sitting quietly right there . . . I wonder if you can enjoy feeling more and more relaxed with each comfortable breath you take. You might notice the relaxation more than the enjoyment . . . or you may being experiencing the enjoyment even more than the relaxation. I don't know, but I can wonder." The effects of indirect suggestions are to obviate resistance and to make trying irrelevant (Barber, 1978). They do not tell the subject what to do; rather, they explore and facilitate what the person's response system can do on an autonomous level without really making a conscious effort to direct itself (Erickson & Rossi, 1979). Erickson & Rossi have devoted a whole volume to classifying and describing different forms of indirect suggestion and their uses in induction and hypnotherapy. Examples of them are:

- "Most people can experience one hand as being lighter than another." (Truism involving an ideomotor process)
- "You already know how to experience pleasant sensations like the warmth of the sun on your skin." (Truism involving an ideosensory process)
- "You don't even have to hold your eyes open . . . You don't know just when those eyelids will close all by themselves." (Not knowing, not doing)
- "We all have potentials we are unaware of, and we usually don't know how they will be expressed." (Open-ended suggestion)
- "Soon you will find a finger or a thumb moving a bit, perhaps by itself. It can move up or down, to the side or press down. The really important thing is to sense fully whatever feelings develop." (Covering all possibilities of a class of responses)

- "Will those lids begin to blink separately or together?" (Question facilitating new response possibilities)
- "Would you like to enter trance now or later?" (Bind based on avoidance conflict)
- "If your unconscious wants you to enter trance, your right hand will lift all by itself. Otherwise your left arm will lift." (Conscious-unconscious double bind)
- "You can make an abstract drawing without knowing what it is. You can later find some meaning in it even though it does not seem related to you personally." (Double dissociation double bind).

A particular induction procedure can be classified as falling on a continuum. There are those which utilize direct suggestion completely and those which are totally indirect. Most inductions, however, are probably a mix. Standardized induction scales such as the Harvard Group Scale of Hypnotic Susceptibility, the Stanford Hypnotic Susceptibility Scale or the Hypnotic Induction Profile (Spiegel & Spiegel, 1978) are mostly based on direct suggestions.

Induction methods, whether direct or indirect, can also be categorized according to the particular activity or process used to focus the subject. According to Ulett & Peterson (1965), these are:

1. Visual fixation on some object leading to sensory restriction, eyelid heaviness, and eye closure.
2. Monotony of voice with suggestions of sleep, drowsiness, relaxation, drifting back, going deeper, and so on.
3. Visualization of an elaborate, interesting, pleasant scene.
4. Arm levitation in which suggestions of lightness and bouyancy are given leading to the lifting of one hand to the cheek.

Typically, a particular induction will employ two or more of these processes. The following examples are given for illustration (from Wolberg, 1948, by permission). The first example illustrates the use of drowsiness and hand levitation:

> "I want you to sit comfortably in your chair and relax. As you sit there, bring both hands palms down on your thighs—just like that. Keep watching your hands, and you will notice that you are able to observe them closely.
>
> What you will do is sit in the chair and relax. Then you will notice that certain things happen in the course of relaxing. They always have happened while relaxing, but you have not noticed them so closely before. I am going to point them out to you. I'd like to have you concentrate on all sensations and feelings in your hands no matter what they may be. Perhaps you may feel the heaviness of your hand as it lies on your thigh, or you

may feel pressure. Perhaps you will feel the texture of your trousers as they press against the palm of your hand; or the warmth of your hand on your thigh. Perhaps you may feel tingling. No matter what sensations there are, I want you to observe them. Keep watching your hand, and you will notice how quiet it is, how it remains in one position. There is motion there, but it is not yet noticeable. I want you to keep watching your hand. Your attention may wander from the hand, but it will always return back to the hand, and you keep watching the hand and wondering when the motion that is there will show itself."

(At this point the patient's attention is fixed on his hand. He is curious about what will happen, and sensations such as any person might experience are suggested to him as possibilities. No attempt is being made to force any suggestions on him, and if he observes any sensations or feelings, he incorporates them as a product of his own experience. The object eventually is to get him to respond to the suggestions of the hypnotist as if these too are parts of his own experiences. A subtle attempt is being made to get him to associate his sensations with the words spoken to him so that words or command uttered by the hypnotist will evoke sensory or motor responses later on. Unless the patient is consciously resisting, a slight motion or jerking will develop in one of the fingers or in the hand. As soon as this happens, the hypnotist mentions it and remarks that the motion will probably increase. The hypnotist must also comment on any other objective reaction of the patient, such as motion of the legs or deep breathing. The result of this linking of the patient's reactions with comments of the hypnotist is an association of the two in the patient's mind.)

"It will be interesting to see which one of the fingers will move first. It may be the middle finger, or the forefinger, or the ring finger, or the little finger, or the thumb. One of the fingers is going to jerk or move. You don't know exactly when or in which hand. Keep watching and you will begin to notice a slight movement, possibly in the right hand. There, the thumb jerks and moves, just like that.

As the movement begins you will notice an interesting thing. Very slowly the spaces between the fingers will widen, the fingers will slowly move apart, and you'll notice that the spaces will get wider and wider and wider. They'll move apart slowly; the fingers will seem to be spreading apart, wider and wider and wider. The fingers are spreading, wider and wider and wider apart, just like that."

(This is the first real suggestion to which the patient is expected to respond. If the fingers start spreading apart, they do so because the patient is reacting to suggestion. The hypnotist continues to talk as if the response is one that would have come about by itself in the natural course of events.)

"As the fingers spread apart, you will notice that the fingers will soon want to arch up from the thigh, as if they want to lift, higher and higher.

(The patient's index finger starts moving upward slightly.) Notice how the index finger lifts. As it does the other fingers want to follow–up, up, slowly rising. (The other fingers start lifting.)

As the fingers lift you'll become aware of lightness in the hand, a feeling of lightness, so much so that the fingers will arch up, and the whole hand will slowly lift and rise as if it feels like a feather, as if a balloon is lifting it up in the air, lifting, lifting,–up–up–up, pulling up higher and higher and higher, the hand becoming very light. (The hand starts rising.) As you watch your hand rise, you'll notice that the arm comes up, up, up in the air, a little higher–and higher–and higher–and higher, up–up–up. (The arm has lifted about five inches above the thigh and the patient is gazing at it fixedly.)

Keep watching the hand and arm as it rises straight up, and as it does you will soon become aware of how drowsy and tired your eyes become. As your arm continues to rise, you will get tired and relaxed and sleepy, very sleepy. Your eyes will get heavy and your lids may want to close. And as your arm rises higher and higher, you will want to feel more relaxed and sleepy, and you will want to enjoy the peaceful, relaxed feeling of letting your eyes close and of being sleepy."

(It will be noticed that as the patient executes one suggestion, his positive response is used to reinforce the next suggestion. For instance, as his arm rises, it is suggested in essence that he will get drowsy because his arm is rising.)

"Your arm lifts–up–up–and you are getting very drowsy; your lids get very heavy, your breathing gets slow and regular. Breathe deeply–in and out. (The client holds his arm stretched out directly in front of him, his eyes are blinking and his breathing is deep and regular.) As you keep watching your hand and arm and feeling more and more drowsy and relaxed, you will notice that the direction of the hand will change. The arm will bend, and the hand will move closer and closer to your face–up–up–up–and as it rises you will slowly but steadily go into a deep, deep, sleep in which you relax deeply and to your satisfaction. The arm will continue to rise up–up–lifting, lifting–up in the air until it touches your face, and you will get sleepier and sleepier, but you must not go to sleep until your hand touches your face. When your hand touches your face, you will be asleep, deeply asleep."

(The patient here is requested to choose his own pace in falling asleep, so that when his hand touches his face, he feels himself to be asleep to his own satisfaction. Hand levitation and sleepiness continue to reinforce each other. When the patient finally does close his eyes, he will have entered a trance with his own participation. He will later be less inclined to deny that he has been in a trance.)

"Your hand is now changing its direction. It moves up–up–up toward your face. Your eyelids are getting heavy. You are getting sleepier, and sleepier, and sleepier. (The patient's hand is approaching his face, his eyelids are blinking more rapidly.) Your eyes get heavy, very heavy, and the hand moves straight up toward your face. You get very tired and drowsy. Your eyes are closing, are closing. When your hand touches your face you'll be asleep, deeply asleep. You'll feel very drowsy. You feel drowsier and drowsier and drowsier, very sleepy, very tired. Your eyes are like lead, and your hand moves up, up, up, right towards your face, and when it reaches your face, you will be asleep. (Client's hand touches his face and his eyes close.) Go to sleep, go to sleep, just asleep. And as you sleep you feel very tired and relaxed. I want you to concentrate on relaxation, a state of tensionless relaxation. Think of nothing else, but sleep, deep sleep."

The following example is an induction making use of visual fixation and drowsiness:

"I am holding an object above your eyes, look at it steadily. You may look at it steadily. You may pick out a spot of light on it, if you desire, and focus on that intently. At the same time relax and do not resist suggestions. Keep concentrating on the idea of sleep and do not permit any other thoughts to enter your mind. Just focus your eyes on the object. You may possibly notice that your eyes may want to travel in one direction or in another direction, but they will always return to a spot on the object. Keep your eyes fixated on this object, keep looking at it as long as you want; and as you keep looking at it, I want you to relax yourself and make your mind passive. Stop resisting; relax.

As you relax you will begin to notice that your arms get heavy, your legs get heavy, your eyes get tired, you get heavier all over. A sense of drowsiness is creeping over your entire body. Keep looking at the object and blink as much as you like. Let your eyes get as tired and drowsy as possible.

You are getting drowsy now. Soon your eyes will tire and water. Wink if you wish. Your lids will get so heavy they will start shutting. Relax and get sleepier. Your eyes are watering. Your lids keep closing. Your eyes get tired, watery, and they burn. They become fatigued. Your eyelids are heavy, and get heavier and heavier. Your eyes are very tired. Soon they will close.

Keep thinking about sleep, how it would feel to be asleep. You notice that you are getting sleepier and sleepier. Keep staring at the object as hard as you can and as long as you can, and you notice that your eyelids are getting heavier and heavier. Your eyes burn, feel tired, and a sense of sleepiness creeps over you. You are getting sleepier and sleepier and sleepier. You are getting very, very sleepy, and your eyelids get heavier and heavier, and they will close and you will go into a quiet restful sleep.

Now your arms and legs are heavy like lead. A warm feeling spreads over your body, a drowsy feeling as if you are floating on a cloud. Let yourself relax and sleep, go to sleep. It is pleasant to relax. Let yourself get sleepy. Sink into a deep, deep sleep. You are relaxed and comfortable. Breathe deeply, very deeply and slowly, just like that. With each breath your sleep gets deeper and deeper. Your eyes have practically closed. You are almost asleep, deeply asleep. Go to sleep, relax and sleep, just sleep, sleep, sleep."

The last example illustrates the use of drowsiness and scene visualization in an induction:

"I should like to have you lie down on the couch and relax yourself all over. I should like to have you become aware of any tensions that exist in your muscles. First concentrate on your forehead, loosen up your forehead. Loosen up the muscles in your face, straighten out your neck, loosen that up too. Now the shoulders. Loosen up your body; stretch out your arms and legs. Let yourself get lazy all over, from your head right down to your feet. Now fold your hands on your chest, and as I talk to you try to visualize things exactly as I talk about them. First become aware of the pressure of the pillow against your head. Concentrate on the back of the head and become aware of how the pillow presses against it. Now the pressure of the pillow against your shoulders, the pressure of the couch against your back. Now shift your attention to your thighs and think of how the couch supports your whole body. It is as if your body sinks into the couch and is supported by it completely. Now I want you to visualize yourself in a comfortable place, the most comfortable place you know, a place where you would like to stretch out, forget your worries and your cares, so you can sleep. Perhaps it will be at the seashore or in the mountains or some other place if you prefer. (The patient here prefers to think of the mountains.)

As you lie there I want you to start breathing deeply and slowly. As you do, relax yourself even more. Make your body limp so that when I raise your arm it will come down limp of its own accord. (The arm is raised, and it falls down unsupported when released.) I want you to relax the rest of your body the same way, from your forehead to your toes. Stretch out and breathe deeply. Good, like that.

Now as you lie there, relaxed, breathing deeply, imagine you are on a mountain top on a sunny day. Everything is peaceful and serene. You are lying in the shade in tall soft grass. You watch the deep blue sky overhead. Perhaps you see one or two billowy clouds floating lazily by. Everything is peaceful and serene like your mind must be now. All around you are tall fir, spruce and pine trees. The scent of pine penetrates your nostrils and makes you feel fresh and relaxed. And in the distance there are lakes, the surface as smooth as glass. Watch the lakes and your mind will become peaceful and quiet like the surface of the water. Your body is relaxed. Your mind is relaxed. Relax and sleep, deeper and deeper. Sleep more deeply, go to sleep.

As you start getting sleepy, your arm, your right arm will get light, like a feather. It will get lighter and lighter, and then it will lift—up—up—up. The sleepier you get, the lighter your arm will feel, and the higher it will lift until it touches your face. As you relax, your hand and arm lift and rise higher and higher, and when your hand touches your face, you will be asleep, deeply asleep. Your arm is rising slowly now, just like a feather—up—up—up—higher and higher and higher. It is getting close to your face, you will be asleep, deeply asleep. Now your hand has touched your face and you are asleep."

Erickson (1980) was well known for his sometimes uncommon techniques for trance induction. These methods grew out of long experience working with a broad spectrum of patients, many of whom were overtly quite resistant to being hypnotized. One of his best known methods is the ***confusion technique***. In speaking, the hypnotist uses homonyms and antonyms (i.e., repeated references to write, right, left, wrong; here, there, this, that) in different contexts, changes in verb tenses, jumps from the present to the future to the past, irrelevancies and non sequiturs in such a way that the subject is kept in a confused state while trying to extract some intended meaning from the talk. The induction talk is delivered in a casual but definitely interested attitude while speaking in a gravely earnest, intent manner expressive of a certain, utterly complete expectation that the subject will understand what is being said. The constant flow of language is delivered in such a way that the subject is just beginning a mental response but is then prevented from getting closure on it because of the presentation of the next confusing idea. Continuation of this process leads to a state of inhibition and a growing need to receive a clear-cut, comprehensible communication which can be readily and fully responded to mentally. As the subject accommodates himself to the seeming confusion of the hypnotist, he unwittingly cooperates in a significant way. Eventually he or she finds himself or herself at such a loss that any positive suggestion is welcomed that will permit a retreat from so confusing a situation. Trance is thereby entered into. Examples of this sort of induction can be found in Erickson (1980) or Haley (1967).

Another of Erickson's inductions is his ***My-Friend-John-Technique***. A subject is asked to pretend that someone by the name of John is sitting in a chair. The subject then gives the imaginary person the suggestions of the hand levitation technique, with much feeling and emphasis, all the while sensing his or her own instructions. The subject makes automatic responses to his or her own suggestions and enters a trance.

Erickson was also well known for employing surprise and pantomime as vehicles for hypnotic induction (see Erickson, 1980).

Besides the notion of indirect suggestion, another major concept in Erickson's approach to induction and hypnotherapy is ***utilization***. Erickson (Erickson & Rossi, 1979) distinguishes between formalized, ritualistic procedures of trance induction, where the same method is applied to everyone and the naturalistic approach, wherein the client's unique personality, attitudes, behaviors, emotions, frames of reference, resistance and/or symptoms are *utilized* to facilitate trance. In this utilization approach the client's attention is fixed on some important aspect of his own personality and behavior in a manner which leads to the inner focus that is defined as therapeutic trance. The client's habitual conscious sets are more or less depotentiated and unconscious searches and processes are initiated and facilitated to produce a therapeutic response. One of the many descriptions of this sort of process comes from Erickson (1980).

Hypnosis had been attempted repeatedly on a dentist's wife but had always been unsuccessful. Each time the woman would become absolutely scared stiff, tearful, and silly. Erickson approached the woman by suggesting to her that for successful trance induction it would really be enough for her to just get stiff without crying. The woman replied that she would get scared stiff and cry. At this point Erickson directed her only to get stiff, stiffer in fact than she had become in response to previous attempts at trance induction. After she had complied by becoming very rigid, he then suggested that she chould next become silly and tearful as she had in the past, but also suggested that it would be much easier for her to take a deep breath and relax fully. She complied with this and further trance-deepening suggestions. The technique of tensing and then relaxing muscle groups is, of course, an integral part of progressive relaxation training. As suggestions for continued relaxation were given, Erickson gave the woman permission at any time to get scared stiff and silly but also suggested that she might not need to since she had learned a new, comfortable response.

One suggestion that has been made regarding approaches based on utilization and indirect suggestion is that they are more effective with resistant clients (Barber, 1978). Since they are based on the individual response style of a given client, however, they may be more difficult to research than standardized, ritualized procedures.

Returning to more traditional modes of trance induction, trance deepening can be achieved in various ways (Cheek & Le Cron, 1968; Ulett & Peterson, 1965; Wolberg, 1948):

1. Indirect challenges can be given such as "When you are sure you can't (open your eyes, lift your hand, etc.), try to make sure you can't" or "If you tried to———, you could, but you won't because you have no desire to."
2. A succession of increasingly difficult suggestions can be given (in line for instance with the Harvard Group Scale induction protocol).
3. Counting interspersed with suggestions of going deeper into sleep or relaxation can also be employed.

4. The subject can also be directed to visualize and imagine himself going down a plush staircase or an escalator which leads to a private room.
5. Stroking the subject's arm or forehead (with forewarning) along with suggestions for more profound trance, heaviness, etc., can also be helpful.

The usual method of awakening is to suggest to the person that she or he will awaken at the count of three (or perhaps five). Counting should be done slowly, allowing time for the person to become awake. The subject should be told that he or she will feel refreshed, relaxed, alert and clearheaded upon coming out of trance.

COMPARATIVE RESEARCH ON HYPNOTIC INDUCTION METHODS

During the past ten years a number of research studies have been published comparing the effectiveness of different induction techniques. These studies have been categorized into four main areas: (1) Duration of induction, (2) Relaxation vs. hypnotic induction, (3) Direct vs. indirect induction, and (4) Comparison of directive methods.

Duration of Induction

Two studies have provided data concerning the duration of hypnotic induction (Klinger, 1970; Gilbert & Barber, 1972). Klinger had each of 68 subjects observe the behavior of a confederate who was being given a hypnotic induction. The confederates acted either responsive or unresponsive to the suggestions. Then subjects were given either a long induction (10 minutes, eye-fixation and relaxation) or a short induction (one minute, eye closure suggestion). After the induction, the Barber Susceptibiility Scale (BSS) was administered. The results did not support the notion that induction length influenced scores on the BSS.

Gilbert and Barber, using 120 subjects, attempted to assess the effect of minimal or extended inductions on cognitive performance. The minimal induction procedure consisted of subjects fixating the eyes on a light blinking in synchrony with the sound of a metronome while receiving suggestions of eye heaviness, eye-closure, relaxation, drowsiness, and sleep for 30 seconds. The extended induction procedure consisted or repeated suggestions for eye heaviness, relaxation, drowsiness, sleep, and deep hypnosis administered for a period of 15 minutes. Half of the subjects were then given motivational instructions. Finally, subjects were tested on four cognitive performance tasks. The extended hypnotic induction produced a marginal trend for higher gain scores on one of the four tasks. Since 28 statistical tests were conducted with respect to four cognitive tasks, this result may have been due to chance.

In sum, there seems to be no experimental evidence to date showing an advantage for using extended as opposed to brief hypnotic inductions. These results are consistent with other research in which subjects given no formal induction scored just as highly afterwards on scales of hypnotic susceptibility as subjects who were given an induction (Barber & Glass, 1962). Since rapid induction techniques have been described and advocated in the clinical literature (e.g., Matheson & Grehan, 1979), continued research could be directed toward determining their effectiveness with clinical problems.

Relaxation vs. Hypnotic Induction

Two studies were found which compared the effects of a hypnotic induction to a relaxation procedure (Dunwoody & Edmonston, 1974; Reyher & Wilson, 1973). Dunwoody & Edmonston recorded electro-oculograms from 12 subjects who were given either relaxation or hypnotic induction instructions. The electro-oculograms were used to determine the rate and number of slow eye movements (SEMs) resulting from the two procedures. SEMs were hypothesized to be more associated with the induction of hypnosis. However, no differences in SEMs were found between subjects given relaxation and hypnosis instructions.

Reyher & Wilson (1973) assigned 20 subjects randomly to one of two groups. The first group read instructions indicating that they would undergo a relaxation procedure. The second group read instructions indicating that they would be receiving a hypnotic induction. As the instructions were read, GSR measures were recorded from S's fingers. Both groups then received the identical procedure administered by an experimenter blind to the subjects' instructions. The procedure consisted of an abbreviated version of the Jacobson progressive relaxation method followed by an altered version of the Stanford Hypnotic Susceptibility Scale (SHSS) in which all references and cue to the word "hypnosis" had been deleted. Results showed that the hypnosis-instructed subjects had higher GSR measures than relaxation-instructed subjects. Mean SHSS scores did not differ between the groups, but hypnosis-instructed subjects showed significantly more variability in their scores than relaxation-instructed subjects. These results were interpreted as suggesting that hypnosis-instructed subjects were either anxious or excited, the former being disruptive, the latter being facilitative. It was also suggested that the progressive relaxation procedure is an effective means of inducing hypnosis.

In sum, there seems to be no evidence to separate relaxation procedures from traditional hypnotic induction procedures in terms of their effectiveness in producing hypnotic behavior. Methods which are not overtly presented as "hypnosis" may be less likely to cause anxiety and may therefore be more effective in certain situations (e.g., Barber, 1978). More research, especially in the clinical area, should be directed toward exploring this question.

Direct vs. Indirect Suggestions

Three studies have investigated direct vs. indirect suggestions in induction procedures and how it influences measures of hypnotic responsiveness. Thorne and Hall (1974) investigated the effects of authoritarian vs. permissive motivational suggestions for amnesia as measured by performance on a word association test (which had been preceded by a paired-associate learning task). Although highly hypnotically susceptible subjects demonstrated more amnesia than less susceptible subjects, the type of sugestion (authoritarian vs. permissive) did not lead to differences in response.

Angelos (1978) studied the effect on analgesic effectiveness of direct vs. indirect hypnotic suggestions. Half of the subjects were administered the Stanford Hypnotic Clinical Scale (the direct method) and the rest were administered the Rapid Induction Analgesia (Barber, 1977) (the indirect method). Analgesia suggestions were framed in a posthypnotic context. After waking, subjects' hand and arm were exposed to cold pressor pain. The success of the analgesia suggestions was determined by taking measures of frontalis muscle tension and subjective pain reports using an open-ended 10-point scale. The indirect method was related to significantly more self-reported analgesia, particularly for subjects having low susceptibility scores. It was suggested that hypnotic analgesia may be made more effective through differential usage of either direct or indirect inductions, depending on the patient's susceptibility score. This notion has yet to be tested out experimentally with clinical populations although it has been discussed in the clinical literature (Barber, 1978).

Alman and Carney (1980) compared the effectiveness of direct and indirect versions of the same induction protocol on the execution of a posthypnotic suggestion. Posthypnotic behavior was scored by observers (objectively) and was rated by the subjects themselves as well (subjectively). The procedure entailed first obtaining Harvard Group Scale Hypnotic Susceptibility Scores from subjects. Subjects then were exposed to one of two taped induction protocols, one with direct, the other with indirect suggestions. Each tape contained suggestions that when asked a cue question, "How are you feeling right now?", the subject would experience a strong itching at the back of the neck and would scratch the itch. Observers then scored the extent to which this behavior was carried out and subjects filled out a questionnaire describing their posthypnotic behavior. The results showed that the indirect induction was more successful in producing posthypnotic behavior as scored objectively. Also, it was shown that low-susceptible subjects receiving the direct induction received lower objective scores than other groups. It was concluded that indirect induction methods seem to be more effective than direct methods in eliciting posthypnotic behavior, particularly from low susceptible subjects.

In summary, although not entirely consistent, there is some interesting evidence that indirect hypnotic induction methods may be more effective than direct methods in producing certain kinds of hypnotic responses, that is, posthypnotic behavior involving somatosensory experience. More research needs to be done in this area, particularly studies using clinical populations.

Comparison of Direct Induction Methods. Banyai and Hilgard (1976) compared the effectiveness of two direct-suggestion induction procedures as measured by responses to items drawn from the Stanford Hypnotic Susceptibility Scale (SHSS). On separate days each of 50 subjects was given a traditional induction procedure (the SHSS protocol), and an "active-alert" induction. In the "active-alert" induction, subjects rode a bicycle ergometer under load while a set of suggestions paralleling those of the SHSS was given. Instead of suggestions for relaxation and drowsiness, substitute suggestions for alertness, attentiveness, and feelings of freshness were given. After the alert and traditional inductions, subjects were tested by eight items drawn from the SHSS. It was found that the two procedures produced no significant differences in SHSS item mean scores. Scores of both groups, however, were significantly higher than a control group which only rode the bicycle ergometer.

Gibbons (1976) compared an induction procedure he termed "hyperempiria" (in which suggestions of increased alertness and mind expansion are given) to a traditional induction of equivalent length containing suggestions of sleep and drowsiness. Separate groups of subjects received the respective inductions and then were administered selected items from the Harvard Group Scale of Hypnotic Susceptibility. It was found that the "hyperempiric" induction (a reading of which indicates that it is a guided visual imagery sort of induction; Gibbons, 1974) resulted in higher HGSHS scores than the traditional induction. It was suggested that suggestions of hyperalertness may be as or more effective as sleep suggestions in inducing trance states.

Friedland (1976) compared the relative effectiveness of three methods for inducing hypnosis: sleeptalk, blackboard visualization, and chiasson. Forty-eight subjects were randomly assigned to each of the three methods, and to one of four hypnotists. The primary dependent variable was depth of hypnosis as measured by a score on a modified version of the Stanford Hypnotic Susceptibility Scale. A measure of mental imagery was also obtained via the revised Betts Questionnaire Upon Mental Imagery. The results indicated that depth of hypnosis did not vary as a function of the induction method utilized. However, vividness of imagery appeared to be positively correlated with depth of hypnosis only when the visualization induction was used.

In sum, two of three studies to date suggest that depth of hypnosis does not vary in relation to the type of induction employed. As Vingol (1968) has argued, it may be that active, alert suggestions seem to produce as adequate a response as more traditional relaxation-oriented methods.

At present, it seems that length of inductions and/or the extent to which they employ relaxation vs. active-alert sorts of suggestions matters little in how effective they are in mediating hypnotic behavior. An interesting question has been the extent to which direct and indirect styles of induction differ in their effectiveness. From a clinical perspective, the indirect method of induction offers the advantages of reducing resistance and increasing the likelihood of establishing a noncompetitive relationship in psychotherapy. Both of these factors would increase the effectiveness of a given intervention.

REFERENCES

Alman, B. M., & Carney, R. E. (1980). Consequences of direct and indirect suggestions on success of posthypnotic behavior. *American Journal of Clinical Hypnosis, 23,* 112–118.

Angelos, J. S. (1978). A comparison of the effects of direct and indirect methods of hypnotic induction on the perception of pain. *Dissertation Abstracts International, 39-B,* 2972–2973. (University Microfilms No. 7822112)

Banyai, E. I., & Hilgard, E. R. (1976). A comparison of active-alert hypnotic induction with traditional relaxation induction. *Journal of Abnormal Psychology, 85,* 218–224.

Barber, J. (1977). Rapid induction analgesia: A clinical report. *American Journal of Clinical Hypnosis, 19,* 138–147.

Barber, J. (1978, August). *Maximizing the effectiveness of hypnosis through indirect suggestion.* Paper presented at the meeting of the American Psychological Association, Toronto, Ontario.

Barber, T. X., & Glass, L. B. (1962). Significant factors in hypnotic behavior. *Journal of Abnormal Psychology, 64,* 222–228.

Cheek, D. B., & Le Cron, L. M. (1968). *Clinical hypnotherapy.* New York: Grune & Stratton.

Dunwoody, R. C., & Edmonston, W. E. (1974). Hypnosis and slow eye movements, *American Journal of Clinical Hypnosis, 16,* 270–274.

Erickson, M. H. (1980). The nature of hypnosis and suggestion. In E. L. Rossi (Ed.), *The collected papers of Milton H. Erickson on hypnosis (Vol. 1).* New York: Irvington Publishers.

Erickson, M. H., & Rossi, E. L. (1979). *Hypnotherapy: An exploratory case book.* New York: Irvington Publishers.

Friendland, M. R. (1976). A comparison of three methods for inducing hypnosis. *Dissertation Abstracts International, 37-B,* 3071–3072.

Gibbons, D. (1974). Hyperempiria: A new "Altered State of Consciousness" induced by suggestion. *Perceptual and Motor Skills, 39,* 47–53.

Gibbons, D. E. (1976). Hypnotic vs. hyperempiric induction procedures: An experimental comparison. *Perceptual and Motor Skills, 42,* 834.

Gilbert, J. E., & Barber, T. X. (1972). Effects of hypnotic induction, motivational suggestions, and level of suggestibility on cognitive performance. *International Journal of Clinical and Experimental Hypnosis, 20,* 156–168.

Gill, M. M., & Brenman, M. (1959). *Hypnosis and related states.* New York: International Universities Press.

Haley, J. (Ed.) (1967). *Advanced techniques of hypnosis and therapy: Selected papers of Milton H. Erickson, M.D.* New York: Grune & Stratton.

Klinger, B. I. (1970). Effect of peer model responsiveness and length of induction procedure on hypnotic responsiveness. *Journal of Abnormal Psychology, 75,* 15–18.

Kroger, W. S., & Fezler, W. D. (1976). *Hypnosis and behavior modification: Imagery conditioning.* Philadelphia: J. P. Lippincott.

Matheson, G., & Grehan, J. F. (1979). A rapid induction technique. *American Journal of Clinical Hypnosis, 21,* 297–299.

Reyher, J., & Wilson, J. G. (1973). The induction of hypnosis: Indirect vs. direct methods and the role of anxiety. *American Journal of Clinical Hypnosis, 13,* 229–233.

Spiegel, H. & Spiegel, D. (1978). *Trance and treatment.* New York: Basic Books.

Thorne, D. E., & Hall, H. V. (1974). Hypnotic amnesia revisited. *The International Journal of Clinical and Experimental Hypnosis, 22,* 167–178.

Ulett, G. A., & Peterson, D. B. (1965). *Applied hypnosis and positive suggestion.* St. Louis: C. V. Mosby.

Vingol, F. J. (1968). The development of a group alert trance scale. *International Journal of Clinical and Experimental Hypnosis, 16,* 120–132.

Wolberg, L. R. (1948). *Medical Hypnosis* (Vol. 1). New York: Grune & Stratton.

Chapter 2

Methodological Considerations in Hypnosis Research

Pamela J. Kebrdle
Nova University

Gregory D. Roeder
University of South Carolina

The motivation for performing research on the influence of hypnosis dates back to the claims of early practitioners that superhuman feats of memory, strength, and the like could be performed by subjects in the hypnotic state. Even the earliest of such claims were met with skepticism, and attempts were made to explain hypnotic phenomena as the result of understandable human qualities and abilities. According to Orne's (1979) history of hypnosis research, it was during the time of Braid's (1847) work that emphasis first shifted away from superhuman explanations to more physiological and psychological definitions of what hypnosis entailed. Perhaps because of its intriguing appearance and apparent divorcement from normal everyday functioning, aspects of the debate over the special or ordinary status of hypnosis have carried through into modern thinking. Hull (1930, 1931) set the stage for an advanced scientific evaluation of hypnotic phenomena by initiating a program of intensive research into their nature. He presented over 100 outlines of experiments and procedures for evaluating hypnotic phenomena. Many of these phenomena are still under investigation today.

The nature of most early research was to compare the effects of hypnosis vs. nonhypnosis treatments and the subsequent behavior changes. Results were reported in terms of gross outcome measures lacking quantitative measurement (i.e., improvement or no improvement).

The emphasis of modern clinical research on hypnosis has been to discover how hypnosis enhances treatment differently from other approaches and to determine the variables that effect hypnotic behavior. It was Barber's work which initiated changes in most research methodology used to resolve these differing views. His reviews (Barber, 1965a, 1966) focused primarily on design and control inadequacies. Barber (1965b) concluded the following: "When sufficient experimental data have accumulated, any simple formula to explain hypnotic behavior will be open to serious question. The influence of any one variable will be found to depend upon the context of other variables. The determinants of response to test suggestions will be found to be multiple and complex" (p. 151). His conclusions have been strongly borne out in the context of advances in methodological design. While some investigators may have resisted his redefinition of hypnosis as a nonspecial condition, they have accepted his methodological challenge: A beginning has been made.

Much attention has been paid to design and control issues in the years since Barber's reviews and early work. The advances in methodology made since the reviews of Barber (1965a, 1966) and Treolar (1967) have been outlined and comprehensively discussed (Coe, 1973; Sheehan, 1973; Sheehan & Perry, 1976). The areas in which these refinements of methodology have been made include: the specification and control of variables not identified as treatments, the specification of subject variables such as susceptibility and sex which may influence performance or interact with treatments, and the specification of details in instructions in order to assess their specific effects in hypnotic and nonhypnotic conditions.

Research publications indicate a current emphasis on the search for a more parsimonious definition of the phenomenon of hypnosis. Before the question as to whether or not hypnosis "works," that is, is effective as a treatment, can be answered definitively, it seems logical that researchers define what (and for some, "if") hypnosis is. That is, does hypnosis indeed contain unique features not present in other procedures? Allowing for the possibility that hypnosis is indeed in some way unique, other researchers seek prerequisites or antecedents to the state.

As experimental investigation continues to delineate and discover variables that may be affecting outcome other than an hypnotic effect, the search for a parsimonious, operational definition of hypnosis has emphasized the need for stricter experimental controls and quantifiable measurement of data. As laboratory research concerning the nature of hypnosis (including antecedents, unique characteristics of, and consequents) uncovers confounding variables, it becomes necessary for clinical studies to account for these variables in order to reasonably justify a claim that a hypnotic induction or a hypnotic experience has influenced or effected a positive outcome of treatment. Gone are the days when a clinician could supposedly induce a supposed hypnotic trance and claim cure. Clinical research demands increased controls, quantitative pretreatment data, more refined statistical design and increased sophistication in the analysis of experimental data. It "has become much more difficult to design a methodologically adequate study today than it was in the 50's and early 60's. Without these laborious controls, however, often ambiguous and even erroneous conclusions can be drawn" (Salzberg & DePiano, 1980, p. 262).

The following paper will describe important factors that current research considers to be possible influences on reported outcomes of treatment utilizing hypnosis. Certain potential confounding variables have been identified experimentally that may call into question the role and efficacy of the clinical application of hypnosis. Such considerations as population, subject variables, experimenter variables, subject-experimenter relationship, situation variables, comparison groups, and experimental design, as they relate to research in the field of hypnosis, will be discussed.

METHODOLOGICAL FACTORS

Statement of Underlying Theory

All scientific research seeks to verify a stated hypothesis based on the assumptions of a theory. The basis of a theory of hypnosis varies according to the beliefs of the researcher. Hypnosis has been defined as an altered state of consciousness (Barber, 1976a) heightened expectancy (Barber, 1976b) increased compliance and belief in the hypnotic state (Wagstaff, 1981), increased suggestibility (Von Dendenroth, 1968), a unique cognitive state (Hilgard, 1977), role-taking (Sarbin & Slagle, 1979), regression (Gill & Brenman, 1961), dissociation (Hilgard, 1977; Nogrady, McConkey, Laurence & Perry, 1983), and heightened imagery (Barber, Spanos & Chaves, 1974). As there are many theories regarding hypnosis today, scientists researching the field must therefore approach their task according to the definition they choose to accept. Good research design necessarily begins with a statement of the researcher's rationale for the experiment. This may seem so obvious as to be an unnecessary reminder, yet many clinical and laboratory studies fail to clearly state their assumptions. "Investigators should become more aware of their underlying paradigms and how paradigms influence every aspect of their research. Investigators should also try to make their assumptions (which derive from their underlying paradigms and associated theories) more explicit" (Barber, 1976b, p. 85).

Population

Though strict random assignment of subjects to treatment groups is most desirable because it allows for greater generalization and extrapolation of the findings, several factors mitigate against its use in the research of hypnosis. Hilgard (1975, Hilgard & Tart, 1966) noted that only 30 percent of the population is highly susceptible to hypnosis and 42 to 45 percent are minimally susceptible.

He argued that the procedure of randomly assigning subjects to independent groups would be insensitive to the small differences in effects expected between a hypnotic treatment group and a comparison group. When an experiment attempts to determine the effects of hypnosis, it is imperative that hypnosis occur, yet many subjects randomly assigned to a hypnotic treatment group would be unable to respond. Thus, any positive effects produced by susceptible subjects would tend to be obscured by the lack of response to hypnosis expected from almost half of the sample unsusceptible to hypnosis. Adhering to strict random assignment necessitates large numbers of subjects in order to assure a sufficient number of susceptible subjects in each treatment cell to verify the effects of treatment. The time and cost constraints are obvious.

For this reason, in order to insure that an adequate number of subjects will indeed experience hypnosis and also to equally insure that nonhypnotic subjects will not inadvertently become hypnotized, much current research utilizes an assignment of subjects by level of susceptibility. Administering the Harvard Group Scale of Hypnotic Susceptibility Form A (Shor & Orne, 1962), or the Stanford Scale of Hypnotic Susceptibility Form A & B, or Form C (Weitzenhoffer & Hilgard, 1959, 1962) allows the experimenter to differentiate between High, Medium, and Low susceptibles according to their scores. Though most studies utilize some form of assessing susceptibility, this control is often rendered deficient by selecting only highly susceptible subjects or failing to include a Medium susceptible group in the design. In addition, any procedure which preselects subjects on the basis of certain characteristics limits the generalizability of the findings.

A random assignment technique using subjects of varying levels of susceptibility, if they are chosen in sufficient numbers to allow for comparisons of meaningful susceptibility categories, may be even superior to stratification because it allows for evaluating moderately susceptible subjects and is easier to perform postexperimentally, thus eliminating its potential reactive effects. Such random assignment does not so restrict generalization and extrapolation to a larger population (DePiano & Salzberg, 1982).

Subject Variables

Clinicians are asking not only for a clarification of when hypnosis is most likely to be effective, but for a clearer definition of what kind of client is most likely to be helped by this procedure. Among the suggestions for improving future research methodology in hypnosis, Wadden and Penrod (1981) state: "Subject characteristics and personality factors should be examined to determine their relationship to treatment outcome" (p. 46). As laboratory research continues factoring out influential variables, they must begin to be accounted for in clinical research.

Subject Attitudes and Beliefs. The subject's attitudes and beliefs concerning the competency of the hypnotist, personal levels of self-efficacy, and expectations as to what behaviors are appropriate or expected in a hypnotic situation can influence outcome (Barber, 1970; Balaschak, Blocker, Rossiter & Perin, 1972; Gruenwald, 1982). Positive outcome data may be enhanced by subjects who have a greater pretreatment belief in the efficacy of the procedure (Johnson & Barber, 1978; Wadden & Anderton, 1982).

A now classic experiment by Orne (1959) demonstrated the potency of expectancy and belief. A group of students were told during a class lecture that hypnotic subjects typically manifest "catalepsy of the dominant hand." A control group was not so informed. Fifty-five percent of the subjects in the experimental group demonstrated hand catalepsy during hypnosis. None in the control group did.

Another type of expectancy effect may be demonstrated when experimenter or situational cues alert the subject to the direction or kind of change that is expected during hypnosis (Spanos, Radtke-Bodorik, Ferguson & Jones, 1979). Spanos, Dubreuil, Saad, & Gorassini, 1983, suggest that their failure to confirm the finding of Wallace and his associates (Wallace & Garrett, 1973, 1975) concerning the displacement aftereffect following prism removal was due to an inadequacy of methodology. They suggest that some subjects may have guessed the experimental hypothesis and responded accordingly. "Future studies [could] vary the extent of preliminary information . . . given about the experimental hypothesis" (Spanos, Dubreuil, Saad, Gorassini, & Petrusic, 1981, p. 332).

Susceptibility Level. Research seems to indicate that level of susceptibility may be related to positive treatment outcome for some people when hypnosis is used in the treatment of some disorders (Wadden & Anderton, 1982). Clarifying for which people with which disorders has been enigmatic. In order to establish or nullify the relationship between various levels of susceptibility and positive treatment outcome, this variability must be accounted for in clinical research.

In order to control for the varying degrees of hypnotic responsivity evidenced by different individuals, standardized measures of behaviors representative of hypnotic performance have been developed. Assignment to High, Medium, or Low levels of susceptibility is determined by the number of items on a scale of increasing difficulty that an individual reports or evidences experiencing. Standardized measures include the following: The Harvard Group Scale of Hypnotic Susceptibility, Form A (HGSHS:A) (Shor & Orne, 1962); the individually administered Stanford Scale of Hypnotic Susceptibility, Forms A and B, and Form C (SHSS:A,B: SHSS:C) (Hilgard, 1965; Weitzenhoffer & Hilgard, 1959, 1962) and the Barber Suggestibility Scale (BSS) which has original and revised scoring procedures (Barber, 1969; Barber & Wilson, 1978–79) and can be administered to individuals or groups. Though recent efforts have been made to enhance susceptibility levels through instruction and practice, it is generally agreed at this time that level of hypnotic susceptibility tends to remain stable over time.

Some research seems to indicate that when the condition being treated is of a volitional nature, such as weight loss (Wadden & Flaxman, 1981) or cigarette smoking, level of susceptibility is unrelated to treatment outcome. However, positive treatment outcome with conditions which are nonvolitional in character such as clinical pain, asthma, or warts seems to be related to susceptibility levels (Perry, Gelfand & Marcovitch, 1979; Wadden & Anderton, 1982).

Wain (1980) states that approximately 50 percent of the patients referred to the Pain Clinic at Walter Reed Army Medical Center receive some form of hypnotic intervention. Further, level of susceptibility in part determines treatment strategy at the Clinic since differences in the effect of hypnosis have been reported by individuals according to their level of susceptibility. When hypnosis is used for pain control, high capacity responders report "numbness," mid-range responders report "tingling," and lower responders report neither and benefit from a greater emphasis on distracting techniques.

Further evidence that level of susceptibility may be indicative of individual differences is the finding that a "hidden observer" effect and duality in age regression is only reported by 40 percent of subjects within high levels of susceptibility (Hilgard, 1979; Laurence & Perry, 1981). The term "hidden observer" is used to represent the part of the subject that is aware of pain during hypnotic analgesia while a part of the subject experiencing hypnosis denies that pain. Duality in age regression refers to the continued awareness of adult identity while experiencing age regression during hypnosis. No relationship has been established experimentally between these two unique experiences and positive treatment outcome. It may be, however, that the "hidden observer" and duality phenomena represent different methods of cognitive processing. The role of differential cognitive processing styles and their relationship to treatment outcome is also as yet undetermined.

High levels of susceptibility have also been associated with shorter estimates of time duration during hypnotic treatment (Bowers, 1979; St. Jean & MacLeod, 1983), yet what effect, if any, time distortion may have on treatment outcome has not been established.

As the search continues for viable correlations between subject variables and positive treatment outcome, verifying subject level of susceptibility according to standardized measures provides comparability across studies and allows inferences to be made that may help develop an accurate profile of subject characteristics that enhance the effectiveness of hypnosis in the treatment of some disorders.

Age and Sex. Both age and sex differences in outcome were reported by Hilgard and LeBaron (1982) in their recent study on the effectiveness of hypnosis in relieving anxiety and pain of young cancer patients who were undergoing bone marrow aspirations. Hilgard and LeBaron reported in this study that greater discrepancies between observer rating and self-reports of experienced pain with children over the age of 10 may be interpreted as an attempt by the older group (age 10+) to conceal pain because of perceived social expectations. Younger children were less skillful at concealing pain or less concerned about social expectations in their expression of pain. Outcome data reflected this difference.

A recent study by Frischolz, Spiegel, Speigel, Balma and Markell (1982) concluded that increasing age is negatively correlated with measures of hypnotic responsivity and absorption. Controlling for such effects should not be overlooked when comparing treatment groups.

Enduring Personality Variables. The conclusions reached by Barber (1964) in his review of research concerning the relationship between enduring personality characteristics and individual differences in hypnotizability have yet to be disproven and remain currently unchallenged. Though several investigators included in this review had reported such a relationship, replication of their findings had failed to confirm their results. Investigators utilized the following measures: Rosenzweis Picture Frustration Test to assess impunitiveness and repression; The Taylor Anxiety Scale, Bills-Vance-McLean Index of Adjustment and Values, the Thematic Apperception Test and others to assess "neuroticism"; self-report inventories, Rorschach, Minnesota Multiphasic Personality Inventory, Edwards Personal Preference Schedule, Leary Interpersonal Check List, California Psychological Inventory, Maudsley Personality Inventory, as well as clinical assessments of personality. All failed to support a relationship between personality factors and susceptibility. Barber concluded that individual differences in hypnotic susceptibility could not be accounted for by "enduring differences among individuals in such characteristics of personality as dominance, extraversion, sociability, neuroticism, etc." (1964, p. 316).

History of the Problem. A complete history of the problem behavior or condition that has been targeted for change is necessary in order to determine the effects of onset, frequency, intensity, or duration on treatment outcome. Such differences in symptomotology are invariably ignored in clinical research on hypnosis. Comparability across studies, even with case histories, is severely compromised. Future investigations should include a complete description of individual data concerning such factors.

Other Subject Variables. Other subject variables that may be relevant in determining the effectiveness of hypnosis include the subject's previous experience with hypnosis, his or her attitude toward the experiment and his or her relationship with the therapist (Gruenwald, 1982; Tart, 1967), his or her motivation for treatment (Barber, 1964; Perry, Gelfand & Marcovitch, 1979; Sheehan & Dolby, 1979), the capacity for imaginative involvement (Hilgard, 1979), or absorption (Tellegen & Atkinson, 1974) and heightened expectancy (Barber, 1976a).

Experimenter Variables

Although many studies indicate that results of an experiment may be influenced by various individual differences of the experimenter, which individual characteristics are significant have yet to be determined (Barber, 1970). Age, sex, and race as well as the perceived prestige, authority, or power associated with the experimenter may increase or decrease expectations and willingness to comply, and thus alter the response of the subject (Small & Kramer, 1969).

The experimenter's own attitude toward the experiment or towards a particular treatment group may also subtly influence subject response (Gruenwald, 1982). It has been demonstrated that the experimenter's expectations influence his or her rate of speech, tone of voice, and paraverbal communications that in turn alter subject response. Utilizing the real-simulator design with the experimenter blind as to which subjects are hypnotized is one way of controlling for such subtle influences (Orne, 1979).

Barber (1976b) further suggests that the experimenter may alter outcome data by failing to follow specific procedures, by misrecording data, by fudging or manipulating data during collection, or by unintentionally communicating experimental biases or expectancies. Research has demonstrated that subjects are likely to exhibit behaviors that fulfill perceived experimenter expectancies (Salzberg & DePiano, 1980).

Designing the experiment to control for these variables may include more rigid control of experimenter behaviors, accounting for the presence of certain experimenter variables and providing for comparisons when such variables are anticipated. Independent observations of the experimental situation may yield significant information concerning these influences.

Subject-Experimenter Relationship

Most relevant research that attempts to demonstrate the unique characteristics of hypnosis and its meaningfulness as a treatment component fails to adequately describe or consider the relationship between the subject and the experimenter (Tart, 1965). Higher levels of hypnotic susceptibility have been correlated with a previously positive relationship with the therapist/hypnotist (Greenberg & Land, 1971; Kramer, 1969; Tart, 1967).

"The capacity for involvement in the hypnotic experience appears to be mediated to a significant extent by S's perception of the hypnotist and the degree of security and alliance which that perception fosters" (Levitt & Baker, 1983, pp. 129–130). Psychoanalytic theorists argue that the hypnotic relationship is characterized by transferential factors. However, they are quick to point out that transference occurs in any relationship to varying degrees and as Chertok (1981) points out: "One can wonder whether the concept of transference makes it possible to account for the specific nature of the hypnotic relationship" (p. 85).

Shor (1979) defines one of the dimensions of hypnotic depth as the "extent of archaic involvement" (p. 126). "Depth of archaic involvement is the extent to which there occurs a temporary displacement of 'transference' of core personality emotive attitudes formed early in life . . . onto the hypnotist" (p. 126). In determining such involvement, Shor recommends a phenomenological measurement which involves investigative cooperation between the examiner and subject. As this method has yet to be investigated experimentally, significance of this phenomenon remains undetermined.

That a positive relationship must exist between hypnotist and subject is generally agreed upon by clinicians. The nature of that relationship as defined by specific characteristics remains illusive. A positive relationship may, in fact, have the unfortunate effect of producing a folie de deux. ". . . the hypnotist is trying his best to make the hypnotic procedures come true for his subjects, and the subjects in return are trying their best to make the hypnotist's fondest theoretical dreams come true—even if to comply sometimes requires that they secretly arrange to cheat and delude themselves" (Shor, 1979, p. 39).

Situation Variables

Most research fails to consider adequately the demand characteristics of the experimental situation. Demand characteristics inherent in hypnotic treatment may determine the nature of the subject's response. Cues may derive from the task, the experimental procedure, the nature of the instructions, or from the experimenter or hypnotist personally. Barber and Calverly (1964) demonstrated that the definition of the experimental situation to the subject influences subject behavior. Subjects were less responsive to hypnotic suggestibility when the situation was defined as a "test for gullibility" than when it was defined as a "test of imagination."

Sarbin and Coe (1979) propose that "the setting identified as hypnosis encourages the subject to engage in actions to achieve or enhance credibility" (p. 524). Subjects may be capable of deception as well as self-deception by becoming involved in not remembering and convincing themselves that they can't remember, thereby satisfying the conflicting demands for honesty along with the demand for the expected response. Highly susceptible subjects may be strongly motivated to verify their hypnotic condition (Orne, 1959; Sarbin & Coe, 1972). Such motivation may alert them to contextual information that would facilitate successfully responding as expected. Spanos, Dubreuil, Saad and Gorassini (1983) recently demonstrated that an apparent effect of hypnotic anesthesia could be eliminated by informing the subjects of an experimental hypothesis to the contrary.

Barber (1970) suggests that a subject may be motivated to deny the experience of pain because of the nature of the hypnotic situation. The subject desires to please the hypnotist and may decide that reporting pain may imply that the therapist's time was wasted. Even though he or she may continue to experience pain, it may be less anxiety-provoking to say that he or she does not. Stam and Spanos (1980) demonstrated that the effectiveness of hypnotic or waking analgesia varied according to the experimental expectations communicated to the subjects. Both self-reports of subjective experience of pain as well as overt behavior conformed to experimentally-induced expectations.

The nature of the experimenter's instruction, behavior, and definition of the task is critically important to the outcome observed. Attention to such detail in the experiment itself as well as in the reporting of the study is necessary in order to assure replicability and comparability. Lack of such attention to detail weakens possible assumptions or conclusions that may be inferred.

COMPARISON GROUPS

As the phenomenon of hypnosis as an effective treatment tool has come under closer scrutiny, alternative explanations have been offered concerning observable results. Any report that claims hypnosis as accounting for change must differentiate the unique contribution of hypnosis as well as demonstrate an increase in treatment effectiveness with hypnosis over other established clinical procedures (Wadden & Anderton, 1982). Further, if the experiment fails to demonstrate the effectiveness of hypnosis, factors that may have accounted for change should be delineated and reported. When using hypnosis in a treatment package, is hypnosis enhancing, effective alone, or in combination with certain other treatment factors, or is it irrelevant? In order to answer these diverse questions, the use of comparison groups in the clinical research of hypnosis becomes unavoidable.

Motivational Comparison Groups

Task Motivational. "Task motivating instructions" were developed by Barber and Calverly (1963a, 1963b) to represent all those elements found in standard inductions which could be considered nonhypnotic (see Barber, 1969, for full text of instructions). According to them such variables include appeal to the subject's self-esteem, the expressed expectation of cooperation, definition of the task as involving imagination, appeal to the subject's desire to help the experimenter, and statements that it is easy to respond. These instructions were developed to test the prediction that nonhypnotic variables could yield effects equivalent to those produced by hypnotic induction and thus provide a more parsimonious alternative explanation for phenomena observed consequent to hypnotic induction. DePiano and Salzberg (1982) stated that "Barber et al's (1974) repeated claim that task motivating suggestions without hypnosis are as effective as hypnotic suggestions has made a 'no hypnosis with task motivating suggestions' group an essential control in studies examining the relationship between hypnosis and performance" (p. 388).

The value of task motivating instructions rests on their equivalence to hypnotic induction in all respects other than their exclusion of elements which are hypnosis-inducing. Bowers (1967), and Sheehan and Dolby (1974) have challenged this necessary equivalency by identifying a factor of "strong social pressure to comply" or "behavioral constraint," respectively. This is represented in the instructions by statements that the value of the experiment and the experimenter's worth depend on the subject's compliance and performance. The social pressure artifact was found to induce subjects to make reports of hypnotic phenomena not truly experienced. These excessive reports were reduced by including demands for honesty in the instructions to subjects. Recently Spanos, Barber, and Lang (1974) published a revised version of task motivating instructions which eliminate the behavioral constraint artifact. Hilgard (1975) recommends them for use in future hypnosis research. Most studies published to date fail to incorporate this procedure or the demand for honesty control suggested by Bowers (1967).

Exhortation Instructions. Exhortation instructions were developed by London and Fuhrer (1961) as a general motivational procedure. These instructions contain content designed to convince subjects that they can exceed their perceived performance limits, that the discomfort of persisting at difficult tasks should be reinterpreted as cues to continue rather than to stop, and that the subject's maximum performance is essential to the experimenter for the successful outcome of the study. The original full procedure was used both alone and with hypnosis and it included brief additional exhortations prior to each task. Improvement as a consequence of rational desire was stressed by these instructions. Exhorting instructions were originally designed for use with physical performance tasks and therefore their use with other tasks would necessitate some changes. The goal of these instructions is similar to that of Barber's task motivational instructions, that is, to control for and/or equate groups motivationally. As with other types of instruction, an effort should always be made to duplicate the original version unless specific justification is given for doing otherwise. Several parts of the exhortation instructions are unique (e.g., to reinterpret experienced discomfort) and may therefore have unique effects. The consequence of using different versions of such instructions is that comparability of results is reduced.

Involving Instructions. Another set of motivational instructions called "involving instructions" was introduced by Slotnick, Liebert, and Hilgard (1965) as an addition to exhorting instructions. The involving instructions are described as different from others because they stress commitment and involvement by the subject in producing increased performance, and because subjects are required to verbally state their intense desire to perform well. Subjects are also instructed to think of their capacity as enhanced. Preliminary results indicated that involving instructions interact with exhortation to enhance performance. Under what conditions and with what tasks they are effective is just beginning to be researched.

Simulating Comparison Group

The search for behavioral characteristics that are intrinsic to hypnosis led Orne (1979) to develop a unique type of comparison group for use in hypnosis research. The simulating procedure provides a group highly motivated to perform exactly as the experiment desires. Thus, a measure of the normal volitional capacity of subjects can be obtained for comparison with hypnotic performance (Sheehan & Perry, 1976). The simulating subject is required to be unsusceptible to hypnosis and is therefore selected from individuals with low scores on susceptibility scales. After being given nonspecific instructions to fake or role play the behavior of a hypnotized person, the simulator is then exposed to the same treatments as the hypnotic subjects. It is crucial that the experimenter remain blind as to the "real" or "simulating" subjects. Orne (1971) has argued that a faking group is an inadequate control unless the fakers believe that the experimenter does not know they are faking. Because of their unsusceptibility to hypnosis and instructions given them to simply role play hypnosis, it is assumed that simulators do not become hypnotized and are responding primarily to experimental cues available to all subjects.

The simulating comparison group controls for such artifacts as (1) subtle cues that alert the hypnotized subject as to the response expected or desired, (2) the differential treatment by the hypnotist of the hypnotized and the nonhypnotized subjects, (3) the effects of information available to the subject about a particular study, (4) the possible effect of hypnosis increasing the motivation of the subject to please the hypnotist, and (5) behavior that is voluntarily engaged in as the result of perceived role expectations of one who has agreed to the role of hypnotized person.

If the simulators are found to perform identically to the hypnotic subjects, the resulting inference is that experimental artifacts such as instructions, interactions, or beliefs rather than a special state called hypnosis may have determined the behavior of the hypnotic subjects as well as that of simulating subjects. It is possible that an alternative explanation other than those already suggested may be necessary to answer the question of why simulators behave as hypnotized subjects. Orne (1979) suggests that the behavior of real and simulating subjects may be mediated by different mental processes.

When the performances of real and simulating subjects differ, it is assumed that the behavior of real hypnotic subjects reflects uniquely hypnotic behavior. This assumption cannot be guaranteed, however, because obtained differences may be due to other artifacts or to the effects of the simulating condition itself (Orne, 1959; Sheehan, 1973). The use of a simulating group provides information regarding behavior during hypnosis that may be attributed to such experimental cues as specific instructions, interaction with the experimenter, or situational cues. Simulating subjects "help establish whether subjects could have figured out from cues in the experimental situation what constituted the expected behavior without having been exposed to the subjective experiences of hypnosis" (Orne, 1979, p. 539).

Though differences are seldom reported between "real" subjects and simulators, Nogrady, McConkey, Laurence and Perry (1983) demonstrated the "hidden observer" effect was unique to approximately one-half of the highly susceptible "reals" who participated in their study. Further, only those subjects who reported a hidden-observer effect reported duality during age regression. Clearly the use of such a control group will help delineate factors unique to a hypnotic experience.

Caution is advised when attempting to utilize this method of comparison. Small differences in the simulating instructions can produce quite different results (Orne, 1979). Orne provides an example of simulating instructions and defines nine requirements for successfully implementing the procedure. Studies which report using simulating groups but fail to specify the procedure or to cite a source for their instructions are considered deficient. Without the use of the standard form of the simulating procedure, comparability with other studies and validity of the procedure's effects is lessened.

Alert Induction Comparison Group

A number of authors have developed nontraditional inductions in order to control for certain effects of the traditional format. Oetting (1964) developed the first "alert" trance induction procedure for use with subjects being assessed on tasks requiring concentration and alertness. He claimed that the suggestions of sleep, drowsiness, and eye closure found in traditional inductions conflicted with subsequent suggestions to achieve a greater state of awareness with the result that these suggestions reduced the level of trance.

Leibert, Rubin, and Hilgard (1965) developed an alert induction for reasons similar to Oetting's. Their procedure consisted of using the traditional Stanford Hypnotic Susceptibility Scale, Form A (SHSS:A) (Weitzenhoffer and Hilgard, 1959) which was altered by the omission of all reference to sleep, drowsiness, or relaxation. Subsequent to this induction, they included suggestions designed to counteract any preexisting expectations of sleep as a part of hypnosis, to induce alertness, and to maintain depth. They used a postexperimental inquiry to verify the presence of alertness and the subjective experience of depth and hypnosis.

Vingoe (1968, 1973) employed a group-administered procedure which begins with a period of establishing rapport followed by the head fall suggestion from the Harvard scale. His alert induction follows and is characterized by concurrent suggestions of mental alertness and bodily relaxation. He defines the experience to subjects as "deep hypnosis" and as dissociation of mind and body. He thereby counteracts any expectations of lethargy subjects have of hypnosis.

The alert induction procedures may suggest different experiences to the subject. It is not clear that they are completely comparable in the states that they may elicit or the effects they have. Oetting's (1964) procedure suggests focusing of attention and fixation of gaze; Liebert, Rubin, and Hilgard (1965) used an altered traditional induction followed by suggestions of alertness and depth; and Vingoe (1968) emphasized mind-body dissociation, alertness, and bodily relaxation. If suggestions or instructions are intended to have specific effects then these inductions may orient subjects to behave differently. The consequence in evaluating studies which use alert induction procedures without direct comparison of procedures using similar specific instructions may be a confusion of the factors attributable to differences in outcome.

Relaxation Comparison Group

Since both relaxation and hypnosis involve changes in voluntary motor response, to claim hypnosis as effecting a change "without also showing that relaxation without hypnosis does not similarly affect the same system is to confound the interpretation of the data" (Edmonston, 1979, p. 442). Therefore, in demonstrating the effectiveness of hypnosis in a clinical setting, it is necessary to differentiate its effectiveness from the use of a standard relaxation procedure. For this reason, a relaxation control group may be utilized. For a thorough review of the similarities of relaxation and hypnosis and current research in this area, the reader is referred to Edmonston (1981).

No Treatment Comparison Group

When there is reason to believe that spontaneous remission may occur without treatment, it becomes necessary to assign similar subjects to a no-treatment or waiting list control group. Success of treatment may then be attributed to the treatment itself without the confounding effects of passage of time, environmental manipulation, or other treatment artifacts.

Attention Control Group

Differences in outcome may be attributed to differences in amount or quality of attention given to subjects in various treatment groups which, in turn, may influence treatment expectancies. "In the absence of an attention control group, differences between conditions are uninterpretable in terms of identifying active components of hypnotic treatment" (Wadden & Anderton, 1982, p. 239). In studies of treatment of migraine, for instance, subjects receiving medication often receive less attention than subjects receiving hypnosis.

Alternative Treatment Comparison Groups

Since the clinician is interested in defining the most effective treatment procedures for a specified problem or disorder, comparing a hypnosis treatment group, hypnosis in combination with other treatment group, and a group receiving only the alternative treatment is required. Such studies have utilized alternative treatments such as behavior therapy (e.g., systematic desensitization, cognitive restructuring, relaxation), acupuncture, pharmacotherapy, biofeedback, and so on.

EXPERIMENTAL DATA COLLECTION

The methods and techniques employed for data collection by clinical researchers often severely compromise inferences that can be made regarding treatment results. The following section calls attention to this facet of research and factors that are frequently overlooked in current clinical studies.

Pretreatment Data

Baseline descriptions of the problem or disorder to be treated are frequently neglected. In order to provide for comparability across studies, this data is of paramount importance. Baseline description should include subject characteristics as well as onset, duration, frequency, and intensity of the behavior. Furthermore, an operational definition of the change desired should be stated.

Baseline testing provides the measure of untreated performance necessary for comparison with treatment conditions (Sheehan & Perry, 1976). Pretesting should be conducted prior to the subjects' becoming aware that an experiment on hypnosis follows and should optimally be conducted in a context divorced from the experimental setting. This allows the measurement to be uncontaminated by subject expectations.

Susceptibility testing should follow pretesting and baseline observation of the problem behavior or condition to be treated. Most studies use a pretest of the dependent variable after susceptibility testing which allows the subject to contaminate initial responding. The measurement of susceptibility may have different effects on high and low susceptible subjects. High and low susceptible subjects have the different experiences of passing and failing most of the items on such scales and this may influence their motivations and attitudes with respect to the rest of the experiment. Susceptibility testing also informs the subject that hypnosis is an important experimental variable. Such knowledge can act as a demand characteristic and may influence subjects to underperform or hold back during pretesting and/or the waking condition in an effort to ensure that the hypnotic performance is superior (e.g., Zamansky, Scharf, & Brightbill, 1964). To control for these effects, susceptibility testing should be done after pretesting on the dependent measure.

Susceptibility testing can also be done on a post hoc basis as Barber and Calverly (1966) have done. This eliminates reactive effects from the experiment altogether. Both procedures require providing some measure and/or treatments to larger subject samples which may make the post hoc procedure impractical. Slotnick and London (1965) used a deception to control for the effects of susceptibility testing and susceptibility. They informed both highly susceptible and unsusceptible subjects that they had performed well on susceptibility testing in an attempt to minimize any perception of the unsusceptible subjects that they were poor subjects. This was done to equalize the motivational sets of both groups of subjects. This is a weaker procedure because, as Sheehan and Perry (1976) note, several studies have shown the experimenter's manipulations to have little effect on the subject's expectancies. A postexperimental inquiry should be included whenever such deceptions are used in order to assess their effectiveness and to assess the subjects' expectations generally. In addition, other effects of selection procedures and/or susceptibility are not controlled by this deception.

Quantitative and qualitative measures of the behavior before treatment will, of course, vary with the type of problem being treated. Performance measures are often task scores; psychosomatic disorders may be scores on questionnaires, undesirable behaviors, or habits. Addictive behaviors or problem behaviors may be scaled according to scores on questionnaires administered to the subject prior to treatment. Self-reports should be verified by ratings of independent observers whenever possible. Any measuring device, task, or questionnaire utilized should be reported in detail in order to provide for replication and comparison across studies.

Treatment Data

An exact report of the treatment procedure utilized with each group or individual is necessary in order to provide for replicability. It is also important to specify all contact with subjects from the time of selection through treatment. The number and length of sessions as well as order of treatment is relevant and frequently unreported. If more than one hypnotic session occurs there may be increasing effectiveness with practice. If not, would the same change have occurred using only one session?

Depth of hypnosis is an important dimension of hypnotic treatment to control for since specific suggestions may succeed or fail and specific hypnotic phenomena may or may not be experienced (e.g., time distortion) depending upon whether the subject has attained sufficient depth for such to occur. Tart (1972, 1978-79) describes depth as referring to the temporal changes in the intensity of various aspects of hypnotic responsiveness and the subjective experience of hypnotic phenomena. He cautions that variations in hypnotic depth can inject sufficient variation into experimental results to hide genuine effects.

Six standard measures of hypnotic depth are discussed by Tart (1979, 1978-79) who recommends their use throughout the period of the hypnotic condition in which the subject is assessed on the dependent variable. He particularly recommends use of the Long Stanford Scale (Tart, 1979) and the regular or extended versions of the North Carolina Scale. See Tart (1979, 1978-79) for a full discussion of these and other scales. Depth procedures are particularly desirable where assessment of the dependent measure is separated in time from the induction and where multiple or continuous assessment of the dependent variable takes place. Most studies do not use a measure of depth or fail to use a standard scale.

A description of the hypnotic experience may be rated by the experimenter, the hypnotist, and an independent observer. Accounting for situational, hypnotist, and interactional differences that may influence results is crucial.

If the treatment uses a combination of self and heterohypnosis it is necessary to specify in what order and with what specific instructions such a combination was activated. Self-hypnosis is usually only verified by subjects' self-reports which may be contaminated by inadvertent duration and frequency. Verification by independent observers in the subjects' environment or by the experimenter may reveal information that could change inferences concerning the use of self-hypnosis.

Post-treatment Data Collection

Orne (1969, 1979) has recommended using a standard inquiry procedure to gain insight into the experimental demand characteristics which may influence subjects' behavior on the dependent variable under study. The postexperimental inquiry can help clarify how the subject perceived the total experimental situation, what the subject believed was expected as the outcome of treatment, and what the subject believed would be the typical responses of others. From this information, the experimenter can learn what the subject perceived as being responses which were desirable in that they represent him favorably and/or please the researcher by validating his experimental hypothesis. Orne (1959, 1979) summarizes literature which indicates that such subject perceptions can significantly influence experimental results. Studies which utilize some form of postexperimental inquiry do so for various reasons including: to assess the effectiveness of specific treatments (Cooper & London, 1973; DePiano & Salzberg, 1982; Sakata & Anderson, 1970), to evaluate a deception procedure (Cooper & London, 1973), or to evaluate demand characteristics (Slotnick et al., 1965).

Among the interesting findings were that subjects provided an alert induction felt less hypnotized than when this was given for their initial susceptibility test (Salzberg & DePiano, 1980) and that exhortation and involving instructions may inhibit the order effects of multiple treatments due to demand characteristics (Slotnick, Liebert, & Hilgard, 1965).

Inquiry procedures clearly have value for evaluating experimental procedures but must be interpreted cautiously. Orne (1969), and Sheehan and Perry (1976) point out that information from inquiry techniques cannot generate direct inferences. There always remains the doubt that the subject's report may reflect the process of reflection or perceived expectation of the desired response rather than the actual experience of the subject. Given this caution, Sheehan and Perry (1976) conclude that the data from such procedures is crucially important and that research on hypnosis should universally include an exhaustive iniqury into the subject's perceptions of experimental procedures.

Immediate evaluation of the hypnotic experience may be obtained by having the subject view a videotape of the session. In this way a subjective description of covert behavior can be correlated with overt behavior during the session. Exact quantitative measures of behavior change should be noted. Such measures may include evaluations of task performance, cognitive performance, recall, anxiety, and so on.

Recording change over time is invaluable in determining the effectiveness of treatment and can verify stability of results. Follow-up data is often neglected entirely or based on self-reports that are returned by mail. Seldom is follow-up data verified by the experimenter, yet results are often based on these self-reports. Post-testing immediately following the experiment as well as at specific follow-up dates would strengthen conclusions.

EXPERIMENTAL DESIGN

Case Study

Many clinicians utilize case studies in reporting successful treatment by hypnosis. Unfortunately, though this design could have heuristic value, data is often so limited in the final report that replicability and comparability is impossible. Attention to the various aspects of data collection previously discussed would improve the value of such reporting. Case studies which are systematic and experimental can set the stage for follow-up research. Insights offered by the author can be enlightening and contribute to resolving the practical problems of research, especially with natural populations.

Own Control Design

In its simplest form, the subject as his own control or "own control" design requires that a single group of randomly sampled subjects be exposed to two successive treatments. These are typically a hypnotic condition and a non-hypnotic comparison condition such as "imagination" instructions, motivating instructions, or a no-treatment waking control. Hilgard (1965; Hilgard & Tart, 1966) has been the major proponent of this design. He recommended its use to overcome problems created by the wide range of hypnotic susceptibility found in the general population. This design allows measurements of individual subject responses to comparison treatments and has the advantage of reducing the estimate of experimental error and increasing sensitivity to treatment effects (Barber, 1967; Hilgard, 1965).

Refined versions of this design have included counterbalancing the treatments. This procedure requires that half of the subjects receive Treatment One first while the second half of the subjects receive Treatment Two first. The responses of subjects to the two treatments are then compared. This procedure was added to control for the possibility that the first treatment might influence responses in the second treatment. Counterbalancing allows for the evaluation of order effects using an analysis of variance statistical design (Coe, 1973).

Despite the use of counterbalancing, however, the presence of order effects cannot be entirely ruled out and may, in fact, manifest in a variety of ways (Campbell & Stanley, 1971; Sheehan & Perry, 1976). The own-control design has been criticized by Barber (1969) on this count. He observed that the subject may respond to experimental demand characteristics perceived as the expectation that performance should be superior in the hypnotic condition. Zamansky, Scharf, and Brightbill (1964) verified this effect by demonstrating that subjects may "hold back" or underperform in the first treatment if they believe that the superior performance is expected in the second, hypnotic treatment.

Sheehan and Perry (1976) have suggested, after a reanalysis of Hilgard and Tart (1966), that subjects might also adjust their performance retrospectively by altering their performance in the second treatment condition. After reviewing relevant literature they conclude that holding back may be only one of many possible order effects pertinent to this design. Subjects may hold back under either treatment condition, respond to demand characteristics for change per se across conditions, or improve across conditions due to a practice effect.

Sheehan and Perry (1976) recommend two procedures to control for such effects. These include counterbalancing with a subsequent analysis for order effects and the systematic manipulation of subjects' expectancies regarding what and how many conditions will occur and what outcomes are expected. They caution, however, that several studies have shown the experimenter's manipulations to have little effect on the subjects' expectancies. A postexperimental inquiry should therefore be included to assess the effectiveness of such manipulations and to assess the subjects' expectations generally.

Interaction Design

The interaction design has a complex format with several requirements. Randomly selected subjects are stratified into two groups of extreme responders on a measure of hypnotic susceptibility. These high and low susceptible subjects are pretested on the dependent variable and randomly assigned from their separate groups to counterbalanced comparison treatments. In this way one half of each group of high and low susceptible subjects receives one of the comparison treatments first while the other half of these subjects receives the remaining treatment first. In its simplest form, four groups are compared on the dependent variable task using an analysis of variance (Coe, 1973; Sheehan & Perry, 1976). This design was developed by London and several coworkers (London, Conant & Davison, 1966; London & Fuhrer, 1961; Slotnick & London, 1965) in order to resolve discrepant findings across a large number of studies in which hypnosis both enhanced and had no effect on performance. Most of these studies manipulated a small number of variables. London and others, however, believed that hypnotic behavior represented an interaction of many factors such as susceptibility, hypnotic treatments, instructions, various sources of motivation, and order of presenting conditions. Using this design they sought to unravel the effects of these variables on performance.

The chief strength of the interaction design lies in the many variables which it formally assesses in their main and interacting effects on performance. Because of their emphasis on refinement of design features as the means to resolve discrepant results, those who have used this design have employed a variety of strong controls now identified with the design itself. Chief among these are the stratification of subjects by susceptibility and baseline pretesting on the dependent measure.

The counterbalanced repeated measures procedure is justified by this design with the same arguments used to support its use in the own-control design. The value of this procedure lies in its ability to increase design sensitivity to hypnotic treatments and to control for order of treatment effects. When baseline testing and counterbalancing are used together a variety of different analyses can be undertaken. As Cooper and London (1973) demonstrate, the first treatments can be compared to the baseline pretest as in the covariance design, and a simple posttest only analysis can be done as in the independent group design. A comparison of these different analyses provides greater insight into relationships between the variables and enhances the validity of inferences obtained from the results. Though counterbalancing of treatments is often employed, most studies fail to report the required formal analyses for order effects. Future studies using this procedure should inform the reader that order effects were clearly ruled out.

The interaction design is considered a superior design when the requirements specified for its use are employed. It is particularly strong because its results can be analyzed in a variety of ways. This enhances the validity of conclusions reached and allows for the identification of unwanted effects. In this respect it is superior to the covariance design.

Covariance Design

The covariance design or "pretest-posttest control group" design (Campbell & Stanley, 1971) requires that a pretest of the dependent variable be taken prior to, or independently from, random assignment of subjects to experimental and control groups (Barber, 1967; Campbell & Stanley, 1971). Any factors which might influence the subject's ability or motivation to respond to the treatments should be controlled (e.g., prior hypnotic experience). Random assignment of subjects generally gives the assurance that such factors are controlled. The use of a no-treatment control group and the inclusion of pretesting also helps to ensure the lack of initial biases between groups (and, beyond this, provides for the control and direct measurement of the effects of repeated testing on the dependent measure). As is true with the practical use of all designs, subjects are often stratified into two groups selected for their extreme scores on measures of hypnotic susceptibility. Pretesting or baseline measures of behavior should be obtained prior to susceptibility testing whenever feasible to prevent contamination of baseline measures.

The particular strength of the covariance design lies in its ability to reduce experimental error and increase sensitivity to treatment effects by assessing the within-subject change on the dependent variables in response to treatments (Barber, 1967). The inclusion of pretesting allows for this. The design came into greater use after the simpler independent groups design was found to be insufficiently sensitive to identify the typically small effect of hypnotic treatments when they might occur. Barber and others chose the covariance design over the equally sensitive own-control design and the counterbalanced designs then in use, because the latter had been found to manifest the potentially serious deficit of allowing subjects to systematically alter their performance across multiple treatments (i.e., demand characteristic and other order-of-treatment effects). By using separate comparison groups the covariance design greatly minimizes these effects.

As distinct from the independent groups design, the covariance design allows for precise inferences to be drawn when differences between treatment group performances are found. This design eliminates the alternative explanation that preexisting group differences may have been responsible for the results obtained. By assessing preexisting differences, this design allows for their analysis and/or future control.

The covariance design is one of the two strongest designs used in hypnosis research. It is both sensitive to the subtle effects of hypnosis and not limited by the order effects found in an interaction design. When treatments are carefully chosen, both the main and interacting effects of variables can be evaluated. Because of these many strengths, its future use in hypnosis research is assured.

Independent Groups Design

In its basic form, this design requires only that unselected subjects be randomly assigned to one or more treatment groups and a no-treatment control group. These groups are then compared on some posttest measure. This design is identical to Campbell and Stanley's (1971) posttest-only control group design and is considered a true experimental design. In hypnosis research, the treatment groups have typically included a formal induction condition and a condition assumed to be nonhypnotic but otherwise equal to induction. Other comparisons have been effectively made, however, and the most widely used of these comparisons have been discussed previously. Barber has been foremost in encouraging the use of this design which he recommends using with a nonhypnotic comparison condition, task motivating instructions (Barber, 1969). The essential comparisons made with this design have the goals of revealing whether hypnotic conditions have effects unique from nonhypnotic conditions, what these effects are, and what components of these treatments and suggestions or instructions are effective. In order for valid comparisons to be made with this design it is essential that any other factors which might discriminate waking and hypnotic subjects, in terms of their ability or activation to respond to treatments, be controlled. The random assignment of subjects and inclusions of a no-treatment control group allows for adequate assurance of lack of initial biases between groups and controls for the effects of testing, although such effects are not measured directly.

This design's chief strength lies in its simplicity. It allows for the uncomplicated isolation of dependent and independent variables and for the assessment of functional relationships between them. The independent groups design is free of many of the weaknesses found in the more complicated designs.

The major criticism of this design has been that it lacks sufficient sensitivity to detect hypnotic phenomena because subjects highly responsive to hypnotic treatments represent only a small proportion of the population randomly assigned by this design. Another limitation of this design has been elaborated by Sheehan and Perry (1976). They point out the inadequacy of this design for allowing precise inferences to be drawn when the performance of subjects in treatment groups differ from the performance of the control group subjects. Random selection and the use of a control group does not guarantee that the differences between groups are not related to preexisting differences in responsivity existing between subjects. They state that inferences about the effects of enhanced suggestibility belong to comparisons within groups and not to intergroup comparisons.

Design Evaluation

A final evaluation of the designs used must find the covariance and interaction designs to be superior. They are developments of simpler designs which incorporate the important controls of pretesting and susceptibility assessment. When used with other controls appropriate to the questions asked, they yield strong inferences.

The design with the greatest capacity to establish the validity of conclusions drawn from its comparisons is the interaction design. Its strength here lies in its capacity to evaluate a wider variety of relationships between the variables manipulated. It allows comparisons identical to those made with the covariance design and the independent groups design in addition to allowing for the assessment of order and interaction effects.

In the final analysis, the strength of any design is dependent upon the ways in which treatment conditions are specified, in what manner they are distinguished, and upon how the control groups are specified as different from the experimental groups (Sheehan & Perry, 1976). "The most important guidelines to the researcher who samples among treatments for the purposes of comparison is that he institutes the means to recognize the essential limitations of the procedures that he employs/controls, as well as experimental" (Sheehan & Perry, 1976, p.292).

SUMMARY

The value of hypnosis as an effective treatment strategy has yet to be demonstrated by scientific research. In order to define when, for what conditions, and why hypnosis can be recommended as a treatment tool, the influence of treatment variables must be assessed. In the case of hypnosis, research is just beginning to exercise the rigorous controls necessary to answer questions of clinical relevance.

Researchers have been reminded of the importance of including a precise statement of their underlying theory. Attention must be given to controlling subject variables such as hypnotic susceptibility, relationship with the therapist, individual differences in such factors as attitudes, motivation, imagination, absorption, and attention, as well as traditional demographic variables. There is a need for more detailed pretreatment descriptions of the condition or disorder including a complete history of the problem in order to increase comparability and generalization to similar populations. Other treatment variables that must be accounted for include experimenter characteristics and behavior, subject-experimenter interactions, and situational variables. The nature of hypnosis frequently necessitates the use of such comparison groups as task motivational, relaxation control, and attention control, simulating subjects as well as alternative treatment groups.

Experimental data reported by investigators in the field of hypnosis research is often insufficient. Care must be exercised to collect and report quantitative baseline data, including both quantitative and qualitative measures of self-report, experimenter observations and independent observer ratings. There is a need for more consistent follow-up and verification of follow-up data in order to verify long-term effectiveness of hypnotic treatment. Several of the experimental designs that have been used most frequently in hypnosis research have been discussed.

Before success can be attributed to any procedure, it must be demonstrated experimentally that treatment results were not produced by factors competing or extraneous to the technique. This paper has attempted to call attention to factors that may contaminate research and hinder the search for answers to questions of clinical relevance in the use of hypnosis. Only when rigorous scientific controls have been applied in the research of hypnosis will recommendations for treatment with hypnosis be possible.

REFERENCES

Balaschak, B., Blocker, K., Rossiter, T., & Perin, C. T. (1972). The influence of race and expressed experience of the hypnotist on hypnotic susceptibility. *International Journal of Clinical and Experimental Hypnosis, 20,* 38–45.

Barber, T. X. (1964). Hypnotizability, suggestibility, and personality: A critical review of research findings. *Psychological Reports, 14,* 299–320.

Barber, T. X. (1965a). The effects of "hypnosis" on learning and recall: A methodological critique. *Journal of Clinical Psychology, 21,* 19–25.

Barber, T. X. (1965b). Experimental analysis of "hypnotic" behavior: A review of recent empirical findings. *Journal of Abnormal Psychology, 80,* 132–154.

Barber, T. X. (1966). The effects of "hypnosis" and motivational suggestions on strength and endurance: A critical review of the research studies. *British Journal of Social and Clinical Psychology, 5,* 42–50.

Barber, T. X. (1967). "Hypnotic" phenomena: A critique of experimental methods. In J. E.Gordon (Ed.), *Handbook of Clinical and Experimental Hypnosis.* New York: Macmillan.

Barber, T. X. (1969). *Hypnosis: A scientific approach.* New York: Van Nostrand and Reinhold.

Barber, T. X. (1970). *LSD, marihuana, yoga, and hypnosis.* Chicago: Aldine.

Barber, T. X. (1976a). *Hypnosis: A scientific approach.* New York: Psychological Dimensions.

Barber, T. X. (1976b). *Pitfalls in human research.* New York: Pergamon Press.

Barber, T. X., & Calverly, D. S. (1963a). The relative effectiveness of task motivating instructions and trance-induction procedure in the production of "hypnotic-like" behaviors. *Journal of Nervous and Mental Disease, 137,* 107–116.

Barber, T. X., & Calverly, D. S. (1964). The definition of the situation as a variable affecting "hypnotic-like" suggestibility. *Journal of Clinical Psychology, 20,* 438–440.

Barber, T. X., & Calverly, D. S. (1966). Effects on recall of hypnotic induction, motivational suggestions, and suggested regression: A methodological and experimental analysis. *Journal of Abnormal Psychology, 71,* 169–180.

Barber, T. X., Spanos, N. P., & Chaves, J. F. (1974). *Hypnosis, Imagination and Human Potentialities.* New York: Pergamon Press.

Barber, T. X., & Wilson, S. C. (1974). Hypnosis, suggestions, and altered states of consciousness: Experimental evaluation of the new cognitive-behavioral theory and the traditional trance-state theory of "hypnosis". *Annals of the New York Academy of Sciences, 292,* 34–47.

Barber, T. X., & Wilson, S. C. (1978–79). The Barber Suggestibility Scale and the Creative Imagination Scale: Experimental and clinical applications. *The American Journal of Clinical Hypnosis, 21,* 84–108.

Bowers, K. S. (1967). The effect of demands for honesty on reports of visual and auditory hallucinations. *International Journal of Clinical and Experimental Hypnosis, 15,* 31–36.

Bowers, K. S. (1979). Time distortion and hypnotic ability: Underestimating the duration of hypnosis. *Journal of Abnormal Psychology, 88,* 435–439.

Braid, J. (1847). Facts and observations as to the relative value of mesmeric and hypnotic coma, and ethereal narcotism, for the mitigation or entire prevention of pain during surgical operations. *Medical Times, 15,* 381–382.

Campbell, D. I., & Stanley, J. C. (1971). *Experimental and quasi-experimental designs for research.* Chicago: Rand McNally.

Chertok, L. (1981). *Sense and nonsense in psychotherapy: The challenge of hypnosis.* New York: Pergamon Press.

Coe, W. C. (1973). Experimental designs and the state-nonstate issue in hypnosis. *American Journal of Clinical Hypnosis, 16,* 118–128.

Cooper, L. M., & London, P. (1973). Reactivation of memory by hypnosis and suggestion. *The International Journal of Clinical and Experimental Hypnosis, 21,* 312–323.

DePiano, F. A., & Salzberg, H. C. (1982). Hypnosis as an aid to recall of meaningful information presented under three types of arousal. *The International Journal of Clinical and Experimental Hypnosis,* 383–399.

Edmonston, W. E. (1979). The effects of neutral hypnosis on conditioned responses: Implications for hypnosis and relaxation. In E. Fromm & R. E. Shor (Eds.), *Hypnosis: Developments in research and new perspectives* (2nd ed.). New York: Aldine.

Edmonston, W. E. (1981). *Hypnosis and relaxation.* New York: Wiley.

Frischolz, E. J., Spiegel, D., Spiegel, H., Balma, D. L., & Markell, C. S. (1982). Differential hypnotic responsivity of smokers, phobics, and chronic-pain control patients: A failure to confirm. *Journal of Abnormal Psychology, 91,* 269–272.

Gill, M. M., & Brenman, M. (1961). *Hypnosis and related states.* New York: International Union Press.

Greenberg, R. P., & Land, J. M. (1971). Influence of some hypnotist and subject variables on hypnotic susceptibility. *Journal of Consulting and Clinical Psychology, 37,* 111–115.

Gruenwald, D. (1982). Problems of relevance in the application of laboratory data to clinical situations. *The International Journal of Clinical and Experimental Hypnosis, 30,* 345–353.

Hilgard, E. R. (1965). *Hypnotic susceptibility.* New York: Harcourt, Brace & World.

Hilgard, E. R. (1975). *Hypnosis, Annual Review of Psychology, 26,* 19–44.

Hilgard, E. R. (1977). *Divided consciousness: Multiple controls in human thought and action.* New York: Wiley.

Hilgard, E. R. (1979). Divided consciousness in hypnosis: The implications of the hidden observer. In E. Fromm & R. E. Shor (Eds.), *Hypnosis: Developments in research and new perspectives* (2nd ed.). New York: Aldine.

Hilgard, J. R. (1979). Imaginative and sensory-affective involvements in everyday life and in hypnosis. In E. Fromm & R. E. Shor (Eds.), *Hypnosis: Developments in research and new perspectives* (2nd ed.). New York: Aldine.

Hilgard, J. R., & LeBaron, S. (1982). Relief of anxiety and pain in children and adolescents with cancer. Quantitative measures and clinical observations. *The International Journal of Clinical and Experimental Hypnosis, 30,* 417-442.

Hilgard E. R., & Tart, C. T. (1966). Responsiveness to suggestions following waking and imagination instructions and following induction of hypnosis. *Journal of Abnormal Psychology, 71,* 196-208.

Hull, C. L. (1930). Quantitative methods of investigating hypnotic suggestion. Part I. *Journal of Abnormal and Social Psychology, 25,* 200-223.

Hull, C. L. (1931). Quantitative methods of investigating hypnotic suggestion. Part II. *Journal of Abnormal and Social Psychology, 25,* 390-417.

Johnson, R. F., & Barber, T. X. (1978). Hypnosis, suggestions, and warts: An experimental investigation implicating the importance of "believed-in efficacy". *American Journal of Clinical Hypnosis, 20,* 165-174.

Kramer, E. (1969). Hypnotic susceptibility and previous relationship with the hypnotist. *American Journal of Clinical Hypnosis, 11,* 175-177.

Laurence, J. R., & Perry, C. (1981). The "hidden observer" phenomena in hypnosis: Some additional findings. *Journal of Abnormal Psychology, 90,* 334-344.

Levitt, E. E., & Baker, E. L. (1983). The hypnotic relationship: Another look at coercion, compliance, and resistance: A brief communication. *The International Journal of Clinical and Experimental Hypnosis, 31,* 125-131.

Liebert, R. M., Rubin, N., & Hilgard, E. R. (1965). The effects of suggestions of alertness in hypnosis on paired associate learning. *Journal of Personality, 33,* 605-612.

London, P., Conant, M., & Davison, G. C. (1966). More hypnosis in the unhypnotizable: Effects of hypnosis and exhortation on rote learning. *Journal of Personality, 34,* 71-79.

London, P., & Fuhrer, M. (1961). Hypnosis, motivation, and performance. *Journal of Personality, 29,* 321-33.

Nogrady, H., McConkey, K. M., Laurence, J., & Perry, C. (1983). Dissociation, duality, and demand characteristics in hypnosis. *Journal of Abnormal Psychology, 92,* 223-235.

Oetting, E. R. (1964). Hypnosis and concentration in study. *The American Journal of Clinical Hypnosis, 7,* 148-151.

Orne, M. T. (1959). The nature of hypnosis: Artifact or essence. *Journal of Abnormal Social Psychology, 58,* 277-299.

Orne, M. T. (1969). Demand characteristics and the concept of quasicontrols. In R. Rosenthal & R. L. Rosnow (Eds.), *Artifact in Behavioral Research.* New York: Academic Press.

Orne, M. T. (1971). The simulation of hypnosis: Why, how, and what it means. *The International Journal of Clinical and Experimental Hypnosis, 19,* 183-210.

Orne, M. T. (1979). On the simulating subject as a quasi-control group in hypnosis research: What, why, and how. In E. Fromm & R. E. Shor (Eds.), *Hypnosis: Research developments and perspectives.* Chicago: Aldine Atherton.

Perry, C., Gelfand, R., & Marcovtch, P. (1979). The relevance of hypnotic susceptibility in the clinical context. *Journal of Abnormal Psychology, 88,* 592-603.

Sakata, K. I., & Anderson, J. P. (1970). The effects of post-hypnotic suggestion on test performance. *The International Journal of Clinical and Experimental Hypnosis, 18,* 61-77.

Salzberg, H. C., & DePiano, F. A. (1980). Hypnotizability and task motivating suggestions: A further look at how they affect performance. *The International Journal of Clinical and Experimental Hypnosis, 28,* 261-271.

Sarbin, T. R., & Coe, W. C. (1972). *Hypnosis: A Social Psychological Analysis of Influence Communication.* New York: Holt, Rinehart & Winston.

Sarbin, T. R., & Coe, W. C. (1979). Hypnosis and psychopathology: Replacing old myths with fresh metaphors. *Journal of Abnormal Psychology, 88,* 506-525.

Sarbin, T. R., & Slagle, R. W. (1979). Hypnosis and psychophysiological outcomes. In E. Fromm & R. E. Shor (Eds.), *Hypnosis: Research developments and perspectives.* Chicago: Aldine Atherton.

Sheehan, P. W. (1973). Escape from the ambiguous: Artifact and methodologies of hypnosis. *American Psychologist, 28,* 983-993.

Sheehan, P. W., & Dolby, R. M. (1974). Artifact and Barber's model of hypnosis: A logical-empirical analysis. *Journal of Experimental Social Psychology, 10,* 171-187.

Sheehan, P. W., & Dolby, R. M. (1979). Motivated involvement in hypnosis: The illustration of clinical rapport through hypnotic dreams. *Journal of Abnormal Psychology, 88,* 53-83.

Sheehan, P. W., & Perry, C. (1976). *Methodologies of hypnosis: A critical appraisal of contemporary paradigms of hypnosis.* Hillsdale, NJ: Erlbaum.

Shor, R. E. (1979). The fundamental problem in hypnosis research as viewed from historic perspectives. In E. Fromm & R. E. Shor (Eds.), *Hypnosis: Research developments and perspectives.* Chicago: Aldine Atherton.

Shor, R. E., & Orne, E. C. (1962). *Harvard Group Scale of Hypnotic Susceptibility, Form A.* Palo Alto, CA: Consulting Psychologists Press.

Shor, R. E., & Orne, E. C. (1963) Norms on the Harvard Group Scale of Hypnotic Susceptibility, Form A. *The International Journal of Clinical and Experimental Hypnosis, 11,* 39-48.

Slotnick, R. S., Liebert, R. M., Hilgard, E. R. (1965). The enhancement of muscular performance in hypnosis through exhortation and involving instructions. *Journal of Personality, 33,* 37-45.

Slotnick, R. S., & London, P. (1965). Influence of instruction: Hypnotic and nonhypnotic performance. *Journal of Abnormal Psychology, 70,* 38-46.

Small, M. M., & Kramer, E. (1969). Hypnotic susceptibility as a function of the prestige of the hypnotist. *The International Journal of Clinical and Experimental Hypnosis, 17,* 251-256.

Spanos, N. P., Barber, T. X., & Lang, G. (1974). Cognition and self-control: Cognitive control of painful sensory input. In H. London & R. Nisbett (Eds.), *Cognitive alterations of feeling states.* Chicago: Aldine.

Spanos, N. P., Dubreuil, D. L., Saad, C. L., & Gorassini, D. (1983). Hypnotic elimination of prism-induced aftereffects: Perceptual effect or responses to experimental demands? *Journal of Abnormal Psychology, 92,* 216-222.

Spanos, N. P., Dubreuil, D. L., Saad, C. L., & Gorassini, D. R., & Petrusic, W. (1981). Hypnotically induced limb anesthesia and adaptation to displacing prisms: A failure to confirm. *Journal of Abnormal Psychology, 90,* 329-333.

Spanos, N. B. Radtke-Bodorik, H. L., Ferguson, J. D., & Jones, B. (1979). The effects of hypnotic susceptibility, suggestions for analgesia, and the utilization of cognitive strategies on the reduction of pain. *Journal of Abnormal Psychology, 88,* 282-292.

St. Jean, R., & MacLeod, P. (1983). Hypnosis, absorption, and time perception. *Journal of Abnormal Psychology, 92,* 81-86.

Stam, H. J., & Spanos, N. P. (1980). Experimental designs, expectancy effects, and hypnotic analgesia. *Journal of Abnormal Psychology, 89,* 751-762.

Tart, C. T. (1965). The hypnotic dream: Methodological problems and a review of the literature. *Psychological Bulletin, 64,* 81-91.

Tart, C. (1967). Psychedelic experiences associated with a novel hypnotic procedure, mutual hypnosis. *American Journal of Clinical Hypnosis, 10,* 65-78.

Tart, C. (1972). Measuring the depth of an altered state of consciousness, with particular reference to self-report scales of hypnotic depth. In E. Fromm & E. Shor (Eds.), *Hypnosis: Research developments and perspectives.* Chicago: Aldine Atherton.

Tart, C.T. (1978-79). Quick and convenient assessment of hypnotic depth: Self report scales. *The American Journal of Clinical Hypnosis, 21,* 186-207.

Tart, C. (1979). Measuring the depth of an altered state of consciousness with particular reference to self-report scales of hypnotic depth. In E. Fromm & E. Shor (Eds.), *Hypnosis: Research developments and new perspectives* (2nd ed.). Chicago: Aldine.

Tellegen, A., & Atlinson, G. (1974). Openness to absorbing and self-altering experiences ("absorption"), a trait related to hypnotic susceptibility. *Journal of Abnormal Psychology, 83,* 268-277.

Treolar, W.W. (1967). Review of recent research on hypnotic learning. *Psychological Reports, 20,* 723-733.

Vingoe, F. J. (1968). The development of a group alert trance scale. *The International Journal of Clinical and Experimental Hypnosis, 16,* 120-132.

Vingoe, F. J. (1973). Comparison of the Harvard Group Scale of Hypnotic Susceptibility, Form A and the Group Alert Trance Scale in a university population. *The International Journal of Clinical Hypnosis, 10,* 194-197.

Von Dendenroth, T.E.A. (1968). The use of hypnosis in 1000 cases of "tobaccomaniacs." *American Journal of Clinical Hypnosis, 10,* 194-197.

Wadden, T.A., & Anderton, C.H. (1982). The clinical use of hypnosis. *Psychological Bulletin, 2,* 215-243.

Wadden, T. A., & Flaxman, J. (1981). Hypnosis and weight loss: A preliminary study. *International Journal of Clinical and Experimental Hypnosis, 29,* 162-173.

Wadden, T.A., & Penrod, J. H. (1981). Hypnosis in the treatment of alcoholism: A review. *The American Journal of Clinical Hypnosis, 24,* 41-47.

Wagstaff, G.F. (1981). *Hypnosis, complicance and belief.* New York: St. Martin.s Press.

Wain, H. J. (1980). Pain control thrugh the use of hypnosis. *The American Journal of Clinical Hypnosis, 23,* 41-46.

Wallace, B., & Garrett, J.B. (1973). Reduced felt arm sensation effects on visual adaptation. *Perception and Psychophysics, 14,* 597-600.

Wallace, B., & Garrett, J.B. (1975). Perceptual adaptation with selective reductions of felt sensation. *Perception,4,* 437-445.

Weitzenhoffer, A.M., & Hilgard, E. R. (1959). *Stanford Hypnotic Susceptibility Scale, Forms A and B.* Palo Alto, CA: Consulting Psychologists Press.

Weitzenhoffer, A.M., & Hilgard, E. R. (1962). *Stanford Hypnotic Susceptibility Scale, Form C.* Palo Alto, CA: Consulting Psychologists Press.

Zamansky, H., Scharf, B., and Brightbill, R. (1964). The effect of expectancy for hypnosis on prehypnotic performance. *Journal of Personality, 32,* 236-248.

PART II

BEHAVIOR MODIFICATION

Chapter 3

Clinical Applications of Hypnosis In the Management of Pain

Kenneth J. Tarnowski
Ohio State University

Robert M. Smith
Nova University

The ubiquity of the experience of pain has generated considerable attention in philosophical, religious, medical, sociological, and psychological realms. The advent of psychological inquiry concerning pain and its management is a relatively recent phenomenon and presently constitutes a rapidly evolving area of investigation and application (Barber, 1982; Hilgard & Hilgard, 1975; Melzack & Dennis, 1978; Turk, 1978). The purpose of this chapter is to examine the utility of hypnotic methods in the management of clinical pain. This chapter is organized into four major sections. The first section provides an overview of pain phenomena. The second section briefly addresses some of the defining characteristics of hypnosis. The third section provides an overview of applications of hypnosis to a variety of problems of clinical significance. Specific applications in the domains of dentistry, surgery, oncology, burn treatment, and obstetrics are discussed. The final section provides the reader with some general comments concerning experimental pain research.

Pain: Conceptual Considerations

What is pain? What is its function? How is pain mediated in the nervous system? Despite an inability to provide definitive answers to all the above questions due to limitations in our current knowledge base, these are questions of importance which need to be addressed before we can intelligibly embark on discussion of treatment.

Historically, conceptualization of pain have varied tremendously and have been the focus of much debate. Initially conceptualized in terms of an emotion, pain lost its affective defining characteristics when the advent of sensory physiology redefined pain in terms of sensory input. As Turk (1978) notes, controversy still revolves around how best to conceptualize the emotional, cognitive, and sensory stimulation contributions to the experience of pain. A unidimensional focus on sensory input is of little utility in terms of treatment, as surgical procedures (e.g., pathway transections) based on this model have produced equivocal results (Melzack, 1973). Recently, a multidimensional focus that emphasizes the subjective experience of pain as defined by the patient as well as stimulus input considerations seems to be gaining momentum (Liebeskind & Paul, 1977; Melzack & Wall, 1965). The multidimensional focus allows for an analysis of the affective and cognitive components of pain and thus necessitates the introduction of psychological variables to augment a heretofore unidimensional medical focus. The multidimensional focus is well-exemplified in a statement by Melzack and Casey (1970):

> The surgical and pharmacological attacks on pain might well profit by redirecting thinking toward the neglected and almost forgotten contribution of motivational and cognitive processes. Pain can be treated not only by trying to cut down sensory input by anesthetic blocks, surgical interventions and the like, but also by influencing the motivational-affective and cognitive factors as well. (p. 435).

As to why we experience pain, a reasonable answer is available. Pain serves an adaptive function for the organism. Specifically, the perception of pain alerts the organism that damage of some type has occurred and localizes the area of insult. Pain functions as a discriminative stimulus which induces the organism to engage in some sort of remedial action. Although it is easy to understand the adaptive function of pain that is perceived upon initial insult, it is exceedingly difficult to understand the function of pain that persists over lengthy periods of time (e.g., chronic pain syndromes).

Briefly, the neural transmission of pain is mediated by two types of peripheral pain fibers–(fibers which are unmyelinated and slow conducting and A-delta fibers which are myelinated and fast-conducting). The spinothalamic tract consists of pain fibers entering the dorsal root of the spinal cord which synapse with secondary neurons ascending to the thalamus. In its ascension, collaterals from this tract branch to the reticular formation (spinoreticulothalamic tract). The trigeminoreticulothalamic and anterior trigeminothalamic tracts serve the head region. The thalamus is thought to be the "end station" for pain since pain perception may continue to occur even in the absence of cortical projections (Carlson, 1977).

Although a number of theoretical models of pain mediation have been proposed, perhaps the most influential has been that described by Melzack and Wall

(1965). The theory, known as gate-control, suggests that interneurons in the substantia gelatinosa of the dorsal horn can effect presynaptic inhibition of both C and A-delta fibers. In essence, this results in a blocking of pain messages to the brain proper. When the interneurons are activated by the A-delta fibers, the "gate" is open." The activity of the C fibers has an inhibitory effect on these interneurons and "closes" the gate, which is sensitive to both the intensity and patterns of impulses in the C and A-delta fibers. Although unspecified in its mode of operation, higher cortical centers are assumed to be able to exert control over this gating system. This assumption is most important in terms of postulating descending cognitive controls of pain phenomenon. Although the theory has mixed support at the moment (Nathan & Rudge, 1974; Wall & Sweet, 1967), it is important in terms of current surgical practice and in stimulating further research on cortical control of pain. In summary, to date no theory is fully acceptable and definitive answers await further research.

The reader interested in the implications of the gate-control theory in relation to the cognitive mediation of pain is directed to Melzack and Wall (1982).

HYPNOSIS: SOME PRELIMINARY COMMENTS

Before embarking on a review of the application of hypnosis to pain management with selected clinical problems it is first necessary to discuss what is meant by the term "hypnosis." Certainly there exists disagreement as to what the term does or should encompass (Hilgard, 1973a). Orne (1977) has addressed this issue by delineating two major approaches to hypnotherapy. The first approach regards hypnosis as a set of antecedent conditions. A defining characteristic of this approach is the use of some formal or informal method of induction. The second approach to hypnotic phenomena does not use therapist behavior per se as its hallmark. Instead, hypnosis is largely defined in terms of a characteristic of the subject that he or she brings to the clinical situation (Hilgard, 1965). In the therapeutic sense, one may take advantage of the individual's hypnotic ability without labeling the activity hypnosis per se. In the first approach, research typically procedes by providing an induction and suggestions to one group of individuals and contrasting outcome on some criteria (e.g., self-reported pain) with subjects receiving either no treatment or alternative treatments (e.g., medication). The second approach typically examines ability (susceptibility), as measured by some preliminary assessment (e.g., Stanford Scales), and relates to this outcome. In what follows, case studies and group analyses are described which employ the above approaches and attempt to relate specific procedures and subject variables to treatment outcome.

DENTISTRY

Efforts to develop effective dental pain management techniques have evolved over the past one hundred years. Ether was first utilized for extraction purposes in 1842 and application of nitrous oxide to dental pain was initiated in 1844. Although a wide array of chemoanalgesics of demonstrated efficacy are currently available and in popular use in modern dental practice, they in no way constitute a panacea to the problem of pain management. Hilgard and Hilgard (1975) cogently point out that chemical interventions do not reeducate the individual in terms of facilitating the acquisition of more adaptive responses to dental treatment. Furthermore, as we all know from firsthand experience, dental treatment is required on a repeated basis throughout the life cycle. Pharmaceuticals by themselves are not extremely effective in the management of anticipatory fears and apprehensions and oftentimes what occurs is an exacerbation or compounding of anxiety as additional treatment sessions ensue. Fear of dental procedures is widespread and perhaps for good reason. Any type of insult to the oral cavity can produce intense pain. Some authors have suggested that the intensity of oral pain is related to the following: (1) proximity of oral neural innervation to the thalamus and cerebral cortex, and (2) the psychological import of the oral cavity (Morse & Furst, 1978; Morse & Wilcko, 1979). Anxieties/phobias centering on dental treatments are quite common and may be acquired through a variety of processes (e.g., aversive conditioning, vicariously generated). Other conditions also exist which necessitate the use of psychological pain management methods (e.g., allergies associated with traditional chemoanalgesics).

Applications of hypnosis to individuals undergoing dental treatment have consisted of two basic approaches: (1) anxiety and pain management procedures, and (2) procedures aimed at more pervasive psychological difficulties revolving around treatment. The latter approach utilizes techniques traditionally described as hypnoanalysis or "uncovering" therapy (Graham, 1974).

Since the 1950s a number of clinical case studies have appeared which document the efficacy of hypnotic procedures applied in the context of a variety of dental procedures. Crasilneck, McCranie and Jenkins (1956) treated an individual who was unable to tolerate procaine as allergenic responses developed with its use. Due to extreme apprehensiveness and fear, general anesthesia was required for minor dental procedures (fillings). Needless to say, the risk of using general anesthesia for minor procedures necessitated alternative means of effecting treatment. Hypnotic procedures were utilized with this individual who was considered to be quite responsive and analgesia was achieved in each of the five dental sessions which followed. More recently, Gheorghiu and Orleanu (1982) reported the successful use of hypnoanalgesia during a dental implant with a patient who was allergic to chemoanalgesics. Interestingly, they also reported the amount of bleeding was comparable to patients receiving vasoconstrictive substances. These studies suggest that hypnotic procedures are useful in achieving analgesia when chemoanalgesics are contraindicated. Other case reports have documented the effectiveness of hypnosis with patients who required multiple extractions and suturing (Radin, 1972; Weyandt, 1972, 1976). Procedures consisted of patient education (e.g., dispelling misconceptions regarding hypnosis), the use of eye fixation and levitation, induction of glove anesthesia and transfer of this phenomenon to the surgical site.

Over the past 25 years many case studies have been reported involving the use of hypnotic procedures to expedite dental treatment (see Hilard & Hilgard, 1975). The procedures have been used in isolation and as adjuvants to traditional chemoanalgesics. Although many of these case studies are rich in clinical information and provide compelling descriptions attesting to the effectiveness of hypnotic procedures they are, in fact, uncontrolled case studies restricted in generality and subject to the limitations inherent in this type of analysis (Chassan, 1967; Hersen & Barlow, 1976). Other case reports have focused on the use of more extensive hypnotic procedures. For example Graham (1974) describes a series of cases in which hypnoanalytic techniques were utilized to "uncover" the deep-seated reasons mediating avoidance/inability to complete dental treatment. Although successful treatment was reported in this series of patients, caution once again must be exercised in extrapolating and generalizing from these uncontrolled case reports. Furthermore, as Graham has noted, the use of these procedures by dental practitioners untrained in psychiatric methods is not advisable and psychiatric consultants should be utilized when such difficult cases are encountered.

Presently, very few comparative analyses are available which contrast hypnoanalgesia with other treatment methods including chemoanalgesia. In a recent study, Gottfredson (1973) compared the effects of hypnosis and local anesthetic in the management of dental pain. Twenty-five subjects elected to participate. Subjects were administered the Stanford Hypnotic Susceptibility Scales and 12 were found to be highly susceptible, 6 medium, and 7 low. Subjects self-reported pain on a 10-point scale by raising the appropriate number of fingers. Hypnotic procedures and local anesthetic were randomly administered across sessions for the first 12 subjects and the inverse order implemented for the remaining subjects. Order of treatment was not found to be significant. Suggestions were provided to relax, enter a deep sleep, and to experience numbness and amnesia for any pain associated with the dental procedures. During hypnosis sessions, local anesthetic was alway available if requested. Results indicated that 75 percent of the high susceptibility subjects managed to complete treatment in the absence of any medication. Thirty-eight percent of the low susceptibility subjects managed without medication. Of interest was the finding demonstrating a -.39 correlation between amount of reported pain and hypnotic susceptibility.

Another recent study examined 100 dental patients who elected to try hypnotic procedures (Barber, 1977). The induction procedure took approximately 10 minutes and five major ideas were communicated to patients: (1) nothing is to be done to the patient, (2) the patient will have awareness of body/environment, (3) reinterpretation of the event may occur, (4) the patient may choose to selectively forget events, and (5) a comfortable feeling may be experienced at any time. Results indicated that 99 out of 100 patients were able to complete dental treatment without the aid of local anesthetics. These are impressive results indeed but a major drawback concerning their interpretation results from Barber's failure to ask patients to self-report degree of experienced pain. Certainly, the results from the above study are encouraging and Barber's "rapid induction analgesia" procedure deserves additional study, but under more well-controlled conditions.

SURGERY

The use of hypnotic procedures in surgery has a reasonably long history (over 100 years). Advances in chemical anesthesia facilitated the demise of hypnotic applications in this area. Since the 1950s however, a significant number of reports have appeared in the medical and psychological literature documenting the use of hypnotic procedures in a variety of surgical applications (see Hilgard & Hilgard, 1975; Kroger, 1963; Marmer, 1959, 1963).

Patient reactions to impending surgery often include anxiety, depression, insecurity, extreme fearfulness, and a host of negative expectations regarding associated pain and prospects for recovery. Hypnotic procedures have been used preoperatively, during surgery proper, and postoperatively.

Perhaps the most dramatic descriptions of hypnotic applications to surgery are contained in case reports by Rausch (1980) and Bowen (1973). Rausch utilized self-hypnotic procedures for major abdominal surgery (cholecystectomy). On the evening preceding surgery Rausch used a variety of techniques to prepare himself for the operation. Progressive relaxation and visualization techniques (going through the steps of the operation) were used until a state of tranquility was achieved followed by a self-reported deep hypnotic trance. No premedication was administered dissociation technique was employed upon the initial incision. Observers reported no facial grimacing or obvious expression of pain and subjective reports denied its presence. Upon the initial incision a rapid blood pressure increase was noted but stabilized shortly thereafter. Feelings of detachment and relation were reported and the operation was completed in 90 minutes with uninterrupted analgesia. Postoperative recovery was brief, painless, and otherwise uneventful.

Bowen (1973) utilized self-hypnosis in a manner similar to that described above for managing discomfort associated with a transurethral resection. Self-suggestions of pleasant warmth were initiated contingent upon the introduction of the urethral dialators and the resectoscope. No discomfort was self-reported nor reported by surgical team observers. Bleeding was also reported to be minimized purportedly, via self-suggestion. The above cited cases are good examples of how hypnotic procedures may be used preoperatively to manage anxiety, operatively to produce analgesia, and post-surgically to minimize discomfort, bleeding, and recovery time. Other factors deemed important in the above cases include positive expectancies for success, complete confidence in the surgical team, and self-confidence in being able to effectively introduce and maintain hypnoanalgesia.

The ability to maintain the hypnotic state is crucial to surgical application and is well documented in a case reported by Scott (1973). A 54-year-old female with a history of coronary heart disease wished to have cosmetic surgery performed to remove large adipose deposits under both upper arms. General anesthesia was contraindicated due to her coronary condition (left bundle branch block). Hypnosis was induced using arm drop and levitation techniques. Analgesia was established by having the patient visualize her right arm being placed into a deep freeze. During her first surgery, analgesia was produced but lightened somewhat at which point she felt a burning sensation. She was coached through the rest of the surgery and apparently was able to reestablish the analgesia. Postsurgical suggestions of no pain, good sleep, and even better success with the next operation were provided. No postoperative pain was reported and analgesic medications were not required. During her second surgical experience on her left arm the same procedures were used and analgesia established. A preoperative test with forceps produced a lightening of the state and subsequent pain. The therapist was unable to reestablish analgesia on this and subsequent trials. An exploration of the reasons for the occurrence of this phenomenon revealed some important information. First of all, during the interim between surgeries, other patients and ward staff apparently ridiculed the patient for subjecting herself to the hypnotic procedures for surgery, told her it was all in her head, and insinuated that she was psychiatrically disturbed. Certainly, this undermined her confidence in the hypnotic proceedings. Furthermore, she associated any discomfort in her left arm with an impending coronary attack and was thus unable to maintain analgesia. The case is important in that it demonstrates the manner in which variables (e.g., social) which are distinct from the hypnotic situation may negatively influence patient confidence and ability to achieve and maintain hypnoanalgesia.

In considering the role of hypnosis in surgical pain management several points deserve mention. First of all, it has been repeatedly demonstrated that the less anxious or fearful the patient, the less he or she tends to rate the intensity of pain (Barber, 1959). It is also important to note in the case of surgery that amount of tissue damage does not correlate significantly with amount of pain. Despite widely held beliefs to the contrary, pain produced by incisions and the like produce less distress than might be expected. For example, Lewis (1942) has demonstrated that it is mainly the external tissues of the body (e.g., skin, mucous membrane of mouth, peritoneum) that result in rather intense pain sensations when cut or subjected to other types of insult. Deeper tissue and organs proper typically generate little or no pain when subjected to surgical insult. In a recent overview of hypnoprocedures applied to surgery, Chaves and Barber (1976) have cited six factors that significantly influence success. The first factor, patient selection, refers to characteristics of the "good subject for hypnoanalgesia. High suggestibility, low anxiety, and positive attitudes concerning the use of hypnosis are critical variables. The second factor concerns the interpersonal relationship between patient and therapist. A close, trusting relationship obviously would facilitate success. The third factor is the nature and extent of preoperative preparatory communication between staff and the patient. Adaptation to the medical environment and learning about the surgical procedures to be implemented can help reduce anxiety substantially. The fourth factor refers to the use of chemical agents (e.g., anesthetics, analgesics). As Chaves and Barber note, most modern-day uses of hypnotic procedures in the context of surgery involve the concurrent use of hypnosis and drugs. Examples of the successful use of hypnotic procedures in isolation were cited previously. The fifth factor concerns the suggestions of analgesia/anesthesia which are to be used. Patients undergoing surgery with the assistance of hypnotic procedures usually maintain rather strong beliefs/expectations regarding the efficacy of these techniques. A variety of direct and indirect suggestions can usually induce analgesia/anesthesia even in the absence of a formal induction (Evans & Paul, 1970; Spanos, Barber, & Lang, 1974). The final factor to be discussed is that of distraction. In both experimental and clinical applications patients are many times specifically requested to engage in some sort of focusing activity (Barber & Cooper, 1972; Spanos, Horton, & Chaves, 1975). Focusing on one's own breathing the hypnotist's voice, music, or anything else that might be effective for the client can be suggested. Although the Chaves and Barber (1976) review is confined to surgical applications, it is likely that the six factors discussed are of equal importance to other areas of application (e.g., dentistry, obstetrics). However, the relative importance of these factors may well vary as a function of the patient populations targeted for treatment.

In summary, hypnotic procedures (direct and indirect suggestions) may be effectively utilized in surgical application even without formal induction methods. Preoperatively, these procedures may be used to decrease anxiety and fear.

Operatively, suggestions may be provided to patients to assist them in achieving analgesia/anesthesia or to control blood loss (Clawson & Swade, 1975). Postoperatively, the use of hypnotic procedures may expedite recovery (Van Dyke, 1970) and promote less dependency on narcotics (Benson, 1971). Results suggest that hypnosuggestive procedures may be of benefit across all phases of medical treatment and recovery. Parenthetically, it should be noted that even patients under general chemoanesthesia may be responsive to comments/suggestions made in the operating theatre. It has been noted that even casual comments (e.g., "let's finish up and get out of here") may have deleterious effects (patients later recall a sense of feeling abandoned) (Cheek, 1966).

ONCOLOGY

Over the past 25 years significant advances have been made in the diagnosis and treatment of cancer patients. Although some of these advances have reduced morbidity and mortality rates associated with various cancers they do not address the psychological distress these patients experience. Anxiety and fears concerning death, feelings of loss of control, intractable pain, and associated narcotic dependence are common concerns.

A number of case studies have appeared in the literature which illustrate the successful application of hypnosis to cancer patients. The Hilgards (1975) described the treatment of a 42-year-old female who was suffering from bone metastasis secondary to primary breast cancer. The treatment was multifaceted and was described as consisting of five general components: (1) therapist support to deal more effectively with the medical crisis, (2) hypnosis for anxiety and pain relief, (3) hypnosis for insomnia secondary to the medical condition, (4) encouragement to maintain and increase activities and interests, and (5) fostering independence via self-hypnotic methods. Like all other applications of hypnosis, the interpersonal relationship between the therapist and client was described as being of critical importance to successful intervention. This point cannot be overstressed particularly in dealing with cancer patients who are in crisis and in need of much support.

As noted by Hilgard and Hilgard (1975) in their review of applications of hypnosis to cancer patients, three basic procedures have been used repeatedly in a number of case reports: conversion, substitution, and displacement. For example, Sacerdote (1970) instructed a patient suffering from a throat lesion that he might substitute the experience of nonaversive electrical tingling for pain in the affected area. Erickson (1967) suggested to an intractable pain patient (secondary to cancer) the experience of a highly distracting itch on the side of the foot which could not be relieved due to the patient's physical immobility. The frequently utilized glove analgesia method has also been employed to help patients transfer hynotically induced sensation loss to painful areas. In an emotionally moving description of the treatment of an 11-year-old with terminal cancer, Gardner (1976) described how the therapist can utilize hypnotically-induced dreamlike states to assist the client with pain management. In this case, the client was taught self-hypnotic methods and visualized that he was an eagle flying to a variety of "safe" places. When in distress, the child used the technique to escape to a place of "safety."

In many cases, repeated medical procedures which are painful and anxiety provoking are required in the treatment of cancer. Frequent blood tests and bone marrow aspirations are commonplace. Hilgard and LeBaron (1982) obtained baseline data from 63 patients (ages 6-19) during bone marrow aspiration. All were offered hypnosis as an aid in the control of pain. A total of 24 patients accepted treatment, 19 of whom were considered highly hypnotizable. Of the 19 susceptible patients, 15 reduced self-reported pain in the first two hypnotic treatments. While the five low-susceptibility patients reported little or no reduction in perceived pain they did experience a reduction in anxiety associated with the procedure.

In a related study, Zeltzer and LeBaron (1982) compared hypnosis and nonhypnotic techniques in the control of pain and anxiety during bone marrow aspiration and lumbar puncture in children and adolescents, ages 6 to 17. The study included both patient and independent observer reports of pain and anxiety for preintervention and intervention procedures. The results of their study indicated: (1) preintervention ratings were similar for both hypnotic and nonhypnotic groups, (2) bone marrow aspiration pain was rated more severe than lumbar puncture pain, (3) bone marrow aspiration pain was reduced to a greater degree by hypnosis than by nonhypnotic techniques and anxiety was significantly reduced by hypnosis alone, (4) pain experienced during lumbar puncture was reduced significantly only in the hypnosis group while anxiety was reduced to both interventions although nonhypnotic techniques had somewhat less impact.

In general, results provided support for the use of hypnosis in the treatment of procedural pain in cancer. Research suggests that the efficacy of hypnotic interventions in the management of pain may vary as a function of the intensity of the perceived pain. While relatively low levels of pain may be treatable directly by hypnosis (e.g., hypnoanalgesia, hypnoanesthesia), as the intensity of the pain increases it may be necessary to alter the focus of intervention toward the anxiety associated with that pain.

In an interesting series of case studies, Schaeffer and Hernandez (1978) describe their experience with patients unresponsive to hypnosuggestions. Even though all patients initially appeared motivated, closer inspection revealed a variety of circumstances which contributed to unsuccessful initial attempts to utilize hypnotic procedures. Schaeffer and Hernandez emphasized the importance of understanding the meaning of pain from the patient's phenomenological perspective. For example, if the patient believes he has had an active role in the genesis of his dysfunction (e.g., cancer due to smoking) he may have an unconscious need to be punished. Secondary gain from the pain syndromes must also be examined (Fordyce, 1976). In some cases the patient is extremely resistent to submitting to the procedures and may do so only after all other alternatives have been exhausted. The case studies are of importance in that they indicate that the therapist should question why a particular individual within a given life context seems unable to benefit from hypnotic pain management procedures when it is obviously to his or her advantage to do so.

An innovative use of hypnosis with cancer patients is found in the application of these procedures to the problem of anticipatory emesis (nausea, vomiting, abdominal pain in anticipation of chemotherapy). Anticipatory emesis is considered a conditioned response in that previously neutral environmental stimuli come to elicit gagging and the like. A number of successful case reports have emerged documenting the success of hypnotic methods in managing these patients (Dempster, Balso, & Whalen, 1976; Hilgard & Hilgard, 1975). A recent study by Redd, Andresen, and Minagawa (1982) used a within-subjects reversal design to evaluate the efficacy of their hypnotic approach in six female cancer patients. Using instructions described by Katz (1979), the therapist explained hypnosis in terms of relaxation and distraction. A three-step hypnotic method was utilized consisting of: (1) fixed point concentration, (2) suggestions of deep muscle relaxation, and (3) verbal descriptions of relaxing imagery. In this study all treatment sessions were mediated by the hypnotherapist. An emphasis was not placed on self-hypnotic strategies. Due to scheduling problems some chemotherapy treatments occurred without a preceding hypnosis session. In essence, this situation constituted a reversal as it was possible to evaluate the response to chemotherapy sessions with and without hypnosis within the same patient. Results were rather dramatic in that anticipatory emesis occurred when hypnosis was not available. Control was reestablished contingent upon the reintroduction of the hypnosis intervention. Parenthetically, it should be noted that control of anticipatory emesis has also been documented with children using hypnotic methods (LaBaw, Holton, Tewell, & Eccles, 1975). This study examined 27 children who were taught how to use self-hypnotic methods. Although the report consists largely of a series of case studies and no statistical analyses were performed it is anecdotally reported that many of these children benefited from the procedures in terms of better sleep, greater manageability during medical treatment, increased food and fluid intake, and decreased fear, anxiety, and anticipatory emesis. In a recent review of psychological interventions for anticipatory emesis, which included hypnosis, Redd and Andrykowski (1982) reported that consistent findings have emerged across studies despite study differences in terms of the type of cancer treated, stage of the disease, type of chemotherapy, and methodology utilized.

As noted by Hilgard and Hilgard (1975), larger scale studies (Cangello, 1961, 1962; Lea, Ware & Monroe, 1960) of hypnotic methods applied to cancer patients typically demonstrate an improvement rate of approximately 50 percent. Certainly, if substantial gains can be obtained with even a portion of the cancer population the methods are worthy of further refinement and more widespread application. The above figure reflects the treatment of patients with a wide variety of medical problems and personal characteristics and thus does not represent intervention with a homogeneous patient population. Nor is treatment standardized across all patients. This last point is important in that the cancer patient must not be approached in a mechanistic manner as someone to be given an invariant hypnotic treatment. Rather, flexibility and a tailoring of treatment is essential in the context of a close, therapeutic relationship. Besides effecting pain control perhaps the major treatment gain consists of the increased sense of self-control the patient may come to realize through the use of hypnotic techniques.

BURNS

The treatments that the burned patient receives while hospitalized are usually quite painful. Routine procedures such as debridement and dressing changes are dreaded experiences which are usually managed with the administration of sedatives. The use of chemical interventions may interfere with consummatory behaviors as well as participation in activities directed towards recovery (e.g., physical therapy Wernick, 1983). Given these constraints it appears that hypnosis may have much to offer the burn patient in terms of pain management and minimization of negative side effects due to medications.

Crasilneck, Stirman, Wilson, McCranie, and Fogelman (1955) conducted the first study which supported the use of hypnotic procedures with burn patients. Of eight patients treated, six were regarded as successes. Increases in consummatory behaviors, cooperation, and positive attitude were noted. These results have been replicated by other investigators (Bernstein, 1965; Dahinterova, 1967; Finer & Nylen, 1961).

In a larger scale study, Schafer (1975) utilized hypnotic procedures with 20 severely burned patients. Assessment of hypnotic depth was conducted on all patients using the Orne and O'Connell (1967) scale. The scale consists of five points where one represents no response and five reflects somnambulistic states.

In line with experimental studies of pain (Evans & Paul, 1970; Hilgard & Morgan, 1975; Knox, Gekoski, Shum, & McLaughlin, 1981; Spanos, Radtke-Bodorik, Ferguson & Jones, 1979), analgesia and subsequent pain management were correlated with depth/hypnotic ability. Fourteen of the subjects (one-half were somnambulists) were considered successes in that they were able to effectively self-manage pain posthypnotically. The six failures with one exception were children and/or adolescents who were described as so panic-ridden that the establishment of adequate rapport was precluded. Subjective ratings of morale, regressive tendencies, and ward adjustment were considered much improved. The use of personalized self-hypnosis tapes for patients' practice was recommended as a useful adjunctive to formal hypnosuggestive procedures.

Wakeman and Kaplan (1978) examined the effectiveness of hypnosis in burn patients as an adjunctive to chemoanalgesics. Self-hypnotic procedures were taught to approximately one-half of the 42 burn patients who elected to participate. Induction techniques varied somewhat but routinely included eye roll, eye fixation, and/or progressive relaxation. Deepening procedures were introduced followed by the development of glove anesthesia. Reduction of anxiety and fear, dissociation procedures, and hynoanalgesia were emphasized repeatedly. Medications (morphine, Tylenol, etc.) were available upon request up to a specified daily ceiling dosage. Two separate studies were performed. The first included patients with burns encompassing up to 30 percent of their bodies in three different age groups: child (7-18), young adult (19-30), and older adult (31-70). The second study examined patients across the same age groups but with more extensive burns (31-60%). Medication-only patient control groups were included for contrast purposes. The dependent variable for all subjects was the amount of medication requested. The results of the first study revealed significant differences between the control and treatment groups in terms of amount of medication requested. The same results were obtained in study II for the more extensively burned patients. That both studies found significant reductions in medication requests for treated groups adds statistical support to previous case report findings (Crasilneck, et al., 1955; Schafer, 1975). Of interest is the fact that younger subjects in both studies did significantly better than the older subjects. This finding is consistent with other reports documenting the greater susceptibility of children (Hilgard & Hilgard, 1975) yet incongruent with the results from the Schafer (1975) study cited previously. The discrepancy in treatment effects for children found in these studies deserves further attention. In general it appears that Wakeman and Kaplan (1978) tailored the hypnotic procedures for the children to a greater extent than did Schafer (1975) (e.g., "television screen" induction, dissociation to favored locations, etc.) and this may partly account for the superior results obtained.

OBSTETRICS

A variety of procedures have been utilized for women undergoing childbirth. The "natural childbirth" method (Dick-Read, 1953), psychoprophylaxis (Chertok, 1959) and the Lamaze technique (Lamaze, 1958) are the methods most widely recognized. It is difficult if not somewhat arbitrary to classify the procedures used in obstetrics as being hypnotic as these approaches usually consist of a variety of techniques (e.g., relaxation, instructions, suggestions, lectures) and inductions and other hallmarks of traditional "hypnosis" may not be employed.

Hilgard and Hilgard (1975) cited eight hypnotic procedural components found to be helpful in managing the pain associated with childbirth: (1) rehearsal (in vivo and imaginal) of events to occur in the process of parturition, (2) relaxation, (3) substitution of mild for severe pain, (4) pain displacement, (5) direct suggestions, (6) indirect suggestions, (7) imaginative separation from current environment, and (8) posthypnotic suggestion. These methods may have been utilized in many of the published reports to date but it is difficult to determine this exactly as explicit description of treatment methods are lacking.

August (1961) described the outcome of 850 deliveries in which hypnotic methods were employed. Of these cases, 58 percent successfully delivered in the absence of any chemoanalgesics. Rock, Shipley, and Campbell (1969) examined 22 subjects receiving hypnosis at time of labor. Controls received approximately equal staff time and attention and no hypnosis. Those subjects receiving hypnosis rated delivery as less aversive than did controls. An additional feature of this study was the inclusion of preliminary measures of susceptibility which were related to treatment outcome. Results indicated that "good" subjects obtained significantly more relief in comparison to the less susceptible subjects.

Werner, Schauble, and Knudson (1982) reported the successful delivery of over 3,000 cases with the aid of hypnosis, the last 1,500 of which were delivered with the hypnoreflexogenous technique first described by Roig (in Werner et al., 1982). This technique assumes and teaches that childbirth is a normal physiological event and, as such, should be free of any pain or discomfort. The fear of delivery is neutralized by reconceptualizing the event in terms of a sublime experience. The pain concept is replaced with one of normal uterine contraction and finally through deep psychological sedation the cerebral cortex purportedly assumes a state of low excitability. The authors indicate that 10 percent of the patients failed to achieve hypnotic trance or just simply gave up during training or sometime during labor. Thirty percent were able to utilize hypnosis with the addition of chemoanalgesics during labor and delivery. With the exception of a few patients requiring a local anesthetic during episiotomy or laceration of the perineum for closure, 60 percent were able to complete labor and delivery without the aid of chemical agents. For a more thorough description and discussion of this technique readers are referred to Werner et al., 1982.

A number of case reports are available which describe innovative applications of hypnotic procedures to shorten labor length (August, 1965) and reduce medication (Pascatto & Mead, 1967). Although the literature supports the use of hypnosis with obstetrical patients, it is difficult to estimate the percentage of patients who are likely to benefit from these procedures, what patient characteristics best predict positive outcome, and what treatment components are actively contributing to the observed effects.

HEADACHE

In recent years there has been an exponential growth in the number of studies examining methods for subjects to self-manage headache pain. These studies are covered extensively in Chapter 8.

A NOTE ON EXPERIMENTAL PAIN RESEARCH

Although a review of the experimental pain literature is beyond the scope of this chapter a few highlights from this literature are worthy of mention here.

Certainly, there exists significant differences between pain that is experimentally produced and that which occurs naturally. Typically, experimental pain is produced by immersion of a limb in iced water for brief durations or by restricting blood flow to a particular body part thus producing ischemic pain (Hilgard & Hilgard, 1975). Thus, the pain produced in these experimental situations is both brief and externally mediated. Barber (1982) noted that despite the differences between experimentally produced and naturally occurring pain, the research from both areas has produced congruent results.

Another consideration of importance concerns suggestions given under "waking conditions" (no induction utilized). Several experimental studies have found equivalent pain reduction for subjects under both "waking" and "hypnotic" conditions (Spanos et al., 1975, 1979). Other studies (Hilgard, Macdonald, Morgan, & Johnson, 1978; Spanos & Hewitt, 1980) have found an advantage in terms of pain reduction for "good" (highly susceptible) subjects provided suggestions under hypnosis in contrast with suggestions given under waking conditions. This finding may be due to the fact that subjects expect to do better under hypnosis (Stam & Spanos, 1980). At any rate, the important point remains that many subjects are able to benefit from suggestions given under "waking" conditions.

Another important area of experimental research concerns subject responsiveness. Experimental findings (Evans & Paul, 1970; Hilgard & Hilgard, 1975) are consistent with the clinical findings cited in this chapter: responsiveness is significantly correlated with ability to effect pain reduction. Although these "good" subjects typically do better than "poor" (those with low responsiveness) subjects, this is by no means a hard and fast rule as "good" subjects may fail to benefit and "poor" subjects may do well. Although numerous studies have attempted to delineate the characteristics of "good" subjects, they have uniformly failed to identify any particular personality correlates (Hilgard, 1975; Spanos & Barber, 1974). The only factor to emerge from these studies attempting to differentiate "good" from "poor" subjects appears to be an ability to fantasize and imagine in a vivid fashion. More research is needed to clarify the role of these imaginal processes as well as research into ways in which we can maximize their usage in the context of clinical interventions.

Much of the pain management research in the reduction of pain through the use of hypnosis is supported only by the verbal report of the subjects, while their physiological responses would indicate that the pain stimulus was percevied (Hilgard, Morgan, Lange, Lenox, Macdonald, Marshall, & Sachs, 1974). This phenomenon led Hilgard (1973b) to invoke the concept of dissociation to explain hypnoanalgesic phenomenon. Hilgard argues that an individual can experience events at different levels of consciousness simultaneously. While a person may be well aware of an event at one level, they are typically not aware of that event on another, unconscious, level. Further, Hilgard suggests that these two levels are separated by what he calls an "amnesic barrier." By this explanation, then, an individual who is hypnotized and given suggestions for analgesia may report experiencing no pain but at another level of consciousness would be completely aware of the pain stimulus. Hilgard proposed that this unconscious level could be accessed by direct suggestion during hypnosis. Hilgard found that these "hidden reports" from his subjects did indeed indicate that the pain stimulus was perceived as more intense at this "unconscious" level (Hilgard, Morgan & Macdonald, 1975). In fact, the hidden reports did not differ significantly from reports of the waking control group. Although these speculations have been well received in some quarters (Chapman, 1978; Weisenberg, 1977), others (Spanos & Hewitt, 1980) have argued that the instructions given in these experiments were sufficient to define a social role which the subjects then enacted. In a recent study, Spanos and Hewitt (1980) employed the same procedures as those used by Hilgard for one group of subjects while subjects in a second group were given identical instructions but in addition were told that the "hidden self" would be less sensitive to the pain stimulus. The subjects expecting high levels of hidden pain reported high levels, however those expecting low levels of hidden pain reported significantly less pain than the "hypnotized self." Instead of postulating a "dissociated state," Spanos and Hewitt propose that the experimental procedures defined a role which the subjects enact in order to remain "good" hypnotic subjects. Additional support for this proposal is found in Hilgard et al. (1978). In this study, "simulators" and "reals" were compared utilizing the same experimental instructions for the hidden reports.

There was no significant difference between the "simulators" and the "real" subjects. The fact that the simulators were able to successfully fake their reports indicated that the procedures contained sufficient clues for appropriate role enactment.

Spanos and Hewitt (1980) further suggested that the differences between hidden reports and overt reports could be the result of selective attention. In other words, when the hidden reports of pain were given the subjects could have focused attention on the painful stimuli whereas attention was diverted from the painful stimuli when "hypnoanalgesic"reports were requested. A recent review by McCaul and Malott (1984) on the effectiveness of distraction as a method of coping with pain lends support to this viewpoint. Although the review purposefully excluded an analysis of those procedures considered to be hypnosuggestive, their conclusions are considered relevant here. Specifically, it was found that those distraction methods which required the most attentional capacity were the most effective in reducing patient distress. Indeed, it may well be that distraction represents a common factor mediating the effectiveness of a broad spectrum of hypnotic procedures which have been applied in the management of pain.

SUMMARY

The preceding overview of clinical applications of hypnotic procedures in the management of pain suggests that these methods may be successfully employed with a variety of patient populations. Although the procedures may be effective for many patients experiencing pain in a variety of contexts, they, like chemical interventions for pain, do not represent a panacea for the problem of pain management. As noted by Barber (1982), hypnotic procedures represent but one facet of a multidimensional approach to dolorology.

Hypnosis is rapidly gaining respect as a legitimate therapeutic tool in diverse clinical specialties (Martin, 1983). The antiquated misconceptions surrounding hypnosis are falling away and its usefulness as an adjunctive technique in a well-rounded, individualized treatment plan is becoming more apparent.

Certainly, much of the literature cited in this chapter consists of uncontrolled case studies. Although clinical case reports offer a basis for optimism they do not constitute an adequate empirical basis for clinical practice. The need for controlled single subject experimentation as well as methodologically sound nomethetic research is obvious.

Since there are many types of pain with varying characteristics (Melzack, 1980) a mechanistic application of "hypnotic" procedures to the pain patient simply will not suffice. A tailored and individualized program that is embedded in a multidisciplinary approach to pain is called for. While its mechanism of effect remains an enigma, neither the refinement of the technique, nor those patients who could benefit from its application, should continue to suffer as a result of the ongoing dialogue of whether or not we can completely understand and explain hypnotic pheonomena.

This chapter has briefly described some hypnosuggestive approaches to the pain patient. For a more detailed description of procedural details including induction methods, preliminary procedures and specific therapeutic suggestions, the reader is referred to Barber, 1982; Erickson, 1967; Hilgard and Hilgard, 1975, and the primary sources cited within this chapter.

REFERENCES

August, R.V. (1961). *Hypnosis in obstetrics.* New York: McGraw-Hill.

August, R.V. (1965). Hypnosis in obstetrics: Varying approaches. *American Journal of Clinical Hypnosis, 8,* 47-51.

Barber, J. (1977). Rapid induction analgesia: A clinical report. *American Journal of Clinical Hypnosis, 19,* 138-147.

Barber, T.X. (1959). Toward a theory of pain: Relief of chronic pain by prefrontal leuctomy, opiates, placebos, and hypnosis. *Psychological Bulletin, 56,* 430-460.

Barber, T.X. (1982). Hypnosuggestive procedures in the treatment of clinical pain: Implications for theories of hypnosis and suggestive therapy. In T. Millon, C. J. Green, & R. H. Meagher (Eds.), *Handbook of Clinical Health Psychology.* New York: Plenum.

Barber, T.X., & Cooper, B. J. (1972). Effects of pain in experimentally-induced and spontaneous distraction. *Psychological Reports, 31,* 674-651.

Benson, V. B. (1971). One hundreded cases of post-anesthetic suggestion in the recovery room. *American Journal of Clinical Hypnosis, 4,* 273.

Bernstein, N. R. (1965). Observations on the use of hypnosis with burned children on a pediatric ward. *International Journal of Clinical and Experimental Hypnosis, 13,* 1-10.

Bowen, D. E. (1973). Transurethral resection under self-hypnosis. *American Journal of Clinical Hypnosis, 16,* 132-134.

Cangello, V. W. (1961). The use of the hypnotic suggestion for relief in malignant disease. *International Journal of Clinical and Experimental Hypnosis, 9,* 17-22.

Cangello, V. W. (1962). Hypnosis for the patient with cancer. *American Journal of Clinical Hypnosis, 4,* 215-226.

Carlson, N. R. (1977). *Physiology of behavior.* Boston: Allyn & Bacon.

Chapman, C. P. (1978). The hurtful world: Pathological pain and its control. In E. C. Carterette & M. P. Friedman (Eds.), *Handbook of perception* (Vol. 7B). New York: Academic Press.

Chassen, J. B. (1967). *Research design in clinical psychology and psychiatry.* New York: Appleton-Century-Crofts.

Chaves, J. R., & Barber, T. X. (1976). Hypnotic procedures and surgery: A critical analysis with applications to "acupuncture analgesia." *American Journal of Clinical Hypnosis, 18,* 217-236.

Cheek, D. B. (1966). The meaning of continued hearing sense under general chemoanesthesia: A progress report and report of a case. *American Journal of Clinical Hypnosis, 4,* 276-282.

Chertok, L. (1959). *Psychosomatic methods in painless childbirth: History, theory, and practice.* New York: Pergamon.

Clawson, T. A., & Swade, R. H. (1975). The hypnotic control of blood flow and pain: The cure of warts and the potential for the use of hypnosis in the treatment of cancer. *American Journal of Clinical Hypnosis, 17,* 160.

Crasilneck, H. B., McCranie, E. J., & Jenkins, M. T. (1956). Special indications for hypnosis as a method of anesthesia. *Journal of the American Medical Association, 162,* 1606-1608.

Crasilneck, H. B., Stirman, J. A., Wilson, B. J., McCranie, E. J., & Fogelman, M. J. (1955). Use of hypnosis in management of patients with burns. *Journal of the American Medical Association, 158,* 103-106.

Dahinterova, J. (1967). Some experiences with the use of hypnosis in the treatment of burns. *International Journal of Clinical and Experimental Hypnosis, 15,* 49-53.

Dempster, C. R., Balson, P., & Whalen, B. T. (1976). Supportive hypnotherapy during the radical treatment of malignancies. *International Journal of Clinical and Experimental Hypnosis, 24,* 1-9.

Dick-Read, G. (1953). *Childbirth without fear.* New York: Harper & Row.

Erickson, M. H. (1967). An introduction to the study and application of hypnosis for pain control. In J. Lassner (Ed.), *Hypnosis and psychosomatic medicine.* New York: Springer-Verlag.

Evans, M. B., & Paul, G. L. (1970). Effects of hypnotically suggested analgesia on physiological and subjective responses to cold stress. *Journal of Consulting and Clinical Psychology, 35,* 362-371.

Finer, B. L., & Nylen, B. O. (1961). Cardiac arrest in the treatment of burns, and report on hypnosis as a substitute for anesthesia. *Plastic Reconstructive Surgery, 27,* 49-55.

Fordyce, W. E. (1976). *Behavioral methods for chronic pain and illness.* St. Louis: Mosby.

Gardner, G. G. (1976). Childhood, death, and human dignity. *International Journal of Clinical and Experimental Hypnosis, 24,* 122-139.

Gheorghiu, V. A., & Orleanu, P. (1982). Dental implant under hypnosis. *American Journal of Clinical Hypnosis, 25,* 68-70.

Gottfredson, D. K. (1973). Hypnosis as an anesthetic in dentistry. *Dissertation Abstracts International, 33,* 7-13: 3303.

Graham, G. (1974). Hypnoanalysis in dental practice. *American Journal of Clinical Hypnosis, 16,* 178-187.

Hersen, M., & Barlow, D. H. (1976). *Single case experimental designs: Strategies for studying behavior change.* New York: Pergamon.

Hilgard, E. R. (1965). *Hypnotic susceptibility.* New York: Harcourt Brace, & World.

Hilgard, E. R. (1973a). The domain of hypnosis, with some comments on alternative paradigms. *American Psychologist, 28,* 972-982.

Hilgard, E. R. (1973b). Dissociation revisited. In M. Henle, J. Janes, & J. Sullivan (Eds.), *Historical conceptions of psychology.* New York: Springer.

Hilgard, E. R., & Hilgard, J. R. (1975). *Hypnosis in the relief of pain.* Los Altos: Kaufman.

Hilgard, J. R., & LeBaron, S. (1982). Relief of anxiety and pain in children and adolescents with cancer: Quantitative measures and clinical observations. *International Journal of Clinical and Experimental Hypnosis, 30* (4), 417-442.

Hilgard, E. R., Macdonald, H., Morgan, A. H., Johnson, L. S. (1978). The reality of hypnotic analgesia: A comparison of highly hypnotizables with simulators. *Journal of Abnormal Psychology, 87,* 239-246.

Hilgard, E. R., & Morgan, A. H. (1975). Heart rate and blood pressure in the study of laboratory pain in man under normal conditions and as influenced by hypnosis. *Acta Neurobiologicae Experimentalis, 35,* 741-759.

Hilgard, E. R., Morgan, A. H., Lange, A. F., Lenox, J. R., Macdonald, H., Marshall, G. D., & Sachs, L. B. (1974). Heart rate changes in pain and hypnosis. *Psychophysiology, 11,* 692-702.

Hilgard, E. R., Morgan, A. H., & Macdonald, H. (1975). Pain and dissociation in the cold pressor test: A study of hypnotic analgesia with "hidden reports" through automatic key pressing and automatic talking. *Journal of American Psychology, 84,* 280-289.

Katz, N. W. (1979). Comparative efficacy of behavioral training, training plus relaxation, and sleep/trance hypnotic induction in increasing hypnotic susceptibility. *Journal of Consulting and Clinical Psychology, 47,* 119-127.

Knox, V. J., Gekoski, W. L., Shum, K., & McLaughlin, D. M. (1981). Analgesia for experimentally induced pain: Multiple sessions of acupuncture compared to hypnosis in high- and low-susceptible subjects. *Journal of Abnormal Psychology, 90,* 28-34.

Kroger, W. S. (1963). *Clinical and experimental hypnosis.* Philadelphia: Lippincott.

LaBaw, W. L., Holton, C., Eccles, D., & Tewell, K. (1975). The use of self-hypnosis by children with cancer. *American Journal of Clinical Hypnosis, 17,* 233-238.

Lamaze, F. (1958). *Painless childbirth: Psychoprophylactic method.* London: Burke.

Lea, P., Ware, P., & Monroe, R. (1960). The hypnotic control of intractable pain. *American Journal of Clinical Hypnosis, 3,* 3-8.

Lewis, T. (1942). *Pain.* New York: Macmillan.

Liebeskind, J. C., & Paul, L. A. (1977). Psychological and physiological mechanism of pain. *Annual Review of Psychology, 28,* 41-60.

Marmer, M. J. (1959). Hypnoanalgesia and hypnoanesthesia for cardiac surgery. *Journal of the American Medical Association, 171,* 152-517.

Marmer, M. J. (1963). Hypnosis in anesthesiology and surgery. In J. M. Schneck (Ed.), *Hypnosis in modern medicine.* Springfield, IL: Thomas.

Martin, J. (1983). Hypnosis gains legitimacy, respect, in diverse clinical specialties. *Journal of the American Medical Association, 249,* 319-321.

McCaul, K. D., & Malott, J. M. (1984). Distraction and coping with pain. *Psychological Bulletin, 95,* 516-533.

Melzack, R. (1973). *The puzzle of pain.* Harmondsworth, England: Penguin.

Melzack, R. (1980). Psychological aspects of pain. In J. J. Bonica (Ed.), *Pain.* New York: Raven.

Melzack, R., & Casey, K. (1970). The affective dimension of pain. In M. Arnold (Ed.), *Feelings and emotions.* New York: Academic Press.

Melzack, R., & Dennis, S. G. (1978). Neurophysiological foundations of pain. In R. A. Sternback (Ed.), *The Psychology of Pain.* New York: Raven Press.

Melzack, R., & Wall, P. (1965). Pain mechanisms: A new theory. *Science, 150,* 971.

Melzack, R., & Wall, P.D. (1982). *Challenge of pain.* New York: Basic Books.

Morse, Dr. R., & Furst, M. L. (1978). *Stress and relaxation: Application to dentistry.* Springfield, IL: C. C. Thomas.

Morse, D. R., & Wilcko, J. M. (1979). Nonsurgical endodontic therapy for a vital tooth with meditation-hypnosis as the sole anesthetic: A case report. *American Journal of Clinical Hypnosis, 21,* 258-262.

Nathan, P. W., & Rudge, P. (1974). Testing the gate-control theory on pain in man. *Journal of Neurology, Neurosurgery, and Psychiatry, 37,* 1366-1372.

Orne, M. T. (1977). The construct of hypnosis: Implications of the definition for research and practice. *Annals of the New York Academy of Science, 296,* 14-33.

Orne, M. T., & O'Connell, D. N. (1967). Diagnostic ratings of hypnotizability. *International Journal of Clinical and Experimental Hypnosis, 15,* 125-133.

Pascatto, R. D., & Mead, B. T. (1967). The use of posthypnotic suggestion in obstetrics. *American Journal of Clinical Hypnosis, 9,* 267-268.

Radin, H. (1972). Extractions using hypnosis for a patient with bacterial endocarditis. *British Journal of Clinical Hypnosis, 3,* 32-33.

Rausch, V. (1980). Cholecystectomy with self-hypnosis. *American Journal of Clinical Hypnosis, 22,* 124-129.

Redd, W. H., Andresen, G. V., & Minagawa, R. Y. (1982). Hypnotic control of anticipatory emesis in patients receiving cancer chemotherapy. *Journal of Consulting and Clinical Psychology, 50,* 14-19.

Redd, W. H., & Andrykowski, M. A. (1982). Behavioral interventions in cancer treatment: Controlling aversion reactions to chemotherapy. *Journal of Consulting and Clinical Psychology, 50,* 1018-1029.

Rock, N., Shipley, T., & Campbell, C. (1969). Hypnosis with untrained, nonvolunteer patients in labor. *International Journal of Clinical and Experimental Hypnosis, 17,* 25-36.

Sacerdote, P. (1970). Theory and practice of pain control in malignancy and other protracted or recurring painful illnesses. *International Journal of Clinical and Experimental Hypnosis, 18,* 160-180.

Schafer, D. W. (1975). Hypnosis on a burn unit. *International Journal of Clinical and Experimental Hypnosis, 23,* 1-14.

Schafer, D., & Hernandez, A. (1978). Hypnosis, pain, and the context of theory. *International Journal of Clinical and Experimental Hypnosis, 26,* 143-153.

Scott, D. L. (1973). Hypnoanalgesia for major surgery: A psychodynamic process. *American Journal of Clinical Hypnosis, 16,* 84-91.

Spanos, N. P., & Barber, T. X. (1974). Toward a convergence in hypnosis research. *American Psychologist, 29,* 500-511.

Spanos, N. P., Barber, T.X., & Lang, G. (1974). Cognition and self-control: Cognitive control of painful sensory input. In H. London & R. E. Nisbett (Eds.), *Thought and feeling: Cognitive alteration of feeling states.* Chicago: Aldline.

Spanos, N. P., & Hewitt, E. C. (1980). The hidden observer in hypnotic analgesia: Discovery or experimental creation? *Journal of Personality and Social Psychology, 39,* 1201-1214.

Spanos, N. P., Horton, C., & Chaves, J. F. (1975). The effects of two cognitive strategies on pain threshold. *Journal of Abnormal Psychology, 84,* 677-681.

Spanos, N. P., Radtke-Bodorik, H. L., Ferguson, J. D., & Jones, B. (1979). The effects of hypnotic susceptibility, suggestions for analgesia, and the utilization of cognitive strategies on the reduction of pain. *Journal of Abnormal Psychology, 88,* 282-292.

Stam, H. J., & Spanos, N. P. (1980). Experimental designs, expectancy effects, and hypnotic analgesia. *Journal of Abnormal Psychology, 89,* 751-762.

Turk, D. C. (1978). Cognitive behavioral techniques in the management of pain. In J. P. Foreyt and D. P. Tathjen (Ed.), *Cognitive behavior therapy: Research and application.* New York: Plenum.

Van Dyke, P. B. (1970). Some uses of hypnosis in the management of the surgical patient. *American Journal of Clinical Hypnosis, 4,* 227.

Wakeman, R. J., & Kaplan, J. Z. (1978). An experimental study of hypnosis in painful burns. *American Journal of Clinical Hypnosis, 21,* 3-12.

Wall, P. D., & Sweet, W. H. (1967). Temporary abolition of pain in man. *Science, 155,* 108-109.

Weisenberg, M. (1977). Pain and control. *Psychological Bulletin, 84,* 1009-1044.

Werner, W. E. F., Schauble, P. G., & Knudson, M. S. (1982). An argument for the revival of hypnosis in obstetrics. *American Journal of Clinical Hypnosis, 24,* (3), 149-171.

Weyandt, J. A. (1972). Three case reports in dental hypnotherapy. *American Journal of Clinical Hypnosis, 22,* 327-334.

Weyandt, J. A. (1976). Hypnosis in a dental patient with allergies. *American Journal of Clinical Hypnosis, 19,* 123-125.

Wernick, R. L. (1983). Stress, innoculation in the management of clinical pain: Applications to burn pain. In D. Meichenbaum and M. E. Jaremko (Eds.), *Stress reduction and prevention.* New York: Plenum.

Zeltzer, L., & LeBaron, S. (1982). Hypnosis and nonhypnotic techniques for reduction of pain and anxiety during painful procedures in children and adolescents with cancer. *Journal of Pediatrics, 101,* 1032-1035.

Chapter 4

A Review and Analysis of Hypnotherapeutic Approaches for the Control of Smoking Behavior

Joseph A. Sandford
Network Services
Richmond, Virginia

INTRODUCTION

Reports by Great Britain's Royal College of Physicians (1962) and the U.S. Surgeon General's Advisory Committee on Smoking and Health have apparently generated many clinical studies evaluating different treatment "packages." As Bernstein (1969) noted, the health scare impact had only a transient effect on the discontinuation of smoking in the United States. Despite the strong medical evidence (USPHS, 1975, 1977, and 1979) linking smoking with an increased risk of lung cancer, cardiovascular disorders, emphysema, and bronchitis, it has proven very difficult for most smokers to stop. In recognition of the problem and in response to the need for services, a wide variety of medical and psychological treatment approaches were developed. Hypnosis was frequently included in many of these treatment plans usually with the belief that it would help facilitate the acceptance and effect of the other treatment techniques (Lazarus, 1973).

In general most treatment approaches which utilized hypnosis tended to be multimodal and used a wide variety of different techniques and procedures (Johnson & Donoghue, 1971). Bernstein (1969) criticized early research efforts for poor methodology and lack of controls, remarking that they contributed little in the way of scientific knowledge. The lack of systematic studies, replication efforts, and a theoretical basis for specific treatments makes assessment of the necessary factors which have contributed to successful outcomes difficult (Holroyd, 1980). In addition, while most studies claimed many successes, limited efforts have been made to explore who fails, when, and why (Johnston & Donoghue, 1971). Nevertheless, rates of abstinence as high as 94 percent (von Dendenroth, 1964a) have provided encouragement about the potential value of hypnosis as part of a therapeutic package.

METHODOLOGICAL QUESTIONS OF INTEREST

Smoking control therapy is generally short-term with clearly definable and observable therapeutic goals. These two factors provide a feasible framework within which experimental hypotheses can be tested. Success rates varying between 4 and 88 percent for 17 (1970–1980) hypnosis and smoking studies (Holroyd, 1980) suggest that there are likely to be a number of independent factors which account for this observed variance in outcome. At this point there are no clear answers about which treatment procedures are best, only partially answered questions.

This review and analysis of current findings will address the "state of the art" in relationship to the following 10 major issues in hypnosis and smoking research.

1. *Theoretical orientation.* A rationale for a learning theory model. The question of whether smoking is an addiction or habit. The need for behavioral analysis.
2. *Measures of success.* Recommended outcome criteria. Measuring long-term maintenance and follow-up. Improving statistical analysis.
3. *Placebo effects.* The placebo effect of attention, demand characteristics, cognitive dissonance, client expectations, and clinical rapport. Comparison of results in terms of placebo effects.
4. *Subject populations.* The issues of using different techniques for different types of clients. Motivation levels of different clients and their effect on results. Ethical issues pertaining to aversive techniques.
5. *Individual in comparison to group treatment.* Comparison of success rates. Group hypnosis and ethical questions. The quality and quantity of therapeutic contact.
6. *Customized and standardized therapy approaches.* The degree of flexibility needed. The benefits of a plan. Making suggestions in the client's own words.
7. *Self-hypnosis.* Is it of any value? Generalizing the treatment. What about tapes?
8. *Number of sessions.* Single-treatment approach explored. The value of additional treatments. If you don't succeed the first time–what then?
9. *Suggestion and trance depth.* Suggestion and motivation. Trance depth and success. Direct versus indirect suggestion.

10. *Hypnosis and behavior therapy.* Behavioral analysis of successful "packages." Hypnosis as a means for facilitating therapy. Behavioral methods for self-control.

Each of the above sections for discussion are presented below. In the last section preferred elements of treatment plans are selected based on this review and analysis. These techniques will eventually need to be evaluated, individually or in combination, to assess their unique contribution to successful outcomes.

THEORETICAL ORIENTATION

Bernstein (1969) was one of the first researchers to propose a learning theory approach as a rationale for treatment procedures. He concluded that cigarette smoking satisfies the World Health Organization's definition of habituation far better than "addiction." This conclusion was based on the observations that smokers did not show a need for a continued increase in the number of cigarettes and that there were no clear-cut withdrawal symptoms. While there may be an element of nicotine addiction for some people, the habitual use of tobacco is primarily related to the complex interaction of psychological, social, as well as physiological needs. In essence, smoking behavior can best be conceptualized as learned behavior. Reinforcing contingencies in the environment which help maintain smoking behavior can be identified with utilization of a learning model approach. As noted by Dengrove (1970), smoking is a mild stimulant and thus, can be rewarding. The stimulating properties of cigarettes can also be combined with alcohol consumption. In this case a person counterbalances the depressant effects of alcohol with a stimulant producing a more pleasurable, euphoric subjective state.

In addition to physiologically reinforcing characteristics cigarettes have socially reinforcing qualities. Smoking behavior often starts in adolescence and as Wright (1970) points out, serves as an initiation or "rite of passage" into adulthood. This social reinforcing attribute is further enhanced by synthetic associations with desirable role models (the macho cowboy and the slim, sophisticated woman) presented in widespread advertisements. This media message creates a social image of the smoker as virile, romantic, sport-oriented, and tranquil (von Dendenroth, 1968). Smoking can also serve in a tension-reducing capacity and thereby become reinforcing in anxiety-producing social situations (Wright, 1970).

Smoking also acquires psychologically reinforcing qualities by association with primary reinforcers. Classical conditioning can occur by the association of smoking after a pleasurable meal and before evacuation of the bowel and bladder. Since the behavior of cigarette smoking and the drinking of coffee are also often contingent in time, the positive reinforcement of this stimulant can produce a conditioned association. In addition, oral gratification (i.e., sucking), and the relaxing quality of long deep breathing of the smoking act may also contribute to the positive reinforcement which maintains smoking behavior.

In contrast to the immediate positive reinforcing qualities of smoking the aversive consequences are delayed. Since the negative health consequences of smoking are not as contingent as the reinforcing characteristics, smoking behavior is maintained unless the environmental influences result in a change in these contingencies. While a learning theory model may provide a useful framework from which to construct logical intervention strategies, it does not dictate the explicit behavioral techniques needed for the individual to develop control (Bernstein, 1969). Behavioral analysis of the reinforcements which exist for a specific individual that maintain smoking need to be identified. Potential reinforcements (e.g., health, cost, social, and personal factors) for strengthening nonsmoking behavior must also be evaluated. Specific intervention strategies can then be devised and implemented which optimize the learning of new behaviors that can help the individual gain self-control.

MEASURES OF SUCCESS

Bernstein (1969) pointed out that researchers in smoking control frequently used different criteria for calculating success. Success can be based on the number of clients who stop smoking as a percentage of the total number of clients who either (1) consider treatment, (2) start treatment, or (3) complete the treatment plan. Thus, success ratios can be expressed in at least three different ways. Consequently, standardization of success criteria was proposed by Bernstein. He selected the denominator in the success percentage to be the total number of clients who completed treatment. This measurement is useful in that it provides for more precise evaluation of the treatment techniques themselves. However, full information with respect to the attrition of clients also needs to be provided, especially if the number of these individuals is relatively large in proportion to the universe of presenting clients.

Holroyd (1980) chose in her review article to compare studies based on the abstinence rates of clients who begin treatment, regardless of whether they finished. The resulting percentage would usually be less (assuming attrition occurs), and, hence, a more conservative measure of success than the first measure described above. This measure, when compared to the success ratio of those completing treatment, reflects the difficulties met in participating in the treatment program itself. This more conservative measure of success was recommended by Holroyd (1980) as a standard for comparison between research studies. As was pointed out in her review, 100 percent abstinence rate is meaningless if 90 percent of those who begin treatment do not complete it. If a treatment is particularly aversive or costly, then expressing success in terms of either those who begin or complete treatment can be misleading. In these circumstances, percentage of success of all those who considered or presented themselves for treatment should also be provided. While this last measure is not often required, the regular report of the two previously mentioned success rates by researchers will enhance the comparison and interpretation of studies in the field.

In measuring success it was recognized by Bernstein (1969) that the most significant problem in the treatment of smoking was not cessation, but long-term maintenance. Thus, success rates need to be provided for both posttreatment and follow-up. Holroyd (1980) recommends using abstinence rates due to the greater reliability of clients' reports versus reductions in the number of cigarettes smoked. Those clients who simply reduce the number of cigarettes they smoke have been found to soon return to pretreatment levels (Barkley, Hastings, & Jackson, 1977; De Paino, Sandford, Cash & Gotthelf, 1983). Since 1970, studies have commonly reported at least six-month follow-up data. Research by Hunt and Bespalec (1974) indicated recidivism most frequently occurred in the first three months following treatment. Based on these factors Holroyd (1980) maintained that a six-month follow-up was sufficient for estimating the permanent effects of treatment.

Generally, measurement periods of at least one week were used during baseline, post, and follow-up assessment. Self-report measures of abstinence have been found to be highly correlated with independent observers' reports and, thus, can be usually accepted as reliable measures (Hoinville & Biggs, 1966). However, careful attention is needed when instructing clients in measurement techniques. Emphasis on reporting accurately should be stressed with clients in order to correct for any tendency on their part to bias the data collected.

Statistical analysis in this area of research can be greatly improved. Few studies analyzed their results for the effects of other independent variables. Researchers seem to primarily be asking if they could do "something" to help resolve the problem, but without knowing what therapeutic techniques work or why. The "state-of-the-art" is now at the point where the treatment package needs to be scientifically analyzed to extract the active elements.

PLACEBO EFFECTS

The use of the term placebo effects in this application refers to all the nonspecific treatment factors which are not usually measured, but are recognized to exist as part of the therapeutic process. Barber, Spanos and Chaves (1974) refer to the demand characteristics of the setting and the expectations of the therapist as well as the client as two major factors contributing to the placebo effect. The effects of initiating a relationship in which one receives the personal attention of a professional, the cognitive dissonance produced by paying fees and the belief in the power of hypnosis are other nonspecific elements of therapy which have been proposed by researchers (Bernstein, 1969; Dengrove, 1970) to be significant factors in motivating clients to stop smoking. Lazarus (1973) even demonstrated how this belief in the power of hypnosis could serve to increase success rates of clients who wanted hypnosis. He found that the success rate was higher (80%) for a group which wanted hypnosis and received it as compared to a similar group that was told they would receive relaxation training (30%) instead of the requested hypnotherapy. The only actual difference in treatment was the inclusion of the term hypnosis in reference to a relaxed state. This issue of the power of suggestion and the use of hypnosis to enhance it will be examined in more detail later.

Medical researchers are particularly aware of the strength of the placebo effects which result when new drugs are first administered. In a section reviewing antismoking drugs, Bernstein (1969) concluded that researchers had failed to demonstrate any difference between these drugs and placebos in controlling smoking. The consideration of success rates achieved in an "attention control" group is very important in evaluating results. This group needs to receive the same degree of therapist contact, attention, and involvement in treatment, while simultaneously excluding active treatment procedures. Evidence exists that an attention-placebo treatment can be at least as effective as clinic programs (Bernstein, 1968; Keutzer, 1968).

Since only a few studies to date have included some type of control group, an estimate of the placebo effect must be viewed as tentative. Three studies (Javel, 1980; MacHovec & Man, 1978; Pederson, Scrimgeour, & Lefcoe, 1979) found 0 percent abstinence in a no treatment control group. A fourth study (Pederson et al., 1975) reported a 12.5 percent abstinence rate in a follow-up for a no treatment group. Though these results provide strong evidence that without treatment very few smokers quit, they are not adequate evaluations of placebo treatment. The counseling group in Pederson, Scrimgeour, & Lefcoe (1975) and the true site acupuncture group in the MacHovec and Man (1978) study appear to be more characteristic of an attention placebo group with a supportive approach. The false-site acupuncture (MacHovec & Man, 1978) and the "cold turkey" attention placebo group in Barkley, Hastings & Jackson (1977) are open too easily to the criticism of experimenter bias. In actuality no definitive study of the placebo effect exists. However, taking a conservative approach, placebo effects alone may account for as much as a 20 percent success rate. Further research in this area is definitely needed.

SUBJECT POPULATIONS

Straits (1966) was one of the few researchers to use a multivariate statistical analysis to predict success. He found that the best predictor of success was mention by the smoker of specific physical ailments or a doctor's advice to quit. This finding was lent further support by the fact that clients in one of the most successful studies (von Dendenroth, 1968) were medically referred. Apparently, the aversive consequences of continued smoking being perceived as life threatening can greatly increase a client's motivation to stop. Since this client population has severe medical problems, techniques which are highly aversive such as rapid-smoking (Barkely, Hastings, & Jackson, 1977) or electric shock (Powell & Azrin, 1968) may produce additional stress that could have undesirable consequences, and hence would be ethically questionable.

On the other hand, volunteer populations who have a presumably lower level of motivation and yet want to stop smoking may benefit safely from aversive conditioning. However, even the covert conditioning of feelings of nausea and bad taste used in most early research (Johnston & Donoghue, 1971) have been reported by Hall and Crasilneck (1970) to apparently produce "notable anxiety" for some clients between treatment sessions.

Evidence lending hope for clients who have failed to stop smoking after previous hypnotherapy was provided in a study by Powell (1980). This study produced a 57 percent (N=7) abstinence rate in clients who had not been helped by previous hypnotherapy. However, none of the six clients who had been unsuccessful with previous hypnotherapy stopped in a study by De Piano, Sandford, Cash, & Gotthelf (1983). Additional follow-up treatments by the same therapist (Kanzler, Jaffee & Zeidenberg, 1976) who initially offered a single treatment package did not help seven clients who requested it to stop. The client and therapist's original expectations in this latter study may have limited the effect of additional treatments. Furthermore, the size of these samples is too small to enable any conclusions to be reached at this time.

Limited research exploring the personality, demographic, and historical variables of smokers related to either success or failure has been generally unfruitful. Keutzer (1968) found no correlations between smoking and ten demographic, history, and personality variables. Bernstein (1968) also failed to correlate smoking reduction with locus of control, extroversion, suggestibility, or emotionality. However, De Piano et al. (1983) have demonstrated that success seems to be related to the perception of their habit. Individuals who feel either positive or negative towards smoking appear to do worse than individuals who feel little affect towards their smoking habit.

Watkins (1976) examined the reasons her clients dropped out of treatment and found that all seven dropouts reported that they used smoking behavior to help control anger. Seven out of eight clients who continued treatment, but did not quit, also reported needing cigarettes to help them handle angry feelings. While this finding of a relationship between emotions and smoking behavior is interesting, it is only anecdotal evidence. At present, population differences which account for success have not been sufficiently studied except for the one finding that the aversive consequences of medical ailments was found to be correlated with the success of therapy.

INDIVIDUAL IN COMPARISON TO GROUP TREATMENT

A group sharing one therapist requires that individuals share their attention, suggestions, recommendations, and support in some equal, but not readily quantifiable way. Consequently, the percent of time client and therapist are engaged in doing individual analysis and psychotherapy as part of a group treatment "package" can vary significantly. Usually direct therapeutic intervention will be much less than would be provided if the individual had the same contact hours in private therapy. The question about individual versus group techniques then becomes how much personal contact with a therapist do clients need and what is the environment in which a particular therapist can best utilize his or her skills and specific techniques.

Holroyd (1980) reached the conclusion that programs with intense personal interactions that focused on establishing individual motivating reasons and provided adjunctive follow-up contact were the most successful. These conclusions apparently indicate that individual therapy would result in higher success rates than group therapy, unless similar conditions were created using group techniques. Three studies (Grosz, 1978a, 1978b; MacHovec & Man, 1978) comparing the use of group and individual treatment with the same hypnotic suggestions and treatment procedures found individual therapy resulted in a higher but nonsignificant abstincence rate. However, successful results have been achieved in two hypnosis and group therapy studies. Kline (1970) treated groups of ten patients who participated in a 12-hour group marathon. His treatment procedure required a 24-hour pretreatment abstinence period. Individualized hypnotic induction was conducted until the entire group was in a trance. Periods of treatment focused on flooding for smoking deprivation followed by relaxation desensitization suggestions. Cigarettes were present and experienced, but not orally contacted. An assistant was also utilized who smoked profusely at times in the group's presence. A remarkable abstinence rate of 88 percent at one year follow-up was achieved. The second successful group study was by Sanders (1977). He increased the frequency of individually tailored suggestions by having hypnotized group members give each other suggestions about problems they brought up. Treatment lasted for four sessions and was conducted in small groups of four or five clients. Treatment procedures included three daily relaxation periods (morning, noon, and night), success visualization, positive self-statements about their ability to make a choice and mental rehearsal of problem situations. A 10-month follow-up found 68 percent of these clients abstinent.

The success rates of these two group studies are comparable to those found in studies where researchers provided at least several treatment sessions utilizing a "package" of techniques administered on an individual basis (Hall & Crasilneck, 1970; Miller, 1976; Nuland & Field, 1970; Watkins, 1976). From one perspective, group and individual treatment studies can be observed to be equally effective if the quality and quantity of therapeutic contact is maximized. The choice of approach therefore is better made on the therapist's predispositions and type of techniques used. Watkins (1976) noted in passing that she did not find her procedures as effective in a group context. Von Dendenroth (1964a, 1964b, 1968) expressed his clinical judgment that individual treatment was better, because it took into account the personal, social, and economic factors of the individual client in therapy. With such little empirical evidence about the relationship of client characteristics and outcome, it is not possible to substantiate von Dendenroth's belief. In fact, individual analysis which suggests that an individual is especially responsive to social reinforcement may lead to a recommendation for group therapy. Likewise, group techniques and exposure could possibly inhibit some individual's potential for success. There is no clear-cut case for the efficacy of either individual or group methods without taking the individual differences of the client, therapist, and selected treatment procedures into account.

To some degree ethical considerations tend to weigh in the favor of individualized treatment. Hilgard (1968) cautions that while the aftereffects in nonpatient populations are very infrequent and generally mild, hypnosis is, for many subjects, a highly charged personal experience that may result in associations of traumatic situations of life. The spontaneous appearance of emotional and personal material when not sought can be disruptive to group therapy, especially in situations where preparations for handling it are limited. Difficulties in arousal, the prolongation of hypnotic effects (e.g. hallucinatory visualizations), and posthypnotic phobias can occur. Though competent professionals can be expected to respond to problems of individuals in a group should they develop, the recognition and ease of instituting specific treatment are greater within an individual counseling situation.

CUSTOMIZED AND STANDARDIZED THERAPY APPROACHES

Some therapists have developed treatment methods which utilize information obtained in a pretreatment interview with the client (Erickson, 1964; Nuland & Field, 1970; Sanders, 1977; von Dendenroth, 1964a; Watkins, 1976). How this information is used varies in each study. Other researchers have chosen to develop a more standardized set of procedures to be administered to all clients (Hall & Crasilneck, 1970; Kline, 1970; Kroger, 1963; MacHovec & Man, 1978; Powell, 1980; Spiegel, 1970; Stanton, 1978). Parts of these standardized "packages" have personalized components. The issue of customized versus standardized approaches can best be examined as a question of the flexibility of treatment. Flexibility relates to the degree that individual differences are considered which maintain smoking behavior. Examination of this issue tends to reveal the implied theoretical orientation (if any) on which the treatment plan is based.

Nuland and Field (1970) hypothesized that the wide range in success rates may be attributable to the degree to which an individualized approach was used. Their success rates for an individualized approach were 60 percent, whereas their previous standardized "package" had only resulted in a 25 percent abstinence rate. Their approach emphasized giving the clients suggestions under hypnosis based on their own reasons for not smoking, maintaining telephone contact, emphasis on increasing personal motivation, and self-hypnosis training. The theoretical value of making a person's own suggestions to them is considered by Erickson (1964) as a means for overcoming resistance. However, for the most part these treatment procedures were selected on the basis of trial and error. Thus, they do not reflect a distinct theoretical rationale guiding the use of specific treatments.

Watkins (1976) developed a rather unique approach: she selected a set of three treatment suggestions and two visualizations for each client from her collection of techniques (i.e., "bag of tricks"). This approach was designed to facilitate cognitive restructuring by giving suggestions to the client while he or she is in a relaxed state. The suggestions are patterned after the client's own reasons for quitting; they attack rationalizations for smoking, provide suggestions for substitute coping behavior, and undermine the client's motives for continuing this behavior. Her suggestions focus on a complex variety of theoretical orientations, including a tension-reduction model via relaxation, ego-enhancing suggestions, catharsis for anger, self-administered monetary reinforcement, aversive conditioning, and deconditioning of the social and personal reinforcing characterisitics of cigarettes. While a typical hypnotic induction is used, clients are told that it is a "concentration-relaxation" technique to avoid preconceptions about hypnosis. The 67 percent success rate at six-month follow-up for those volunteers who completed five treatment sessions suggests that some of this plethora of techniques works, but it does not suggest which ones. In addition, her approach—because of its exceedingly flexible structure—would be difficult to replicate.

Von Dendenroth (1964a, 1964b, 1968) tailors a specific set of treatments which focuses on many behavioral techniques that gradually enable the client to experience successful control of smoking behavior. Treatment is conducted for three sessions over 21 days during which time clients prepare themselves for "Quit Day." Behavioral components include changing to a less desirable brand of cigarettes, not smoking before and after meals for increasing periods of time, engaging in behavior incompatible with smoking when the desire to smoke arises, covert aversive conditioning to the act of smoking, avoiding smoking when drinking alcohol, and keeping an ongoing notebook of reasons for not smoking. Hypnosis is utilized with the rationale that it is a physiological tool that renders the client more susceptible to positive suggestion. Follow-up abstinence rates of 94 percent for 1,000 clients treated in the last six years stand out as the best achieved of all large-scale studies. These results are impressive, but, as mentioned before, these clients were highly motivated by the aversive consequences of medical ailments which alone may account for part of this high rate of success. Interestingly enough, von Dendenroth (1968) takes an "addiction" model approach to account for the maintenance of smoking behavior, referring to his clients as "tobaccomaniacs." He cites the appearance of withdrawal symptoms (agitation, anxiety, anorexia, nausea, vomiting, and tremors) in support of this viewpoint. However, he appears to contradict himself somewhat when he also refers to his clients as "psychologically enslaved." Consequently, though his theoretical model seemingly reflects his medical orientation, he practices predominantly behavioral techniques in conjunction with hypnosis.

The group study by Sanders (1977) was described in the last section. His unique contribution was to use mutual hypnosis and have clients give each other individually oriented suggestions and social reinforcement. This approach illustrates techniques to provide individualized attention with the economy of cost provided by group therapy.

Kline (1970) used a standardized group marathon desensitization treatment for his clients. The therapeutic rationale was to enable clients to experience the tension of smoking deprivation without anxiety. The treatment details of this study were presented in the last section. The follow-up success rate in this study of 88 percent indicates that the adverse consequences of smoking cessation may be a critical factor that prevents individuals from stopping smoking. Thus, a treatment which helps reduce the anxiety usually encountered in deconditioning the smoking habit warrants further study.

Hall and Crasilneck (1970) were also successful in using a standardized approach that helped 64 percent of their clients stop smoking without symptom substitution. Elements of their "package" included screening of the need for additional counseling, increasing incompatible exercise behavior, substitution of another oral gratification (e.g., increased fluid intake, gum, or mints), and the utilization of hypnosis to demonstrate mental control of physical processes. Thus, the procedures they used in general reflected a behavioral rationale. Of their successful noncigarette smoking clients, 22 percent manifested symptom substitution (i.e., now smoked a pipe or cigars, or used gum or candy on a regular basis). MacHovec and Man (1978) and Kroger (1963) both used covert aversive sensory conditioning. MacHovec and Man (1978) also emphasized the value of relaxation in their treatment approach. Covert aversive conditioning to the taste and smell of smoking was often used in many of the early studies (Johnston & Donoghue, 1971). Frequently the emphasis was on training the client to actively generate and experience a slight state of nausea when the desire to smoke arose. Kroger's (1963) other treatment components included gradual reduction, holding the cigarette in the opposite hand, and the use of peppermint lifesavers to help satisfy oral desires. These behavioral techniques produced a 60 percent abstinence rate for Kroger's clients.

Spiegel (1970) popularized a one-session standardized treatment approach which stressed health-oriented, self-preservation suggestions and self-hypnosis training. His use of suggestion stressed making the urge not to smoke more reinforcing by association with positive thoughts about being *for* the survival and health of the body. The client was also instructed in the extinction principle of conditioning as a rationale for treatment. They were told that if they ignore any urge, biological or psychological, its frequency of occurrence subsides to very little and eventually loses all controlling influence. Clients were instructed to practice making a three-part suggestion to themselves that smoking is a poison, you need your body to live, and you owe your body respect and protection. They were encouraged to practice these three suggestions after doing a self-hypnotic induction as much as 10 times a day, every one to two hours. The client was also instructed how to practice these suggestions when total privacy is not available using a very brief and socially unobtrusive induction. A 20 percent abstinence rate was achieved at follow-up of the 615 clients treated.

Spiegel (1970) notes that his program is targeted for the hard-core smoker who wants to stop but cannot do so despite repeated efforts. He excludes the group of smokers who acknowledge the danger yet continue to smoke from being suitable candidates for this treatment. Spiegel's (1970) consideration of matching client characteristics to treatment modalities is an important concept to consider further. However, in this case no mention was made of operationally defining criteria for selection nor of any recorded effort that such a screening was made. There appears to be the assumption that one can readily identify clients who have a conscious or unconscious wish to use cigarettes as a slow means of suicide. While it was not specifically mentioned by Spiegel, it seeems logical to assume that clients with a "death wish" would be by implication those who did not find the suggestions for body survival positive and reinforcing.

The value of Spiegel's concept of selection is in making the step to take individual differences of reinforcers into account. His approach implies the need to match clients selectively with specific therapeutic approaches. Likewise, the weakness of standardized approaches involves the assumption that certain common positive and negative reinforcements can be manipulated to help bring about behavioral change in a substantial number of clients. Thus, the underlying theoretical rationale of the standardized approach would be to identify a group of people that smoke for a similar reason or reasons. The specific characteristics which differentiate general "types" of smokers could then be used to select a treatment package best suited for each unique group. Of course this rationale assumes that therapeutically relevant groups actually exist.

The techniques or combinations of techniques discussed in this section generally lack a consistent theoretical rationale for their application as a "package." Different elements of each "package" may work for different types. Therefore, therapy can be optimized by either matching based on a behavioral analysis and inventory the treatment(s) to the client ("customized" approach) or the client to the treatment(s) ("standardized" approach).

SELF-HYPNOSIS

The value of self-hypnosis has not been empirically demonstrated (Holroyd, 1980) though variations of the technique have been a substantial part of many studies (Berkowitz, Ross-Townsend, & Kohberger, 1979; Spiegel, 1970; Watkins, 1976). Self-hypnosis' value is often perceived as a means for helping the client to generalize treatment effectiveness. Holroyd (1980) criticizes the use of self-hypnosis as being inadequate when it is used in single session therapy (Berkowitz et al., 1979; Spiegel, 1970) to shift responsibility for success outcome to the client. Her conclusion was that self-hypnosis training did not seem critical for success. De Piano et al. (1983) have added support to this position. In their study no differences were found between those receiving instruction/training in self-hypnosis and those receiving in-office treatment only. A single study by Stanton (1978) did not include self-hypnosis and yet achieved a higher success rate (42%) than Spiegel (1970) or Berkowitz et al. (1979), rates of 20 percent and 25 percent, respectively.

None of the above studies looked at the correlation between the practice of self-hypnotic techniques taught and success rates. Also, no experiment has taken a relatively standardized "package" and assessed whether self-hypnosis practiced in a regular, systematic way has any clinically significant value. The use of self-hypnosis tapes to facilitate the generalization of treatment has not been reported. Tapes may have the value of enhancing therapeutic treatment at a substantially lower cost to the client. At present the lack of the necessary research in this area makes the assessment of the possible contribution of self-hypnosis towards successful outcomes not possible. It may have value, but current evidence indicates that its effect is at best a moderate one.

NUMBER OF SESSIONS

Spiegel's (1970) claim in this field was that he had developed a one-session treatment using hypnosis that achieved a 20 percent success rate. Berkowitz et al. (1979) replicated Spiegel's results. They recalculated Spiegel's (1970) follow-up data and reassigned a percentage of clients who did not respond to mail questionnaires to the nonsmoking group. This estimate of abstinence in noncontacted follow-up clients was derived based on Kanzler's et al. (1976) findings that 27 percent of the clients who did not respond to mail queries reported having stopped smoking when contacted by telephone. This adjustment increased Spiegel's (1970) percent of success to 25 percent. The success rate of the Berkowitz et al. (1979) study was also 25 percent. Thus, the effect of one session of hypnotic suggestions with a convincing therapist can help 20 to 25 percent of clients seeking to stop smoking through hypnosis at minimal cost.

With additional types of suggestion Stanton (1978) was successful in raising the single session abstinence rate to 45 percent. His treatment included suggestions for body survival and health needs (Spiegel, 1970), confidence building, increased mental control of physiological processes (von Dendenroth, 1968), ego enhancement (Hartland, 1971), the red balloon visualization (Walsh, 1976), and a success visualization. Stanton (1978) believes that one of the most powerful factors in effective therapy is the level of belief, expectation, and hope fostered by the therapist that the patient will be successful in achieving his or her goals. Javel (1980) also achieved a comparable success rate of 50 percent using Stanton's (1978) methods, replicating his findings. These positive feelings about successful results are related to and facilitated by therapeutic rapport. This factor of belief engendered by the therapist is part of the placebo effect that exists.

Treatment success rates can be compared to the rough estimate of 20 percent success attributed to the reinforcing effect of behaviors and beliefs related to "being in therapy" (i.e., the placebo effects). In effect a percentage of success can be subtracted from the overall success rate. The amount of success left over reflects the "true" effect of the combination of treatments used. Based on this assumption of a 20 percent placebo effect Spiegel's (1970) "true" success rate is much lower (0-5%), indicating little or no real effect. Stanton (1978) used a wider variety of suggestions and with this very conservative criterion, a success rate of 25 percent can be considered to be achieved. Many multiple treatment studies with multimodal techniques have achieved abstinence rates usually in the 60 to 90 percent range (Holroyd, 1980) which when adjusted for placebo effects means a 40 to 70 percent "true" success rate. These studies indicate that four to six individual therapy contact hours are sufficient to achieve maximal success rates. Additional therapy contact hours are associated with higher success rates (Holroyd, 1980) and may benefit clients who failed to succeed after only one session. While Nuland and Field 1970) reported 73 percent of the clients who stopped did so in the first session, Nuland (1970) expressed the belief that with several sessions clients are more likely to remain nonsmokers than with a single treatment.

SUGGESTION AND TRANCE DEPTH

The general public conceives of hypnosis as a state of mind like sleep, but in which one can more easily accept suggestions (Webster, 1981). The general professional viewpoint concurs that hypnosis provides a milieu which facilitates behavioral change (Erickson, 1960; Hilgard, 1977) and suggestions for changes in memory, perception, and personality (Lazarus, 1973). As mentioned before, von Dendenroth (1968) considers hypnosis as rendering the individual more suggestible to positive suggestion. Hypnosis is purported to also achieve positive effects by relaxing the individual, heightening imagery, and focusing attention (Sanders, 1977; Stanton, 1978). Hypnosis has been recognized by Wickramsekara (1976) as a state in which 1) the effects of cognitive processes on bodily functions are amplified, 2) the locus of control is more internally oriented, and 3) distractibility is lower.

Hypnosis can also have therapeutic benefits, because of its mystique as a special state. Hunt and Bespalec (1974) contended that it enhances the client's feeling that sometihing special is happening to him or her which will be of considerable value. Lazarus (1973) demonstrated that just adding the word hypnosis to a relaxation treatment for clients requesting hypnosis produced significantly higher success rates. In other words, if the client believes in the "power" of hypnosis, this belief contributes to the placebo effect of hypnotherapy.

Depth of trance is clinically reported not to be important (Perry, Gelfand & Marcovitch, 1979; Perry & Mullen, 1975; Spiegel, 1970; von Dendenroth, 1968; Watkins, 1976). However, von Dendenroth (1968) found that the few clients who were not hypnotizable were not suitable for treatment. Since most studies reported were clinically and not experimentally designed, hypnotic susceptibility has not usually been measured with a standardized method. Perry and Mullen (1975) found some relationship between hypnotic susceptibility and reduction in cigarettes consumed. Deyoub and Wilkie (1980) noted how trance depth has been found to be related to successful outcome in their weight control study and in other studies using hypnosis to facilitate control, asthma relief, and pain control. King and McDonald (1976) provided evidence linking high suggestibility and a greater propensity for verbal conditioning and, thus, a more cooperative and willing attitude towards suggestion. Thus, corrollary evidence indicates that depth of trance as measured by suggestibility may correlate significantly with successful outcome. In addition, two researchers have remarked how indirect suggestion was useful in overcoming resistance (von Dendenroth, 1964b; Erickson, 1964). Yet, direct evidence to confirm or refute that the more suggestible clients are the more successful ones is limited (Perry, et al., 1979).

A recent study (De Piano et al., 1983) did find a significant relationship between hypnotic suggestibility and successful smoking cessation. A major difference between this study and previous ones was the use of a standardized instrument to measure susceptibility, the Stanford Hypnotic Susceptibility Scale, Form C (Weitzenhoffer & Hilgard, 1962). Forty-one percent of the clients who achieved a scale score of eight or higher stopped smoking. However, none of the clients with a scale score of four or below stopped. Follow-up was conducted at four months following treatment. At one week follow-up, client's ratings of hypnotic trance depth significantly discriminated between smokers and nonsmokers. However, this effect was not observed at the four-month follow-up. These findings suggest that it may be useful to screen clients for suggestibility, but that such screening would need to utilize a standardized instrument.

HYPNOSIS AND BEHAVIOR THERAPY

Behavioral analysis of the reinforcing contingencies which operantly condition and the discriminative stimuli that classically condition cigarette smoking provides a practical and testable theoretical orientation to guide the selection of appropriate therapeutic treatments (Dengrove, 1970). This learning theory approach predicts that smoking behavior stops when the majority of the strongest reinforcers that act to maintain it, lose effectiveness, or are prevented by other stronger reinforcers which maintain incompatible responses when smoking (Bernstein, 1969). Thus, a behavioral approach towards helping an individual to stop smoking will involve a combination of unlearning old responses and replacing them with newly learned behaviors.

Hypnosis can be used to enhance the acceptance and impact of a variety of therapeutic techniques. The effect of the techniques which have shown the most promise can be analyzed, regardless of the therapist's orientation, in behavioral terms and techniques.

The behavioral techniques that were used in successful studies with hypnosis are listed below:

1. Aversive covert suggestions of bad taste, smell, and slight feelings of nausea were conditioned, rehearsed, and to be actively applied by clients when the desire for a cigarette occurs. Hypnosis facilitates this technique

to the degree that it enhances the vividness of the aversive covert associations and the client's desire to practice the exercise.

2. Desensitization to the aversive feelings of desiring a cigarette. Hypnosis helps here through its relaxing qualities. This technique helps the client extinguish the desire for cigarettes.
3. Substitution of some other less harmful or nonharmful oral gratification. This technique can be useful as a first step in developing control of the smoking impulse.
4. Indirect and direct suggestions have been used to help the client cognitively restructure his or her perceptions of the aversive contingencies associated with continuing to smoke and the positive benefits which will be accrued through not smoking. Hypnosis can increase the client's acceptance of these suggestions as his or her own. Feedback of the individual's own suggestions has been used to help promote this acceptance. In this case the client's perception of the environment was manipulated in order to change the impact of reinforcing contingencies.
5. Hypnosis exercises have been used directly to strengthen the client's belief in the power of his mind to control the body in new ways.
6. Behavior changes in the contingencies which make the act of smoking less reinforcing (e.g., changing brands), and no longer temporally contingent with other reinforcing behaviors (e.g., meals, drinking alcohol, socializing) were applied to reduce smoking's reinforcing qualities.
7. Maintenance of follow-up contact by telephone with the therapist provided opportunities to receive positive social reinforcement (i.e., praise) for success or aversive consequences for failure. Hypnosis may have enhanced the effect of these telephone contacts through posthypnotic techniques.
8. Visualizations of the desired outcome and its benefits have been used as a means to reinforce positive expectations. Hypnosis' facility to enhance the lifelike quality of imagery helps in this approach.
9. Mental rehearsal of problematic situations in which new behavior was practiced. Individualized solutions and coping skills can be rehearsed in this way to help facilitate the maintenance of self-control.

A therapist can develop an integrated package from the above techniques, selecting those best suited for the individual client. These techniques are tools which can be used to restructure the environmental and subjective contingencies so that smoking behavior is no longer reinforced and maintained.

CONCLUSIONS

Hypnosis can be used to enhance the acceptance and impact of a variety of therapeutic techniques. The effect of the techniques which have shown the most promise can be analyzed in a comprehensive way within the context of a behavioral learning theory. Essentially, it appears that the techniques work by enabling the client to change the reinforcing contingencies of smoking behavior. At present the overall results indicate that when a group of these techniques is used as a "package" with properly motivated and supported clients, about two-thirds of those who complete several sessions of treatment can be expected to be abstinent at six-month follow-up. However, it is not possible to determine the extent to which the client's motivation to stop has contributed to this success rate. It should also be noted that as selection procedures become less stringent, and mild or poorly motivated clients enter into a program, success rates are reduced dramatically. In fact, it is suggested that outcome may be more related to the motivation/disposition of the client than to the treatment procedures themselves.

Motivation is related to an individual's expectation. If we expect very little, minimal effort is put forth. In this regard, individuals placed in groups may expect less, thus influencing their general motivation to put forth the effort necessary to stop smoking. Again outcome is not related to the therapeutic technique per se but rather to the general predisposition of the client.

When comparing individual programs to packages ones, it seems that the greater success rate seen in the individualized treatment programs are more a function of the quantity and quality of time spent with clients in this type of format. When contact time with the client is controlled for, little difference between these approaches is found.

Finally, it does not appear that the addition of self-hypnosis has contributed to the success rate of smoking cessation programs. However, it should be cautioned that few studies have attempted to assess the extent to which individuals in self-hypnosis programs have actually employed/practiced this techniques. It may be that self-hypnosis programs have little effect because the clients are not actually engaging in its use to an appreciable degree.

Continued research in this area is clearly warranted. In particular, evaluation of the effects of self-hypnosis, and the number of sessions employed would be most useful to the practitioner. In addition, from a research point of view, it is extremely important that attempts be made to determine the relative contributions made by the individual's predisposition (especially motivation and expectation) and that made by the treatment techniques themselves. In this way we can attempt to ferret out the "true" therapeutic gain versus those ascribed to "placebo" effect.

SUMMARY

This review and analysis of hypnosis and smoking control studies addresses the "state-of-the-art" in terms of theoretical orientation, measures of success, placebo effects, subject populations, individual vs. group treatment, customized vs. standardized therapy, self-hypnosis, number of sessions, trance depth, and behavior therapy. Almost all treatments involved a composite of several techniques, making it difficult to discern the specific active elements of therapy. Basically, these treatment "packages" work, but the factors accounting for their effectiveness are unclear. The successful treatment procedures used were analyzed based on a behavioral learning theory in an attempt to account for the observed changes. Hypnosis was examined as a means for enhancing the acceptance and impact of the various therapeutic techniques used. In general, successful therapy seemed to be accounted for by enabling the client to change the reinforcing contingencies and conditioned discriminative stimuli which maintained smoking behavior. At present the overall results indicate that when a group of these techniques is used as a "package" with properly motivated and supported clients, about two-thirds of those who complete several sessions of treatment can be expected to be abstinent at six-month follow-up. A list of promising techniques was provided in order to help therapists develop their own integrated "packages." Research efforts now need to be directed in a more systematic way towards identifying the relative contribution of each of these techniques.

REFERENCES

Barber, T. X., Spanos, N. P., & Chaves, J. F. (1974). *Hypnotism, imagination and human potentialities.* New York: Pergamon.

Barkley, R. A., Hastings, J. E., & Jackson, T. L. (1977). The effects of rapid smoking and hypnosis in the treatment of smoking behavior. *International Journal of Clinical and Experimental Hypnosis, 25,* 7-17.

Berkowitz, B., Ross-Townsend, A., & Kohberger, R. (1979). Hypnotic treatment of smoking. The single treatment method revisited. *American Journal of Psychiatry, 136,* 83-85.

Bernstein, D. A. (1968). *The modification of smoking behavior.* Unpublished doctoral dissertation, Northwestern University, Evanston, IL.

Bernstein, D. A. (1968) Modification of smoking behavior: An evaluative review. *Psychology Bulletin, 71,* 418-440.

Cohen, S. B. (1969). Hypnosis and smoking. *Journal of the American Medical Association, 208,* 335-337.

Dengrove, E. (1970). A single-treatment method to stop smoking using ancillary self-hypnosis: Discussion, *International Journal of Clinical and Experimental Hypnosis, 18,* 251-256.

De Piano, F., Sandford, J., Cash, J., & Gotthelf, C. (1983). *Hypnosis and smoking: A comparison of individualized versus packaged suggestions with and without self-hypnosis.* Submitted for publication.

Deyoub, P. L., & Wilkie, R. (1980) Suggestion with and without hypnotic induction in a weight reduction program. *The International Journal of Clinical and Experimental Hypnosis, 28,* 333-340.

Erickson, M. H. (1960). Breast development possibly influenced by hypnosis: Two instances and the psychotherapeutic results. *American Journal of Clinical Hypnosis, 2,* 157-159.

Erickson, M. H. (1964). The burden of responsibility in effective psychotherapy. *American Journal of Clinical Hypnosis, 6,* 269-271.

Grosz, H. J. (1978). Nicotine addiction: Treatment with medical hypnosis, part 1. *Journal of the Indiana State Medical Association, 71,* 1074-1075. (a)

Grosz, H. J. (1978). Nicotine addiction: Treatment with medical hypnosis, part 2. *Journal of the Indiana State Medical Association, 71,* 1136-1137. (b)

Hall, J. A., & Crasilneck, H. B. (1970). Development of a hypnotic technique for treating chronic cigarette smoking. *International Journal of Clinical and Experimental Hypnosis, 18,* 283-289.

Hartland, J. (1971). Further observations on the use of ego-strengthening techniques. *American Journal of Clinical Hypnosis, 14,* 1-8.

Hilgard, E. R. (1968). *The experience of hypnosis.* New York: Harcourt.

Hilgard, E. R. (1977). *Divided consciousness: Multiple control in human thought and action.* New York: Wiley.

Hoinville, G. W., & Biggs, H. W. (1966). Establishing smoking habits in retrospect. *The Statistician, 16,* 23-43.

Holroyd, J. (1980). Hypnosis treatment for smoking: An evaluative review. *International Journal of Clinical and Experimental Hypnosis, 28,* 341-357.

Hunt, W. A., & Bespalec, D. A. (1974). An evaluation of current methods of modifying smoking behavior. *Journal of Clinical Psychology, 30,* 431-438.

Javel, A. F. (1980). One-session hypnotherapy for smoking: A controlled study. *Psychological Reports, 46,* 895-899.

Johnston, E., & Donoghue, J. R. (1971). Hypnosis and smoking: A review of the literature. *American Journal of Clinical Hypnosis, 13,* 265-272.

Kanzler, M., Jaffe, J. H., & Zeidenberg, P. (1976). Long and short-term effectiveness of a large scale proprietary smoking cessation program: A 4-year follow-up of Smokenders participants. *Journal of Clinical Psychology, 32,* 661-669.

Keutzer, C. S. (1968). Behavior modification of smoking: The experimental investigation of diverse techniques. *Behavior Research and Therapy, 6,* 137-157.

King, D. R., & McDonald, R. D. (1976). Hypnotic susceptibility and verbal conditioning. *The International Journal of Clinical and Experimental Hypnosis, 24,* 29-37.

Kline, M. V. (1965). Hypnotherapy. In B. B. Wolman (Ed.), *Handbook of Clinical Psychology.* New York: McGraw-Hill.

Kline, M. V. (1970). The use of extended group hypnotherapy sessions in controlling cigarette habituation. *International Journal of Clinical and Experimental Hypnosis, 18,* 270-282.

Kroger, W. S. (1963). *Clinical and expermental hypnosis.* Philadelphia: Lippincott.

Lazarus, A. A. (1973). "Hypnosis" as a facilitator in behavior therapy. *International Journal of Clinical and Experimental Hypnosis, 31,* 25-31.

MacHovec, F. J., & Man, S. C. (1978). Acupuncture and hypnosis compared: Fifty-eight cases. *American Journal of Clinical Hypnosis, 21,* 45-47.

Martin, J. E., & Frederiksen, L. W. (1980). Self-tracking of carbon monxide by smokers. *Behavior Therapy, 11,* 577-587.

Miller, M. M. (1976). Hypnoaversive treatment in alcoholism, nicontinism, and weight control. *Journal of the National Medical Association, 68,* 129-130.

Nuland, W. (1970). A single-treatment method to stop smoking using ancillary self-hypnosis: Discussion. *International Journal of Clinical and Experimental Hypnosis, 18,* 257-260.

Nuland, W., & Field, P. B. (1970). Smoking and hypnosis: A systematic clinical approach.

International Journal of Clinical and Experimental Hypnosis, 18, 290-306.

Pederson, L. L., Scrimgeour, W. G., & Lefcoe, N. M. (1975). Comparison of hypnosis plus counseling, counseling alone, and hypnosis alone in a community service smoking withdrawal program. *Journal of Consulting and Clinical Psychology, 43,* 920.

Pederson, L. L., Scrimgeour, W. G., & Lefcoe, N. M. (1979). Variables of hypnosis which are related to success in a smoking withdrawal program. *International Journal of Clinical and Experimental Hypnosis, 27,* 14-20.

Perry, C., Gelfand, R., & Marcovitch, P. (1979). The relevance of hypnotic susceptibility in the clinical context. *Journal of Abnormal Psychology, 88,* 592-603.

Perry, C., & Mullen, G. (1975). The effects of hypnotic susceptibility on reducing smoking behavior treated by an hypnotic technique. *Journal of Clinical Psychology, 3l,* 498-505.

Powell, D. H. (1980). Helping habitual smokers using flooding and hypnotic desensitization technique: A brief communication. *International Journal of Clinical and Experimental Hypnosis, 28,* 192-196.

Powell, J., & Azrin, N. (1968). The effects of shock as a punisher for cigarette smoking. *Journal of Applied Behavior Analysis, 1,* 63-71.

Royal College of Physicians of London. (1962). *Smoking and health.* New York: Pittman.

Sanders, S. (1977). Mutual group hypnosis and smoking. *American Journal of Clinical Hypnosis, 20,* 131-135.

Spiegel, H. (1970). A single-treatment method to stop smoking using ancillary self-hypnosis. *International Journal of Clinical and Experimental Hypnosis, 18,* 235-250.

Stanton, H. E. (1978). A one-session hypnotic approach to modifying smoking behavior. *International Journal of Clinical and Experimental Hypnosis, 26,* 22-29.

Straits, B. C. (1966, August). *The discontinuation of cigarette smoking: A multiple discriminant analysis.* Paper presented at the annual meeting of the American Sociological Association, Miami Beach, Florida.

United States Public Health Service. (1975). *The health consequence of smoking.* Washington, D. C. : United States Department of Health, Education & Welfare.

United States Public Health Service. (1977). *The Smoking Digest.* Washington, D. C. : United States Department of Health, Education & Welfare.

United States Public Health Service. (1979). *The health consequence of smoking.* Washington, D. C.: United States Department of Health, Education and Welfare.

von Dendenroth, T. E. A. (1964). The use of hypnosis with "tobaccomaniacs." *American Journal of Clinical Hypnosis, 6,* 326-331. (a)

von Dendenroth, T. E. A. (1964). Further help for the "tobaccomaniacs" *American Journal of Clinical Hypnosis, 6,* 332-336. (b)

Walsh, S. L. (1976). The red balloon technique of hypnotherapy: A clinical note. *International Journal of Clinical and Experimental Hypnosis, 24,* 10-12.

Watkins, H. H. (1976). Hypnosis and smoking: A five session approach. *International Journal of Clinical and Experimental Hypnosis, 24,* 381-390.

Webster's new collegiate dictionary. (1981). Springfield, MA: Meriam.

Weitzenhoffer, A. M., & Hilgard, E. R. (1962). *Stanford Hypnotic Susceptibility Scale, Form C.* Palo Alto, CA: Consulting Psychologists Press.

Wickramasekara, I. (1976). Effects of "hypnosis" and task motivational instructions in attemping to influence the "voluntary" self-deprivation of money. In *Biofeedback, behavior therapy and hypnosis.* Chicago: Nelson-Hall.

Wright, E. M. (1970). A single-treatment method to stop smoking using ancillary self-hypnosis: Discussion. *International Journal of Clinical and Experimetal Hypnosis, 18,* 261-267.

Chapter 5

Hypnosis and Weight Management

Michael J. Simon

Arkansas Mental Health Services Division,
Little Rock

Obesity can be considered one of the most prevalent and serious disorders in modern society. Estimates of its prevalence among American adults range from 15 to 50 percent (Bray, 1976; Van Itallie, 1977), while approximately 25 percent of all children are overweight (Forbes, 1975). The problems faced by obese individuals are really twofold. First is the fact that the obese person is stigmatized in our slim-conscious society. They are often not accepted socially and may find that they are discriminated against in many areas of their lives. Compounding this situation is the fact that, unlike individuals with other physical disabilities, they tend to be blamed for their condition and are labeled in terms that imply personal responsibility (weak, lazy, etc.). Second, and more important, are the many health risks associated with obesity. For example, cardiovascular disorders have been conclusively linked with obesity (Cappon, 1973). Also many illnesses such as diabetes, gastrointestinal disorders, cancer, and bone and joint disorders have been found to occur with increased frequency in obese individuals. Thus, it is not surprising that studies done for insurance companies consistently show that a person's mortality rate increases as his or her weight increases above the norm (Hafen, 1975).

The psychosocial consequences and medical problems associated with obesity insure that a large percentage of overweight individuals will attempt to look for some way to overcome their affliction. Most of these individuals have already tried various self-help approaches without long-term success. Thus they tend to be very susceptible to commercially packaged treatments that promise a quick and easy solution for their problem. In the past several years there has been a proliferation of "hypnosis clinics" which are aimed at attracting this clientele. These clinics typically claim high rates of success and make their treatment appear easy and appealing. Thus one purpose of this paper is to realistically assess the research evidence regarding the effectiveness of hypnosis in treating obesity. This will allow professionals who are considering the use of hypnosis in treating their overweight clients to be aware of the strengths and limitations of this procedure. In addition it will provide the public with information they can use to make an informed choice about what type of treatment would be best for them.

The second and primary purpose is to familiarize the practicing clinician with some of the specific hypnotic procedures which appear to have utility in the treatment of overweight individuals. This chapter extrapolates information from the various clinical reports, case studies, and research studies reported in the literature in an attempt to come up with a list of the most effective procedures in the treatment of obesity.

CLINICAL TREATMENT REPORTS

Some of the most respected names in the field have used hypnosis to treat obese clients (Kroger, 1970; Erickson, 1960; Spiegel & Debetz, 1978). Several of these, as well as other clinicians, have provided detailed descriptions of how they employ hypnosis in the treatment of obesity in their respective clinical practices.

Kroger (1970) describes a comprehensive treatment program which he employs in treating obesity. He recommends that his patients follow a well-balanced, high protein and potassium, low-carbohydrate, low-fat, and low-sodium diet of between 1000 to 1350 calories. He also advises that they take 0.5 to 1 gram of enteric KCL after meals and drink at least two quarts of water each day. With some refractory obese patients he prescribes two to three gram doses of desiccated thyroid. However, the bulk of his program involves the utilization of a variety of hynotic techniques. Early in treatment the patients, while under hypnosis, are taught how to develop satiation or aversion to certain foods in response to revolting thoughts or feelings. The patient is also shown how to produce "glove anesthesia" and told to transfer this numbness to his stomach whenever he suffers hunger pangs. In addition a variety of techniques, first introduced by Erickson (1954), are employed by offering the appropriate posthynotic suggestions. *Symptom Substitution* allows the patient to "trade down" eating high calorie foods for other eating behaviors such as chewing gum. *Symptom Transformation* allows the patient to trade the symptom of overeating for more appropriate behaviors such as exercising or shopping. *Symptom Amelioration* involves reducing overeating behavior by initially having the patient deliberately increase food consumption. This operates under the supposition that this helps the patient to see that eating is under his or her control. *Symptom Utilization* consists of encouraging activity which interferes with faulty eating patterns. Other techniques used include visualization of oneself as thin, setting a deadline for weight loss, and suggestions for eating slowly, focusing on, and enjoying each morsel of food eaten. Kroger recommends treating obese individuals in a group rather than individually.

Herbert Spiegel (Spiegel & Spiegel 1978; Spiegel & Debetz, 1978) describes his approach to treating obese patients. His treatment is generally limited to one or two sessions, although he indicates that grossly obese individuals may require periodic reinforcement sessions. He begins the treatment by presenting several basic principles, which he feels his patients must understand if they are to lose weight. The patients are then taught self-hypnosis and asked to concentrate on three "critical" points:

1. For your body overeating is, in effect, poison.
2. You cannot live without your body.
3. To the extent that you want to live your life to the fullest you owe your body this commitment to respect it and protect it.

The patients are then informed that they should practice this simple self-hypnosis exercise every 1 to 2 hours. After the patients are taught the above exercise the difference between "thin-eating" and "fat-eating" are explained to them. Included in this are instructions to begin eating like a gourmet. In other words, they are told to begin paying close attention to each and every swallow they take and to make each swallow a "total encounter" with food. In this way the fulfillment and enjoyment of each morsel of food is greatly enhanced eliminating the need to overeat in order to get satisfaction.

Erickson (1960) reports three case studies in which widely disparate, individual hypnotic approaches were used in treating three obese women. In case 1, time distortion was used to expand and lengthen the patient's perception of time so that after she ate for a short period of time she would feel satisfied and satiated as if she had been eating for hours. Case 2 involved a patient who had a history of successful weight loss followed by immediate weight gain. Under hypnosis she was told that she would be allowed to lose weight only after she had gained between 15 and 25 pounds. Thus her previous "lose-then-gain" cycle was replaced by a much more adaptive "gain-then-lose" cycle. Finally, in Case 3 an overweight woman who weighed 270 pounds was told to overeat enough to support 260 pounds. When she reached this goal she was told to overeat enough to support 255 pounds, and so on until she weighed 190 pounds after six months. It is clear that Erickson emphasizes the need to individualize treatment in order to meet the needs of the particular person being treated. While there certainly is some truth to this argument, it is felt that, at this point in time, an emphasis should be placed on developing standardized procedures which can be replicated by other researchers in this area. This will be discussed in more detail in the next section.

REVIEW OF THE LITERATURE

Two comprehensive reviews of the hypnosis and obesity literature have been published in the past six years (Mott & Roberts, 1979, Simon & Salzberg, 1982). Mott and Roberts state that the published studies in this area consist of anecdotal reports and uncontrolled studies of selected cases. They point out that the literature is very difficult to interpret for many reasons. For example, there was no standardization of induction techniques or suggestions across studies and consequently there was little evidence of attempts to replicate findings. Follow-up evaluations of outcome were generally lacking and in most cases no attempt was made to determine which aspects of a particular treatment program were most important. In addition, no attempt was made to measure hypnotizability objectively and relate this to treatment success. In conclusion, Mott and Roberts point out that the results of the reviewed studies suggest that hypnosis may have a place in weight control programs. However, they stress that the extent of its usefulness and how it can be best used cannot be assessed until controlled research is conducted in this area.

Simon and Salzberg (1982), after referring to the Mott and Roberts review, summarize several controlled studies published since the earlier review. Deyoub (1979a) found hypnosis to be significantly more effective than a no-treatment control group in treating obese females. However, no relationship between suggestibility and weight loss was found. Deyoub (1979b), in an uncontrolled study, also found no relationship between hypnotizability and weight loss. In contrast to the above findings, Deyoub and Wilkie (1980) found hypnosis to be no more effective than task-motivating instructions or no-treatment control, but did find a relationship between suggestibility and weight loss.

Bornstein and Devine (1980) assessed the utility of combining hypnosis with a behavioral approach known as covert modeling in treating obese volunteers. The results indicated that a covert modeling/hypnosis condition was significantly more effective than a no-model control group, but no more effective than covert modeling alone or a minimum treatment group. Wadden and Flaxman (1981) compared the effectiveness of hypnosis, covert modeling, and a relaxation-attention control. All three treatments resulted in statistically significant weight losses, although they did not differ significantly from each other in effectiveness. In addition, a positive relationship between suggestibility and weight loss was not found. Finally, Goldstein (1981) reported that hypnosis with proof (i.e., a suggestion for hand levitation to "prove" that the induction was successful) was more effective than both behavior modification and hypnosis without "proof" in treating obese females.

A review of the recent literature (since Simon & Salzberg, 1982) appears to indicate that no additional controlled studies have been done. However, the above studies signify a dramatic improvement in the quality of research which will hopefully continue. These studies have begun to correct some of the earlier methodological flaws outlined by Mott and Roberts (1979). For example, several of the more recent studies have attempted to assess the relationship between hypnotizability and weight loss. Preliminary data suggest that hypnotizability is not an important variable in treatment success although more research is needed. Several authors have presented their induction techniques and specific suggestions in sufficient detail to allow replication by future researchers (Deyoub, 1979a; Goldstein, 1981; Wadden & Flaxman, 1981). In addition one author (Deyoub, 1978; 1979a; 1979b; Deyoub & Wilkie, 1980) has done a series of studies in which attempts at replication were made. Finally, several authors (Deyoub, 1979a; Devine & Bornstein, 1980; Wadden & Flaxman, 1981) have incorporated more sophisticated measures of weight loss (change in percentage overweight, weight reduction quotient, etc.) rather than simply presenting data in terms of absolute weight loss. These measures allow the results of different studies to be compared in a meaningful fashion even though the subjects may vary greatly with regard to their degree of obesity.

Despite these improvements there are still methodological problems which need to be addressed. The most serious is the continued reluctance of researchers to provide long-term follow-up data (i.e., 6 months to 1 year). This is of central importance because a failure to maintain weight loss is the most critical shortcoming of most weight management programs. A related problem is the tendency of researchers to focus on the statistical significance of their findings, while disregarding the question of whether the treatment was clinically significant. In other words, as discussed by Simon and Salzberg (1982), a five pound weight loss in a treatment group which on the average started treatment at 50 pounds overweight may be statistically significant, but clearly has little clinical significance. A final problem, which was discussed by Mott and Roberts (1979), is the fact that many authors have tended to include subjects who vary greatly in their degree of obesity in the same study. Evidence suggests that extremely obese patients manifest considerably more psychopathology than mildly obese individuals, and thus the hypnotic procedures applicable to these two groups may be very different.

It should be pointed out that the fact that much of the research in this area has serious methodological problems in no way suggests that hypnosis is not effective in treating obesity. It should simply serve as a warning to the practitioner that the positive results presented by most authors cannot always be taken at face value. The preliminary data suggests that hypnosis has a place in the treatment of obesity. However if hypnosis is to gain wider acceptance in the scientific community it is essential that the quality of the research improve.

RECOMMENDATIONS FOR THE CLINICAL PRACTITIONER

Simon and Salzberg (1982) recommend the use of a systematic dismantling strategy (Lang, 1969) to assess the effectiveness of the various components of the hypnotic treatment approaches employed in treating addictive behaviors including obesity. Unfortunately the research in this area has not yet reached this level of sophistication and thus it is difficult to assess exactly which hypnotic techniques are most useful in treating obese patients. Despite this the present article offers an attempt to outline some of the specific techniques and procedures which appear to have the greatest utility. The decision to include a particular technique was based both on intuitive judgment and the apparent effectiveness of the procedure in the studies in which it was employed.

Before determining what specific techniques should be incorporated in treatment, the clinician must first make a decision with regard to the format in which treatment will be offered (i.e., individual vs. group). Slightly less than half of the studies reviewed by Simon and Salzberg (1982) employed a group approach to treatment. Although the results of the studies are difficult to assess because of the methodological problems discussed above, individual treatment did not appear to be significantly more effective than group treatment. This in itself would suggest the preferability of a group approach because of its obviously greater cost effectiveness. In other words, the group format allows the clinician to offer treatment to a far greater number of patients than would be possible if treatment was offered on an individual basis, with little or no adverse effect on treatment results. In addition there are several factors which suggest that the group approach may be preferable to individual treatment from a purely clinical standpoint. The group provides social support, encouragement, and reinforcement to individuals who have more typically encountered social ostracism and/or ridicule because of their weight problem. They are likely to develop a sense of comaraderie and belongingness with other individuals who have encountered similar problems. Thus the group becomes a forum where they can discuss their common difficulties in attempting to lose weight in the past. In addition, it becomes a social event which, unlike most in our society, does not center around eating. Along the same line, with regard to future maintenance, the group provides individuals the opportunity to develop friendships whose future socializing can focus on things other than food and eating.

Before discussing some of the hypnotic techniques that appear to be most useful in treating obesity, it may be helpful to identify two well-known procedures that do not appear very effective. The first is the use of *direct suggestions* for change. Few contempory researchers appear to put much credence in the use of this technique. In other words, simply giving hypnotized subjects the suggestion that they will lose weight or eat less is not likely to result in weight reduction.

Another well recognized procedure that does not appear to have much utility in treating obesity is hypnoaversion. This refers to the use of hypnosis to create a conditioned aversion to a particular substance. While the effectiveness of this type of procedure in treating any type of addictive behavior is questionable (Simon & Salzberg, 1982) it seems particulary ill-suited for treating overweight individuals. Whereas with smoking, drug abuse, or alcholism, treatment can be aimed at extinguishing the behavior completely, this is not the case with obesity since eating cannot be eliminated if the patient is to survive. Thus instead the treatment is aimed at eliminating certain "problem foods." However, it appears that most cases of obesity are not due simply to an in ability to avoid certain high caloric foods. In fact, studies have shown that reducing the desirability of certain target foods does not necessarily result in a corresponding loss of weight (Elliot & Denny, 1975). It could be argued that the adjunctive use of this approach in a more comprehensive weight loss program may be of some benefit. However, it is felt that the negative aspects of using an aversive approach outweight any benefits it might produce. It is obviously not a pleasant experience to imagine oneself vomiting or becoming nauseous in the presence of desirable foods. Thus the use of this approach with some patients will likely lead to a deterioration of the therapeutic relationship, if not outright termination of therapy.

One important component in the majority of treatment studies reported in the literature is the use of "ego-enhancing suggestions." These are typically aimed at increasing the patient's sense of self-worth and their belief in their own ability to overcome their weight problem. Patients are helped to develop a sense of pride in their own bodies and shown how overeating is a threat to their very existence. This technique seems expecially well suited for overweight patients since they are frequently lacking in self-esteem and often feel rather hopeless because of their past failures in achieving and/or maintaining weight loss.

One specific technique which is used by a majority of authors who report their results in the literature and which seems to have a great deal of utility is the use of hypnotic suggestions to alter the patient's perceptions with regard to eating. In other words, suggestions are aimed at altering the way these individuals typically respond to food or food ingestion. According to Brodie (1964), patients are taught to eat like "gourmets." For example, they are given suggestions that they will be more aware of what they are eating than they have ever been before. They are told to focus on the taste, texture, and consistency of the food they eat and to slowly savor each bite they take. They are typically informed that their appetite will be satisfied by the quality of their eating experience rather than the quantity that they eat. The effectiveness of this procedure is enhanced by the fact that the incorporation of these suggestions will result in a change in eating habits, something typically seen as a necessary component of almost all weight loss programs. In other words, patients who are taught to savor each bite will necessarily eat in a slower more appropriate fashion. This type of procedure will hopefully be self-reinforcing since it should increase the pleasure and enjoyment of the eating experience. Another example of altering perceptions, reported in the literature, simply involves suggesting to patients that they will find themselves feeling full and satisfied after eating a small portion of food. This suggestion can certainly be used in conjunction with the above procedure.

A helpful component of many programs involves having hypnotized patients visualize themselves at their ideal weight. They are typically told to picture themselves looking "slim and trim," wearing the type of clothes they would like to wear, and/or engaging in an enjoyable activity which they find difficult or impossible at their present weight. Suggestions are given that this imagery will come to mind several times a day, particularly when they are about to eat a meal. Maltz (1967) has discussed the importance of "target imagery" in treating various problem behaviors. According to Maltz, when a patient imagines a desired end product, the subconscious mind will direct the individual's behavior so that the target will be achieved without any conscious effort on the part of the patient. Stanton (1975) supports Maltz's formulation in discussing his own use of the imagery technique with obese patients stating that most of his patients report surprise at the ease and lack of effort involved in their weight loss.

One aspect of treatment that is agreed on by many of the researchers in the field is that self-hypnosis should be a integral part of treatment. It seems rather clear that it will be difficult to attain a significant change in behavior if the patient's treatment is limited to the typical 50 minute weekly session. Teaching the patient self-hypnosis early in treatment enables the patient to practice several times a day the specific procedures he has undergone in the office. Not only does this reinforce what has occured in the session, but it also gives patients the sense that they are actively involved in their own treatment rather than just passive participants. In this way it may help ease the strong sense of dependency often exhibited by obese patients. Clinicians vary with regard to how often patients should engage in self-hypnosis outside of the session. However, most seem to agree that the amount of time actually spent in autohypnosis need not be long and should generally be in the area of five to fifteen minutes. Thus it does not seem unreasonable to expect patients to practice at least twice a day. With some patients who are in need of structure it may be advisable to set aside specific times for autohypnosis such as in the morning and at bedtime or before meals.

Only a handful of authors (Deyoub & Wilkie 1980; Dyoub 1979; Brodie,

1964) have incorporated exercise or increased physical activity into their hypnotic treatment programs. Although it is well documented that exercise alone will not result in a significant loss of weight, it is felt that it can be a useful adjunct to treatment. Brownell (1982) discusses five reasons why exercise is important for weight reduction: it may 1) increase energy expenditure, 2) counteract the ill effects of obesity, 3) suppress appetite, 4) decrease basal metabolism, and 5) minimize the loss of lean tissue. In addition, by incorporating suggestions for increased exercise the clinician can begin the process of changing the obese individual's lifestyle so that it is more conducive to maintaining an ideal weight. If the individual already has a favorite sport or activity which involves muscular activity, suggestions are given that encourage him or her to engage in it more regularly. If not, the clinician and patient should come up with a suitable activity or exercise program together.

The procedures outlined above represent a summary of the techniques used by various authors which seem to have a reasonable amount of utility in the treatment of obese patients. The procedures which have been outlined should serve only as a guide to the clinician and should not be considered as etched in stone. The particular procedures employed by individual clinicians will depend on their own particular orientations and what is most comfortable for them. Also additional research is still needed to help determine which procedures are most useful. In addition to the above procedures some clinicians may feel more comfortable including more structure in their treatments such as having patients monitor their caloric intake. Although this would seemingly be of great benefit to many obese clients, a majority of the authors who report their findings in the area do not seem to feel this necessary for treatment success.

SUMMARY

This chapter provides an overview of the use of hypnosis in weight management. First the specific treatment programs of three of the most respected individuals in the field were outlined. Next an overview of the research literature in the area was provided. This suggested that the quality of the research in this area has improved in the last few years, but that more good research is still needed before definitive conclusions can be drawn. Finally, some of the most widely used and apparently effective hypnosis procedures were outlined and discussed.

REFERENCES

Bornstein, P. H., & Devine, D. A. (1980). Covert modeling hypnosis in the treatment of obesity. *Psychotherapy: Theory, research and practice, 17,* 272–276.

Bray, G. A. (1976). *The obese patient.* Philadelphia, PA: Saunders.

Brodie, E. I. (1964). A hypnotherapeutic approach to obesity. *American Journal of Clinical Hypnosis, 6,* 211-215.

Brownell, K. D. (1982). Obesity: Understanding and treating a serious, prevalent, and refractory disorder. *Journal of Consulting and Clinical Psychology, 50,* 820–840.

Cappon, D. (1973). *Eating, loving, and dying: A psychology of appetites.* Toronto: University of Toronto Press.

Deyoub, P. L. (1978). Relation of suggestibility to obesity. *Psychological Reports, 43,* 175–180.

Deyoub, P. L. (1979). Hypnosis in the treatment of obesity and the relation of suggestibility to outcome. *Journal of the American Society of Psychosomatic Dentistry and Medicine, 26,* 137–149. (a)

Deyoub, P. L. (1979). Hypnotizability and obestity. *Psychological Reports, 45,* 974. (b)

Deyoub, P. L., & Wilkie, R. (1980). Suggestion with and without hypnotic induction in a weight reduction program. *The International Journal of Clinical and Experimental Hypnosis, 28,* 333–340.

Elliot, C. H. & Denny, D. R. (1975). Weight control through covert sensitization and false feedback. *Journal of Consulting and Clinical Psychology, 43,* 841–850.

Erickson, M. H. (1954). Special techniques of brief hypnotherapy. *Journal of Clinical and Experimental Hypnosis, 2,* 109–129.

Erickson, M. H. (1960). The utilization of patient behavior in the hypnotherapy of obesity: Three case reports. *American Journal of Clinical Hypnosis, 3,* 112–116.

Forbes, G. B. (1975). Prevalence of obesity in childhood. In G. A. Bray (Ed.), *Obesity in perspective (Vol. 2).* (DHEW Publication No. (NIH) 75-708). Washington, D. C.: U. S. Government Printing Office.

Goldstein, Y. (1981). The effect of demonstrating to a subject that she is in a hypnotic trance as a variable in hypnotic interventions with obese women. *International Journal of Clinical and Experimental Hypnosis, 29,* 15–23.

Hafen, B. Q. (1975). *Overweight and obesity: Causes, fallacies, treatment.* Provo, UT: Brigham Young University Press.

Kroger, W. (1970). Comprehensive managment of obesity. *American Journal of Clinical Hypnosis, 12,* 165–170.

Lang, P. J. (1969). The mechanics of desensitization and the laboratory study of fear. In C. M. Franks (Ed.), *Behavior therapy: Appraisal and status.* New York: McGraw-Hill.

Maltz, M. (1967). *Psycho-Cybernetics.* New York: Essandess.

Mott, T., & Roberts, J. (1979). Obesity and hypnosis: A review of the literature. *American Journal of Clinical Hypnosis, 22,* 3–7.

Simon, M. J., & Salzberg, H. C. (1982). Hypnosis and related behavioral approaches in the treatment of addictive behaviors. In M. Hersen, R. M. Eisler, & P. M. Miller (Eds.), *Progress in behavior modification (Vol. 13),* New York: Academic Press.

Spiegel, H., & Debetz, B. (1978). Restructuring eating behavior with self-hypnosis, *International Journal of Obesity,* 287–288.

Spiegel, H., & Spiegel, D. (1978). *Trance and treatment: Clinical use of hypnosis.* New York: Basic Books.

Stanton, H. E. (1975). Weight loss through hypnosis. *American Journal of Clinical Hypnosis, 18,* 94–97.

Van Itallie, T. B. (1977). *Testimony before Senate Select Committee on Nutrition and Human Needs.* Washington, D. C.: U. S. Government Printing Office.

Wadden, T. A. & Flaxman, J. (1981). Hypnosis and weight loss: A preliminary study. *International Journal of Clinical and Experimental Hypnosis, 29,* 162–173.

Chapter 6

Hypnosis in the Treatment of Phobias

Gerald F. McKeegan
Nova University

Fear is an innate emotional response which has obvious adaptive and survival value to the human species. With fear, an individual experiences feelings of discomfort, agitation, and an anticipation of possible painful or aversive consequences. As a result, the "fearing" individual attempts to avoid the situation or object which is generating this emotional response in order to escape from possible aversive outcomes. Without such an emotional signal of potential danger, it is debatable whether the human species could have survived. One can imagine that without fear, our simian forefathers would have probably been rather tasty morsels to many of the larger carnivores in the environment.

There are instances, however, in which the fear response is either disproportionate to the situation or socially disturbing to either the individual or others in the environment. It is at these times that society has placed the label of "phobia" on such a reaction (Ullman & Krasner, 1975). A phobia has been defined as

> a clinical condition in which the patient suffers from and complains about one or more intense fears that are in lesser or greater degree interfering with at least some aspect of the patient's life. (Mavissakalian and Barlow, 1981, p. 1)

In an attempt at a rather concise description of a phobia, the American Psychiatric Association (1981) has recently stated that a phobia is a

> persistent and irrational fear of a specified object, activity, or situation that results in a compelling desire to avoid the dreaded object, activity, or situation . . . The fear is recognized by the individual as excessive in proportion to the actual dangerousness of the object, activity, or situation. (p. 225)

In summary, for a fear reaction to be classified as a phobia it must have three essential conditions: (1) a severe reaction involving physiological changes usually associated with anxiety to a stimulus society deems as relatively nonthreatening, (2) the individual's awareness of the "irrational and absurdity" of the reaction, and (3) in order to reduce the frequency of the reaction, avoidance of the feared stimulus by the individual which usually results in some impairment in that person's normal functioning; this avoidance may be so extensive as to even include one's "thinking" about the stimulus. Resultantly, a phobia involves all response systems of an individual: autonomic, cognitive-linguistic, and motoric.

The phobias have been differentiated in various ways using different criteria. The American Psychiatric Association (1981) in its third edition of the *Diagnostic and Statistical Manual (DSM-III)* has subdivided the phobic disorders into three types: (1) agoraphobia, which is a pervasive fear reaction to various situations outside the person's home, (2) social phobia, which is an avoidance of being scrutinized in public places, and (3) simple phobia, which includes all non-social well-circumscribed fears.

Mavissakalian and Barlow (1981) have divided the phobias according to their major themes. The types of phobias were: (1) monosymptomatic, which included phobias to simple objects and situations usually deemed as nondangerous, (2) somatic-oriented phobias related to blood, illness, or bodily injury, (3) social-oriented phobias which involved interpersonal situations, and (4) agoraphobia.

Despite these general classifications, there are about as many phobias as there are stimuli in the environment. To list all the phobias encountered in clinical casework would be a mind-boggling enterprise; Scott (1970) has stated that there are 275 phobias listed by name in medical dictionaries but even this number does not substantially cover all of them. No matter what type of phobia an individual has, there are two elements in common: anxiety and avoidance. It is usually these two elements upon which all therapies focus.

Historically, the term phobia comes from the name of the Greek god "Phobos" who instilled fear, terror, and panic into one's enemies. The word phobia was first used to describe an irrational fear by the first century Roman encyclopedist, Celsus, who described a fear of water (hydrophobia) as part of the symptomatology of rabies (Marks, 1969). Beginning with Hippocrates, phobias have been described throughout the centuries. Not only does it seem that phobias have existed since the emergence of humankind but that it effected individuals in all strata of society. It has been reported that Henry III of France had a cat phobia while James I of England had panic attacks at the sight of an unsheathed sword (Marks, 1969).

The first comprehensive study of phobias was done by Robert Burton in 1621 in the classic *Anatomy of Melancholia* (Marks, 1969). Several other studies of the phenomena followed in other countries.

It was not until 1801, however, that the term phobia was used to describe the clinical syndrome. The term syphilophobia was coined in 1848 by Dunglison in describing the morbid fear of contacting the disease of syphilis. The use of the word phobia increased with dramatic frequency after the publication of a clinical description of agoraphobia in 1871. Phobias then became the realm of psychiatric study and became a clinical entity as it is known today at the turn of the century (Marks, 1969).

With the recognition of phobias as a psychological phenomenon in the early 1900's, the psychoanalytic school was the first to attempt to study it. Through the writings of Freud and his associates, phobias were viewed as an outward symptom of an underlying unconscious conflict. Through the defense mechanisms of repression and displacement, the phobic individual

> keeps the original, more threatening source of anxiety from awareness but becomes doubly shielded against such awareness by attributing this anxiety to a more manageable cause or situation. (Mavissakalian & Barlow, 1981, p. 12)

As a result, the major means of treatment was through years of psychoanalysis. As the use of hypnosis had fallen into disfavor with Freud and his associates at this time, it can be said that if it was used in the treatment of phobias by a "wayward disciple" it was not reported. Such uses of hypnosis would be seen as merely a means of relieving the individual from the symptom without resolving the "real unconscious conflict" which was the primary cause of the phobia; without resolution, this conflict would lead to other symptom developments.

Hypnosis as a technique to be utilized in therapy did not disappear with its falling into disfavor among the "hard line" Freudian psychoanalysts. As psychoanalysis became popular, it began to be modified by a number of its adherents. As a result, hypnosis was incorporated into the new "psychoanalytic psychotherapy." Hypnotic phenomena such as age regression and revivification of traumatic events through imagery were utilized to assist in uncovering, corrective emotional experiences (abreaction), and the enhancement of archaic involvement (transference). Presently, the advocates of hypnosis in psychoanalytically-based therapies support its use as a facilitating and positive influence on treatment outcome (Frankel, 1981; Mott, 1982). The support for using "hypnoanalysis" in treating phobic disorders has been presented in the literature by case reports. In fact, it has been hypothesized that the unconscious and conscious functionings needed for a good hypnotic subject may be identical to the type of processes which are common to those individuals who display phobic behaviors (Frankel, 1974, 1981; Frankel & Orne, 1976).

With the application of learning and reinforcement principles to clinical problems in the 1920's, phobias were defined according to a conditioning model. In the 1930's, Mowrer (cited in Mavissakalian et al., 1981) postulated a two-factor theory of phobic disorders in which (1) the physiological "emotional" reaction has been acquired through classical conditioning and, through the process of generalization, the control of the original eliciting stimulus has disseminated to other stimuli of similar characteristics; and (2) the avoidance of various phobic stimuli has been maintained through the reduction of the arousal of the "fear" response (negative reinforcement).

The treatment of phobias under a behavioral model sought to control or "recondition" the "fear" response and attendent avoidant behaviors. In 1958, Wolpe's *Psychotherapy by Reciprocal Inhibition* provided one of the most effective means of alleviating phobias. The procedure was named "systematic desensitization." The treatment involved the graduated presentation of anxiety-provoking images while the client was deeply relaxed; the client was trained in deep muscle relaxation and requested to imagine the scenes of the "fear hierarchy" as presented by the clinician. In this way, the relaxed state of the client was incompatible with the anxiety produced by the "fear" response. Through a process of extinction and reconditioning the client was able to overcome a phobia.

Hypnosis found better reception in the behavioral treatment of phobias than it did in the psychoanalytic school. Wolpe (1958, 1973, 1976) has made numerous references to the use of hypnosis in systematic desensitization. Wolpe has postulated that hypnosis enhances relaxation and imagery through hypnotic suggestion and that it is particularly effective in rather difficult cases. He has mentioned a case (1973) in which a business executive was relieved of aerophobia of 10 years duration in a single session through the use of direct suggestion. Wolpe related this "cure" to the counter-conditioning of the anxiety response by the suggestions of pleasant sensations while flying. Dengrove (1973), Kroger and Felzer (1976), and Lazarus (1973) also supported the use of hypnosis as a facilitator of the techniques used in behavioral therapies. There is, however, some confusion as to exactly what are the enhancing effects of behavioral therapy when hypnosis is employed. This question will be discussed in a later section of this paper.

In summary, hypnosis has been and is being employed in both psychoanalytic and behavioral treatments for the alleviation of phobias. The following two sections will review the data—both clinical and experimental—which support or do not support the application of hypnosis in the treatment of phobias. Subsequent sections will attempt to identify those factors in the hypnotic phenomenon which may contribute to the treatment of phobias. Finally, methodological recommendations and considerations for future research in the area of hypnosis and phobias will be addressed.

REVIEW OF THE EVIDENCE: CLINICAL

The use of hypnosis in effectively alleviating phobic disorders has been well documented through single case reports. A total of 34 cases have been reviewed in the literature since 1970. These cases are summarized in Table 6.1; the information included author, year reported in the literature, age and sex of the client (if reported), type of phobia treated, and the theoretical rationales behind the effectiveness of hypnosis in that specific case.

As can be seen from Table 6.1, hypnosis has been employed with clients ranging in age from 4½ (Lawlor, 1976) to 68 years (Seif, 1982). The phobias have included rather common ones such as aerophobia (Deyoub & Epstein, 1977; Miller, 1979; Schneck, 1975; Speigel, Frischolz, Maruffi, & Speigel, 1981) to idiosyncratic fears such as the phobia to the mating calls of cows and bulls (Cohen, 1981) and substances such as mayonnaise (Van Dyke & Harris, 1982).

One type of phobia which has not received a great deal of attention in the hypnosis literature over the past decade has been agoraphobia, perhaps the most debilitating and hardest to treat of all the phobias. Gruenewald (1971) has reported that there has been little confirmation of success in the treatment of this disorder with hypnosis. She goes on to report the moderate reduction in agoraphobia in a 58-year-old woman using modified hypnotic suggestions. With a 43-year history of the phobia, the client was not able to undergo systematic desensitization due to an inability to hold an imaginary scene. Instead, the author instructed the client to "free associate" after having undergone a hypnotic induction which consisted of several minutes of progressive relaxation suggestions interspersed with suggestions of strength and tranquility, all verbalized in a warm, supportive manner. In this manner, the client was allowed to undergo emotional reactions to disturbing, freely occurring thoughts while in a relaxed state. The author accounted for the partial success of the treatment by this modified "cathartic" procedure and the relaxation produced by hypnosis. In this way, the client was partly able to control her panic attacks and engage in more behaviors which were previously avoided.

Several authors of the psychodynamic orientation have reported the use of age regression in hypnosis as an aid in uncovering long repressed fears and conflicts (Epstein & Deyoub, 1981; Gustavson & Weight, 1981; Lawlor, 1976; Miller, 1979; Scott, 1970; Van Dyke & Harris, 1982). Scott (1981) has reported on the effective use of such a procedure in the treatment of a long standing phobia of "flying things" by a 27-year-old female. In what the author has labeled as "psychic desensitization," the patient was regressed back to a younger age in order to uncover the original trauma which has produced the phobia. While in the generally relaxed state of the hypnotic trance, the client was given suggestions to relive or revivify in imagination the causal fear; the

Table 6.1 Clinical Cases Treated With Hypnosis

Author (Year)	Age/Sex	Type of Phobia	Technique and Rationale
Baker & Boaz (1983)	30/female	Dental work	Age regression, abreaction, counterconditioning through positive imagery
Cohen (1981)	64/male	Bovine sounds	Relaxation and shaping behavior through suggestions
Daniels (1975)	4th year graduate student	Performance reprimands	Relaxation during in vivo desensitization
Danels (1976)	24/female	Needles, injections	Relaxation and counterconditioning through imagery
Dieker & Pollack (1975)	49/female	Chlorine bleach (agoraphobia)	Relaxation and counterconditioning through imagery in conjunction with systematic desensitization
Deyoub & Epstein (1977)	30/female	Aerophobia	Relaxation and suggestion
Epstein & Deyoub (1981)	47/male	Swallowing	Uncovering, relaxation, and suggestion of symptom remission
Frutiger (1981)	26/female	Intercourse	Suggestions used in conjunction with systematic desnsitization
Golan (1971)	29/female 29/female	Dental work Dental work	Relaxation and suggestion
Golan (1975)	22/female	Dental work	Suggestion
Gruenewald (1971)	58/female	Agoraphobia	Abreaction and relaxation
Gustavson & Weight (1981)	21/female	Slugs	Age regression and uncovering of real fear
Lawlor (1976)	5/male 4½/female 6/female	School phobia School phobia School phobia	Age regression and uncovering of real fear
Miller (1979)	39/female 21/female 30/female Graduate student/ male	Aerophobia Being assaulted Aerophobia Hydrophobia	Flooding; relaxation and extinction through imagery
O'Donnel (1978)	29/female	Contracting cancer	Implosion; relaxation and extinction through imagery
Ritow (1979)	21/female	Vomiting	Paradoxical statements
Schneck (1975)	45/female	Aerophobia	Relaxation and counterconditioning through suggestions
Scott (1970)	27/female	Birds & insects	Age regression, abreaction, and relaxation
Scrignor (1981)	23/male 47/female	Contamination Contamination	Flooding; relaxation and extinction through imagery and suggestions

Table 6.1 (continued) Clinical Cases Treated With Hypnosis

Author (Year)	Age/Sex	Type of Phobia	Technique and Rationale
Seif (1982)	68/male	Urinating in public facilities	Relaxation and shaping of behavior through imagery
Surman (1979)	47/male 57/female	Sleeping, death Agoraphobia	Relaxation and counterconditioning through imagery
Van der Hart (1981)	24/female	Dead birds	Systematic desensitization, relaxation, and counterconditioning through imagery
Van Dyke & Harris (1981)	36/male	Mayonnaise	Age regression and corrective emotional experience
Wijensighe (1974)	24/female	Vomiting	Flooding; relaxation and extinction through imagery
Yamauchi	51/male (schizophrenic)	Dental work	Relaxation and modified systematic desensitization procedure

client underwent a cathartic experience in which she abreacted to the repressed fear and thus was able to resolve it. The client was able to "successfully" overcome her phobia after five months of treatment! Although slightly different in terminology, the procedure used by Scott seems hauntingly similar to the flooding technique of the behaviorists after a careful and thorough analysis was done in order to confirm what was the genuine fear(s) to be treated.

The behavioral school has employed hypnosis in the treatment of phobias in a variety of ways: (1) facilitation of relaxation, (2) increased visual imagery, and (3) providing techniques which aid in the management of the difficult client (Dengrove, 1973). The case studies have presented hypnosis being used as an adjunct to systematic desensitization (Cohen, 1981; Daniels, 1975, 1976; Dieker & Pollack, 1981; Frutiger, 1981; Van der Hart, 1981; Yamauchi, 1981), flooding (Scrignor, 1981; Wyensighe, 1974), and implosion (O'Donnell, 1978).

Dieker and Pollack (1975) reported on the case of a 49-year-old woman with the unusual fear of chlorine bleach. Such a fear severely limited her sojourns from the house since the sight or smell of bleach would cause a panic attack. Hypnosis was used to increase the muscle relaxation and imaging of the items in the fear hierarchy during the desensitization process. Using three outcome measures of compulsive hand washings, anxiety attacks, and approach to a bottle a bleach, the authors stated that the first two measures decreased significantly while the third increased during treatment. Although successful, the authors concluded that "while no new problems or fears developed, she (the client) reported that she remained anxious when using bleach" (p. 173). Dieker and Pollack postulated that perhaps the systematic desensitization techniques used only eliminated the avoidant operant while leaving the classically conditioned fear response intact.

Van der Hart (1981) reported on the use of hypnosis alone with no instructions from the clinicians to the client as to deep muscle relaxation or hierarchy construction. The suggestion was given to the client for her to construct her own "personal" hierarchy and progress through it as in the regular procedure. In such a way, a 24-year-old female client reduced her phobia of dead birds.

Flooding has been described as the prolonged, high-intensity exposure to the phobic stimuli through imagination or in reality (Lazarus & Wilson, 1976). In combining hypnosis with flooding, Astrip (1974) has stated that

> Flooding in hypnosis seems to involve complex mechanisms of which desensitization of psychological and physiological structures in the Pavlovian sense may be the most important. (p. 704)

He went on to say that hypnosis could be used with the flooding technique in the same way as in systematic desensitization.

Following on this advice, several authors treated phobias with flooding and hypnosis. Scrignor (1981) used both in the modification of two cases of fear of contamination. Employing a hypnotic induction as a means of facilitating relaxation and the acquisition by the client of positive suggestion and corrective information, the author presented scenes in which the client was covered with mucus from other people's noses and lungs. In both cases the incident of self-reported anxiety decreased.

Building upon the augmentation of imagery, suggestibility, and relaxation during hypnosis, several authors have used this characteristic in restructuring cognitions through covert techniques. Covert conditioning is a term used to describe the conditioning procedure "in which the stimuli and responses are presented in imagination" (Cautela, 1975, p. 15). Several authors have used covert conditioning procedures alone (Deyoub & Epstein, 1977; Epstein & Deyoub, 1981; Golan, 1971, 1975; Schneck, 1975; Speigel et al., 1981) or in conjunction with other behavioral techniques previously mentioned (Daniels, 1975; Dieker & Pollack, 1975; Surman, 1979).

One technique which has been used was covert reinforcement. Daniels (1975) treated a female fourth-year graduate student in medical school with a fear of performing in front of others. While hypnotized, the client was instructed to imagine herself presenting in front of her professors and colleagues. As soon as she became anxious, she was to switch to a scene from her own hierarchy of reinforcement. By such repeated pairings, she was able to gradually overcome her fear and successfully perform in the avoided situations.

Dengrove (1973) has explained a useful technique of hypnotic time distortion which could be employed in behavioral therapies. Dengrove has stated that in time distortion:

> One can project a patient into the future and have him live through an anxious situation as if it were happening in the present, but in a relaxed

> manner. On awakening, he can be left with the feeling that he has been through all of this before and has progressed adequately. (p. 15)

This method is similar to Erickson's (1980) "pseudo-orientation in time" which has been employed by some authors in their case reports. By projecting the client into the future in which he or she could imagine the completion of a desired goal, Erickson stated

> The patient was enabled to achieve a detached, dissociated, objective, and yet subjective view of what he believed at the moment he had already accomplished, without awareness that those accomplishments were the expression in fantasy of his hopes and desires. (p. 397)

Deyoub and Epstein (1977) reported on the case of a 30-year-old female with aerophobia. Using hypnotic time distortion, the client imagined a successful flight beginning with her preparation, her arrival at the airport, her boarding and listening to the confident tone of the pilot's voice, and finally her landing and disembarkment. Shortly afterwards, the client was successful in such an activity. The authors contended that the use of hypnotic time distortion led to a "unitary" and more effective change in how the individual perceived the situation, rather than the incremental process of relearning which is present in the traditional desensitization techniques.

Dengrove (1973) has mentioned the use of a post-hypnotic suggestion of dreaming the competent completion of the phobic task or behavior. Although no case reports have been found using this technique, a group study comparing this technique with systematic desensitization has been reported (O'Brien, Cooley, Ciotti, & Henninger, 1981) and will be reviewed in a later section of this presentation.

Speigel et al. (1981) reported on 178 cases of aerophobia in which all were given one 45-minute session of hypnosis and "cognitive restructuring suggestions" in which the probability and possibility of plane disasters were explored as well as the catastrophizing effects by our society about such occurrences. Fifty-two percent of the clients reportedly had a decrease in self-reported phobic reactions in a follow-up study six months to 10.5 years after treatment. One must question the enthusiasm of the authors for the effectiveness of the treatment as Agras and his associates (cited in Mavissakalian & Barlow, 1981) have reported a 43 percent natural improvement rate in a five-year follow-up of phobic patients.

Although seemingly effective through case reports and research employing traditional covert conditioning techniques, Cautela (1975) has exclaimed that the use of hypnosis in these procedures have not been empirically supported. His main contention has been that until studies comparing the effectiveness of covert conditioning procedures with and without hypnotic induction have been done, then it is more parsimonious not to employ hypnosis.

REVIEW OF THE EVIDENCE: EXPERIMENTAL

Although the case report literature amply supported the use of hypnosis in the treatment of phobias, the research data has been equivocal at best.

Horowitz (1970) reported that the first experimental study in hypnotherapy and phobias was reported in 1947 by Clyde. In this unpublished masters thesis, phobic participants were asked to recall the earliest traumatic experience in either a relaxed or hypnotized condition. Using a cathartic abreaction explanation from the psychodynamic orientation, all subjects showed a decrease in anxiety as measured by respiration rate.

Since the introduction of systematic desensitization (Wolpe, 1958), only one study has directly compared hypnosis with this effective technique (Marks, Gelder, & Edwards, 1968); several others have studied the effects of hypnosis as an adjunct to relaxation and imagery in systematic desensitization (Lang & Lazovik, 1963; Lang, Lazovik, & Reynolds, 1965; Schubot, 1967).

HYPNOSIS VERSUS SYSTEMATIC DESENSITIZATION

Marks, Gelder, and Edwards (1968) compared the effects of systematic desensitization with those of hypnosis in 28 outpatients with varying types and severities of phobias. The progress of intervention was assessed on (1) ratings on symptomatology by the patient, therapist, and an independent psychiatric assessor; (2) three questionnaires on symptoms, personality change, and social adjustment; and (3) an interview by a psychiatric social worker. If the patient was rated as showing no improvement by two out of three raters after 12 sessions of either systematic desensitization or hypnotic suggestions of relaxation and unspecified fear removal, then these patients were "switched over" for an additional 12 sessions of the alternative intervention after a six-week delay.

Although the results revealed that both treatments significantly improved phobias across all groups, only the patients' ratings significantly judged systematic desensitization as leading to more symptom relief than hypnosis. No other measure reached significance as differentiating the two procedures as to effectiveness.

Despite the positive results of this study in regard to hypnosis, many methodological and conceptual problems existed which may call the results into question. The authors reported that several patients in all groups were receiving medication at the time of the study; the medication, although given as an additional uncontrolled intervention for the phobic symptoms, may have facilitated or inhibited either or both treatments. No mention was made in the study as to the expertise of the therapist nor as to whether the two independent assessors were blind as to the treatment received by each participant. A final criticism could be made that the dependent measures were all self-reports by either the patients, the therapists, or another assessor. No checks as to their reliabilities were made. Furthermore, self-reports are notoriously susceptible to biases of the reporter. An objective measure of a phobia such as a physiological or behavioral approach measure could have been added to assess other parameters of phobic reactions (Agras & Jacob, 1981).

HYPNOSIS WITHIN SYSTEMATIC DESENSITIZATION

Hypnosis has been used as a methodological tool in exploring the different intervention factors which comprise the process of systematic desensitization. Hypnotic induction has been employed to study the effects of relaxation (Lang & Lazovik, 1963; Schubot, 1967) and suggestibility (Lang et al., 1965) in systematic desensitization.

Controlling for susceptibility by administering one of the Stanford Hypnotic Susceptibility Scales (SHSS), Lang and his associates studied the effects of relaxation with that of the desensitization process. The subjects were assessed as to their fear of snakes using two self-report measures—the Fear Survey Schedule and a "fear thermometer"—a behavioral approach task, and an interview and ratings by independent experimenters. Hypnosis was used to increase the degree of relaxation after training and practice in a progressive deep muscle relaxation procedure.

The results revealed that relaxation by itself does not lead to any significant decrease in self-reported or observed fear. The authors concluded that the desensitization process in which the feared stimuli was presented in a graduated fashion while in a relaxed state accounted for significant improvement in the experimental group. Schubot (1967), however, found that with highly anxious participants, hypnosis as an aid in relaxation facilitated a reduction of phobic behavior. In a secondary finding, Schubot found that vividness of imagining the phobic scenes and hypnotic susceptibility were positively and significantly correlated with how quickly an individual could overcome their fear through systematic desensitization.

In further studies by Lang and his colleagues (1965), hypnosis was used as a measure of suggestibility in systematic desensitization. Using the same dependent measures as in the previous study, subjects were balanced for susceptibility in the control and experimental groups by their scores of the SHSS. The results revealed that increased suggestibility did account for some fear reduction but that the change was not significant. The authors concluded

> While a significant part of the control subjects' fear change is attributable to SHSS, no similar relationship between the scale and fear reduction was found for the experimental group. For desensitization subjects the positive effects of treatment were so overriding as to render undetectable any variance assignable to suggestibility. (p. 401)

Unlike the research in comparing hypnosis with other treatments, these studies must be cited for their relative methodological precision such as controlling for susceptibility, intensity of fear, therapists' expertise across conditions, the use of comparable empirically derived hypnotic induction procedures, and the employment of multiple measures of the phobia. A suggestion for further clarification of the degree of improvement in the phobia would be to include several physiological measures as objctive indices of anxiety and its reduction.

Although praised for their precision, the results of these studies must be inspected with some uncertainty as to their generality. The subjects employed were college students who were chosen for their fear of snakes. This was not a clinical population which may be characterized by more intense and debilitating reactions to more than one discrete stimulus. Schubot's (1967) findings that hypnosis facilitated improvements among highly anxious subjects may be indicative of a differential effectiveness of hypnosis among clinical cases of phobias. Perhaps as postulated by Frankel (1974, 1981) and Frankel and Orne (1976), the use of hypnosis in clinical cases of phobia may be more effective than other treatments because of (1) differences in responsiveness to suggestions among clinical phobias, and (2) similarities between hypnotic capacities and the acquisition of phobic behavior among this population group. Although theoretically important, no data have yet been produced to support these contentions. From the evidence now available, one must conclude that perhaps hypnosis should not be considered as a treatment for phobias by itself, but as an aid or adjunct in other more effective procedures (Lang et al., 1965). Speigel et al. (1981) has stated that there is "nothing inherently therapeutic about the hypnotic experience per se" (p. 240) but should be used as "a method of disciplined concentration which can be used adjunctively with a primary treatment strategy" (p. 239).

Despite this challenge to the adherents to the effectiveness of hypnosis as a valid treatment modality, few studies have been done which further explored this issue.

As previously reviewed in the case reports, hypnosis has been used in a variety of ways to reduce fear. The three major ways or reducing fear via hypnosis seem to be : (1) inducing a cathartic experience by a revivification of the feared situation, (2) inducing relaxation while imaging the feared behavior or experience, and (3) positive suggestions in which perception and cognitions were structured.

Horowitz (1970) investigated the effectiveness of these three uses of hypnosis in the reduction of the "standard" fear of snakes against a nonhypnotized control group. Dependent measures were similar to the controlled studies by Lang et al. (1963, 1965). The three hypnotic groups all went through induction by one of the Stanford Scales (SHSS:A, SHSS:B, or SHSS:C); the three groups consisted of (1) suggestions of relaxation while recalling a fear event, (2) recalling a feared event and reexperiencing the panic, and (3) after controlling for time in hypnosis, suggestions as to the harmlessness of the phobic object and that the fear would go away. There were no differences among groups as to their scores on the SHSS.

After nine successive days of the assigned treatment, the participants in the relaxed and posthypnotic suggestion group significantly differed from the controls on the behavioral approach task with the relaxed condition having the greatest gain; all groups improved significantly across trials on measures of self-reported anxiety. At follow-up, the relaxation group continued to show the greatest improvement on all measures. The author concluded that the effectiveness of hypnosis was due to (1) a substitution of relaxation responses to imaginal cues formerly evoking fear, and (2) a learning to discriminate prior learning experiences from the present situation.

In another study utilizing the various techniques within hypnosis, O'Brien et al. (1981) investigated the efficacy of the suggestion of a positive or coping dream with systematic desensitization against a standard systematic desensitization procedure. The posthypnotic susggestion of dreaming was explained as a vivid fantasy in which the client was successfully interacting with the phobic object; the phobia could be eliminated through the dual procedures of covert rehearsal and extinction.

The results indicated that the combined use of hypnotic dream induction alternating with systematic desensitization was more effective than systematic desensitization alone in decreasing avoidant behavior; there were, however, no significant differences between groups on self-reports of anxiety.

The findings of this research were unclear, nevertheless, because of the nonrandom selection of subjects from each group. Those in the hypnotic dream induction group were chosen because of their scores on the SHSS:A; the desensitization group had unknown levels of susceptibility. The authors were aware of such a methodological shortcoming and concluded that:

> The inability to equate for susceptibility could indicate that the control subjects were simply worse desensitization subjects. The uncontrolled differences in attention between groups and the use of the same therapists for both treatments and for measurement are other possible biasing factors. (p. 238)

If one takes into account the finding of other researchers that hypnotic susceptibility was positively related to reduction in fears using either systematic desensitization (Schubot, 1967), or hypnosis alone (Horowitz, 1970), then one must look with some questions as to the conclusion that hypnotic dream induction facilitated the alleviation of phobic behavior.

HYPNOTIC FACTORS IN THE TREATMENT OF PHOBIAS

The hypnotic phenomenon is composed of complex processes involving all aspects of the individual. Any attempt to simplify what takes place in hypnosis will of course fall short in fully explaining what is occurring during a hypnotic induction. Likewise, it is difficult to explain exactly what occurs during hypnotherapy for phobias. Three components of hypnosis which have been identified as possible mechanisms of change in the treatment of phobias will be reviewed. These components were: (1) imagery, (2) relaxation, and (3) suggestibility.

Imagery

Bell (1972) has stated that hypnotherapy is no longer the simple use of suggestions that an individual's symptom will disappear. By the use of hypnosis in desensitization procedures, the client can maximally reexperience the phobic situation through imagery. One significant feature of the hypnotic state is the facilitation of imaginal activity (Kroger & Felzer, 1976; Mott, 1982; Sheehan, 1978).

Although it is usually thought to involve only visual phenomenon, imagery during hypnosis has been related to the ability to relive an experience in any or all sensory modalities including haptic, auditory, kinesthetic, taste, and olfactory (Kroger & Felzer, 1976). The ability to image also has been found to be related to positive experiences in an individual's life history (Hilgard, 1978).

In reviewing the literature before 1978, Sheehan has found that although few controlled studies have been performend "to test the assumption that there is actual enrichment of imagery experience in hypnosis" (p. 338), those studies which have been done have been generally of a positive nature. One confounding factor, however, has been the relationship between imagery ability and hypnotizability. It has been evident that those individuals who were "good imagers" were also "good" hypnotic subjects. It seemed likely that those subjects who had imagery ability also reached greater depths in hypnosis. It was also determined that an individual's ability to image was better predicted on those items of a standard hypnotic susceptibility scale which required the production of an experience (i.e., the visual hallucination on the SHSS:C) than on those items requiring the inhibition of an experience (i.e., the amnesia item on the SHSS:C). From the results of this experimental literature, Sheehan has concluded that a certain type of mentation is brought to the hypnotic setting which influences both hypnotic abilities and imagery abilities. Positive correlations between these two phenomenon have been positive and significant (Hilgard, 1978; Sheehan, 1978); it should be noted also that this relationship between imagery production and susceptibility to hypnotic induction is not a direct linear relationship (Hilgard, 1978; Sheehan, 1978). Studies have found that although producing imagery does not predict hypnotizability, the absence of reported imagery by individuals seem to predict their lesser degree of responsivity to hypnotic induction procedures (Hilgard, 1978; Sheehan, 1978).

Imagery itself should not be viewed as a unidimensional construct, but as being comprised of many different processes. Three measures of imagination which assess different properties of this ability are (1) vividness, (2) control, and (3) effortlessness in imaging. Vividness in imagery could be described as the extent of detail, realism, and perceptual clarity in the imagined scene; control, on the other hand, would be the extent to which the individual could change and modify various aspects of the scene (i.e., changing the color of a car, etc.); effortlessness in imaging would be related to the ease of producing and maintaining an image. Vividness of imagination would expedite the desensitization procedure by making the feared imagined scenes more realistic to the client; control of imagery would be advantageous to a technique such as time distortion by assisting the client in successfully projecting himself or herself through the phobic situation. Effortlessness would facilitate an individual's elicitation and holding of an image while in a relaxed hypnotic state; this ability would enhance the extinction or counterconditioning processes in such behavioral treatments as flooding and systematic desensitization, respectively.

In regard to the experimental literature on these parameters of imagery in hypnosis, Sheehan (1978) and Hilgard (1978) both have reported an increase in vividness during hypnosis; however, most increases in vividness of imagery as reported on various self-report questionnaires have been positively correlated for males only with the number of items passed on standard scales of hypnotic susceptibility (Sheehan, 1978). T'Hoen (1978), likewise found a small but significant relationship (r=.28) between vividness of imagery and the ability to be hypnotized.

Research which has explored vividness and control of imagery in hypnosis has recently found that hypnosis could increase vividness but not control (Coe, St. Jean, Burger, 1980; Spanos, Valois, Ham, & Ham, 1973); there was, however, no correlation between suggestibility as measured on empirically derived measures and imagery ability in either dimensions although Coe et al. (1980) found a significant positive correlation (r=.52) between vividness of imagery and suggestibility for males only.

Regarding the parameter of effortlessness of imagery during hypnosis, Gale, Morris, Lucas, and Richardson (1972) found a suppression of EEG alpha activity when subjects produced images with effort. Since alpha activity has been associated with a relaxed state (Edmonston, 1981), the use of effort in producing images would suggest an inhibition of relaxation as seen in hypnosis. Therefore, effortlessness in imaging should be related to the ability to enter into hypnosis.

Recent research in the area of effortless experiencing of imagery has supported this contention. The results have generally found a significant relationship between effortlessness of imaging for both externally evoked imagery and susceptibility (Bowers, P., 1978, 1982; McConkey & Sheehan, 1982). Susceptibility and effortlessness also has been predicted by the ratings of subjects' vividness of produced images (Bowers, P., 1982; McConkey & Sheehan, 1982).

It seems that before any definite statement can be made about hypnosis and the enhancement of imagery, further research must be done which controls for some of the factors mentioned by Sheehan (1978). These factors included: (1) homogenity of samples tested with respect to sex, socioeconomic status, and control of imagination; (2) the nature of the technique of investigation, either correlational or analyses of variances; (3) adequacy and comparability of imagination measures (which are usually nonstandardized, self-report instruments); (4) cues given to subjects via instructions as to the most appropriate response; and (5) the efficacy of single versus multiple predictors of hypnotizability. Consideration of one or more of these factors may clarify the issue at hand.

Relaxation

Several authors have supported the assumption that hypnosis is an aid in the inducement of relaxation (Benson, Arns, & Hoffman, 1981; Edmonston, 1977; Korger & Felzer, 1976; Mott, 1982; Todd & Kelley, 1970; Wolpe, 1958). It was assumed that the hypnotized client easily enters into a physiological state which is marked by a decrease in muscle tonus, electrodermal responses, heart rate, and oxygen consumption. The assumed enhancement of relaxation in hypnosis would facilitate the counterconditioning of the fearful responses associated with phobias; the counterconditioning procedure is common to many of the behavioral therapies which have proven successful in treating this disorder.

Benson et al. (1981) and Edmonston (1978, 1981) have pointed out that the physiological changes one experiences in hypnosis are similar to those experiences in the "relaxation response;" the "relaxation response" is a term for a physiological state characterized by a generalized reduction in the arousal of the sympathetic nervous system. These authors also have referred to the similarities between the hypnotic induction and the traditional methods used in eliciting such a response. The similarities in the procedures included limitations of sensory reception and bodily activity, restriction of attention, narrow and monotonous stimulation, and an altering of bodily awareness.

In an experimental study of this assumption, Paul (1969) contrasted hypnotic and progressive muscle relaxation groups with a "quiet" control group on several physiological and subjective measures of relaxation. Although both groups significantly differed from the control group on measures of enhanced relaxation, Paul concluded that the muscle relaxation group achieved the results in only one session while the hynotic group did not.

Although Paul did not employ an empirically derived induction procedure in his study, one must conclude that no differences can be found between progressive muscle relaxation and hypnosis. In fact, all attempts at differentiating hypnosis from relaxation by some physiological measure have not been productive (Mather & Degun, 1975).

Suggestibility

Woody (1973) has argued that an important component which is often "downplayed" in hypnotherapy—and especially in systematic desensitization—is the use of suggestions and persuasion in overcoming the fear. Woody has stated that hypnosis offers

> a purposeful induction of heightened suggestibility usually through promoting a hypnotic trance-like state. The term "clinical suggestion" included techniques which are sometimes part of hypnosis, via serving as the communication vehicle for the suggestion that will hopefully alter post-hypnotic behavior, as well as techniques, used with hypnosis, that offer overt or subtle shaping suggestions, such as might be present in verbal conditioning. (p. 252)

Several authors (Barrios, 1973; Bowers, K. S., 1982; Kroger & Felzer, 1976, Mott, 1982) have stated that suggestions in hypnosis could potentiate the reduction and alleviation of many different types of disorders, both somatic and psychological. In regard to the treatment of phobias, hypnotic suggestions possibly could be employed to: (1) reduce the overt symptoms associated with the phobia, such as anxiety and avoidance; (2) change irrational covert self-statements, cognitions, and attitudes about the fear-eliciting stimulus; and (3) enhance the induction of relaxation and imagery during systematic densensitization.

Suggestibility in hypnosis and verbal conditioning has been proposed as abilities involving the same process of higher-order conditioning as initially stated in 1927 by Pavlov (1927/1960) and later by Barrios (1970) and Salter (1961). Support for this contention has been supplied by several researchers, King and McDonald (1976) obtained positive correlations between high suggestibility and greater ability to condition both operantly and respondently (classically). Mather and Degun (1975) also found heightened susceptibility to suggestion in a hypnotized group than under a relaxed condition. Barrios (1970) was able to condition salivation (an automatic response) in a hypnotized group to a previously neutral stimulus by the simple use of a suggestion that involved imagining a sour lemon candy in the participant's mouth; the same suggestion given to a nonhypnotized control group did not produce the conditioned response. An unpublished doctoral dissertation by Coleman in 1976 (cited in Edmonstron, 1981), however, found no difference between relaxed and hypnotized groups responding to standard challenges (i.e., items on the SHSS:C) usually offered to hypnotized individuals. A control group which sat quietly in their chairs differed from the relaxed and hypnotized groups by their failure to respond to these standard suggestions. In a review of the literature between 1960 and 1964, Barber (1965) concluded that suggestions designed to change physiological responses were equally effective in both hypnotized and waking control conditions.

Further studies must be conducted before any conclusions can be reached as to whether hypnosis increases responsivity to suggestions. Controlling for some of the same variables mentioned by Sheehan (1978) for future research endeavors in imagery abilities in hypnosis, systematic studies should investigate the relationship between suggestibility and hypnotizability as well as the "non-volitional" aspect of responsivity which has been hypothesized to occur within the hypnotic context (P. Bowers, 1982).

METHODOLOGICAL CONSIDERATIONS

A review of the recent literature on the use of hypnosis in the treatment of phobias has indicated substantial support from the case histories for its continued employment; results from the experimental research studies have questioned the validity of this proposition. Several factors have arisen from this review which have been singled out as pertaining to the interpretation of the results from both case studies and research. Consideration of one or more of these factors may alter the findings of the studies previously presented; these findings may be altered to nullify significant results or explain the absence of positive data.

Subjects

The controlled studies generally used samples of college students with varying degrees of a specific phobia, such as a snake phobia. One may question the severity of such a fear in that it had not debilitated the phobic participants. Clinical phobias usually are chronic and severe phobias which have generalized to many situations in the environment and greatly limit adaptive behavior. Although on the surface seemingly easier to attentuate, the circumscribed phobia of volunteer subjects may be qualitatively and quantitatively different from the clinical population. As a result, the research which has shown hypnosis to not be an effective intervention must be reinterpreted in light of the rather limited population sampled. Clinical phobias may be complex phenomena which may be more effectively treated through hypnosis.

Several controlled studies which have found positive results for hypnosis have not controlled for suggestibility in their treatment groups. From this deficit, one cannot be certain if hypnosis is effective with the general phobic population or only with the relatively select group of high or moderately susceptible individuals who also happen to be phobic. Perhaps with further research some basis to Frankel and his colleagues' (1974, 1976, 1981) assertion that individuals who are phobic and highly suggestible may have learned a conditioning process which facilitates the acquisition of a phobia and the ability to be hypnotized. Such a relationship may determine subgroups of phobic individuals who may benefit from hypnosis in relieving their phobic disorder.

Dependent Measures

As noted previously, a phobic reaction involved all response systems of an individual: cognitive, emotional or physiological, and behavioral. As such, when assessing the intensity of a phobia and its purported alleviation, multiple measures from these response systems should be assessed. The clinical and experimental studies fail to do this; generally, one or two responses were measured in pretreatment and posttreatment. The validity of the results either for or against hypnosis must be opened to question especially if the treatment may independently effect or not effect one of the response systems not assessed. It is suggested that self-reports, behavioral tasks, and multiple physiological measures be made during the assessment phases.

As always, if the studies involve independent raters, these individuals should be "blind" to what treatment is being assessed. In this way, uncontrolled bias and prejudice could be adequately controlled.

Independent Variables

One of the major weaknesses with the literature on the clinical application of hypnosis to the phobias was a nonstandardization of induction procedures. Personally developed induction methods were employed in several case reports whereas, in some of the controlled studies, empirically derived hypnotic scales were not in evidence. Such a lack of standard induction procedures could lead to a noncomparability of methodological procedures. It is suggested that the well-known empirical scales be used in future research to ensure comparability of results.

In the research literature, several shortcomings in procedure have been noted. The first one was a lack of control in length of treatment between conditions; without such control one could not be sure if the results were due to the temporal effect of being in treatment. The second deficit was a lack of control for the theoretical beliefs and expertise in the treatment being presented. Studies have shown that the therapist's belief in the procedure used as well as his or her facility in using it lead to significant positive outcomes (Garfield & Bergin, 1978). Even in such well-controlled studies as those as Lang and his colleagues (1963, 1965), the orientation and beliefs of the therapists involved in administering the procedure were not mentioned.

Finally, an important aspect of using hypnosis in the treatment of phobias seems to be the specificity of the suggestions used in the removal of fear. Although well employed in the clinical studies in which the suggestions were all directed towards the reduction of the specifics of the fear, the experimental research basically employed a general nonspecific suggestion of fear removal or relaxation. The less-than-significant positive results for hypnotherapy in these studies must be questioned. In the comparison treatments (usually systematic desensitization), the parameters of the technique were specifically designed to "decondition" the fear to the particular stimuli. Perhaps the degree of effectiveness between the case studies and group comparison studies could be the "generalized" suggestions used in the latter and the "tailor-made" ones of the former.

CONCLUSION

The conclusion to the effectiveness of hypnotic procedures in the treatment of phobic disorders must be held in abeyance. Further research must be performed in order to clarify this issue; hopefully, such research will be better controlled and perhaps take one or more of the above-mentioned factors into consideration. Finally, research must be focused not only on the comparable effectiveness of hypnosis vis-a-vis other more traditional techniques, but methods within hypnotherapy should be further explored in an attempt to delineate those which are efficacious and beneficial to the clinical population.

REFERENCES

Agras, W. S., & Jacob, R. G. (1981). Phobia: Nature and measurement. In M. Mavissakalian & D. H. Barlow (Eds.), *Phobia: Psychological and pharmacological treatment.* New York: Guildord Press.

American Psychiatric Association. (1981). *Diagnostic and statistical manual* (3rd ed.). Washington, D. C.: Author.

Astrip, C. (1974). Flooding therapy with hypnosis. *Behavior Therapy, 5,* 704-705.

Baker, S. R., & Boaz, D. (1983). The partial reformulation of a traumatic memory of a dental phobia during trance: A case study. *International Journal of Clinical and Experimental Hypnosis, 31,* 14-18.

Barber, T. X. (1965). Physiological effects of "hypnotic suggestions": A critical review of recent research (1960-1964). *Psychological Bulletin, 63,* 201-222.

Barrios, A. A. (1970). Hypnotherapy: A reappraisal. *Psychotherapy: Theory, Research, and Practice, 7,* 2-7.

Barrios, A. A. (1973). Posthypnotic suggestion as higher-order conditioning: A methodological and experimental analysis. *International Journal of Clinical and Experimental Hypnosis, 21,* 32-50.

Bell, G. K. (1972). Clinical hypnosis: Warp and woof of psychotherapies. *Psychotherapy: Theory, Research, and Practice, 9,* 276-280.

Benson, H., Arns, P. A., & Hoffman, J. W. (1981). The relaxation response and hypnosis. *International Journal of Clinical and Experimental Hypnosis, 19,* 259-270.

Bowers, K. S. (1982). The relevance of hypnosis for cognitive-behavioral therapy. *Clinical Psychology Review, 2,* 67-78.

Bowers, P. (1978). Hypnotizability, creativity, and the role of effortless experiencing. *International Journal of Clinical and Experimental Hypnosis, 26,* 184-202.

Bowers, P. (1982). The classic suggestion effect: Relationships with scales of hynotizability, effortless experiencing, and imagery vividness. *International Journal of Clinical and Experimental Hypnosis, 30,* 270-279.

Cautela, J. R. (1975). The use of covert conditioning in hypnotherapy. *International Journal of Clinical and Experimental Hypnosis, 23,* 15-27.

Cohen, S. B. (1981). Phobia of bovine sounds. *American Journal of Clinical Hypnosis, 23,* 266-268.

Coe, W. C., St. Jean, R. L., & Burger, J. M. (1980). Hypnosis and the enhancement of visual imagery. *International Journal of Clinical and Experimental Hypnosis, 28,* 225-243.

Daniels, L. K. (1975). The treatment of psychophysiological disorders and severe anxiety by behavior therapy, hypnosis, and transcendental meditation. *American Journal of Clinical Hypnosis, 17,* 267.

Daniels, L. K. (1976). Rapid in-office and in-vivo desensitization of an injection phobia utilizing hypnosis. *American Journal of Clinical Hypnosis, 18,* 200-203.

Deiker, T. E., & Pollack, D. H. (1975). Integration of hypnosis and systematic desensitization techniques in the treatment of phobias: A case report. *American Journal of Clinical Hypnosis, 17,* 170-174.

Dengrove, E. (1973). The uses of hypnosis in behavior therapy. *International Journal of Clinical and Experimental Hypnosis,* 21, 13-17.

Deyoub, D. L., & Epstein, S. J. (1977). Short-term hypnotherapy for the treatment of flight phobia: A case report. *American Journal of Clinical Hypnosis, 19,* 251-254.

Edmonston, W. E. (1977). Neutral hypnosis as relaxation. *American Journal of Clinical Hypnosis, 20,* 69-75.

Edmonston, W. E. Jr. (1978). The effects of neutral hypnosis on conditioned responses: Implications for hypnosis as relaxation. In E. Fromm & R. E. Shor (Eds.), *Hypnosis: Developments in research and new perspectives* (Rev. 2nd ed.). New York: Aldine Press.

Edmonston, W. E. Jr. (1981). *Hypnosis and relaxation: Modern verification of an old equation.* New York: Wiley & Sons.

Epstein, S. J., & Deyoub, P. R. (1981). Hypnotherapy for fear of choking: Treatment implication of a case report. *International Journal of Clinical and Experimental Hypnosis, 19,* 117-127.

Erickson, M. H. (1980). Pseudo-orientation in time as a hypnotherapeutic procedure. In E. L. Rossi (Ed.), *The collected papers of Milton H. Erickson* (Vol. IV). New York: Irvington.

Frankel, F. H. (1974. Trance capacity and the genesis of phobic behavior. *Archives of General Psychiatry, 31,* 261-263.

Frankel, F. H. (1981). Short-term psychotherapy and hypnosis. *Psychotherapy and Psychosomatics, 35,* 236-243.

Frankel, F. H., & Orne, M. T. (1976). Hypnotizability and phobic behavior. *Archives of General Psychiatry, 33,* 1259-1261.

Frutiger, A. D. (1981). Treatment of penetration phobia through the combined use of systematic desensitization and hypnosis: A case study. *American Journal of Clinical Hypnosis, 23,* 269-273.

Gale, A., Morris, P. E., Lucas, B., & Richardson, A. (1972). Types of imagery and imagery types: An EEG study. *British Journal of Psychology, 63,* 525-531.

Garfield, S. L., & Bergin, A. E. (1978). *Handbook of psychotherapy and behavior chance.* New York: Wiley & Sons.

Golan, H. P. (1971) Control of fear reactions in dental patients by hypnosis: Three case reports. *American Journal of Clinical Hypnosis, 31,* 279-284.

Golan, H. P. (1975). Further case reports from Boston City Hospital. *American Journal of Clinical Hypnosis, 18,* 55-59.

Gruenewald, D. (1971). Agoraphobia: A case study of hypnotherapy. *International Journal of Clinical and Experimental Hypnosis, 19,* 10-20.

Gustavson, J. L., & Weight, D. G. (1981). Hypnotherapy for a phobia of slugs: A case report. *American Journal of Clinical Hypnosis, 23,* 258-261.

Hilgard, J. R. (1978). Imaginative and sensory-affective involvements in everyday life in hypnosis. In E. Fromm & R. E. Shor (Eds.), *Hypnosis: Developments in research and new perspectives* (Rev. 2nd ed.). New York: Aldine Press.

Horowitz, S. L. (1970). Strategies within hypnosis for reducing phobic behavior. *Journal of Abnormal Psychology, 75,* 104-112.

King, D. R., & McDonald, R. D. (1976). Hypnotic susceptibility and verbal conditioning. *International Journal of Clinical and Experimental Hypnosis, 24,* 29-37.

Kroger, W. S., & Felzer, W. D. (1976). *Hypnosis and behavior modification: Imagery conditioning.* Philadelphia: J.B. Lippincott.

Lang, P. J., & Lazovik, A. D. (1963). Experimental desensitization of a phobia. *Journal of Abnormal and Social Psychology, 66,* 519-525.

Lang, P. J. , Lazovik, A. D., & Reynolds, D. J. (1965). Desensitization, suggestibility, and pseudotherapy. *Journal of Abnormal Psychology, 70,* 395-402.

Lawlor, E. D. (1976). Hypnotic intervention with "School Phobic" children. *International Journal of Clinical and Experimental Hypnosis, 24,* 74-86.

Lazarus, A. A. (1973). "Hypnosis" as a facilitator in behavior therapy. *International Journal of Clinical and Experimental Hypnosis, 21,* 25-31.

Lazarus, A. A., & Wilson, G. T. (1976). Behavior modification: Clinical and experimental perspectives. In B. B. Wolman (Ed.), *The therapist's handbook: Treatment methods of mental disorders.* New York: Van Nostrand Reinhold.

Marks, I. M. (1969). *Fears and phobias.* New York: Academic Press.

Marks, I. M., Gelder, M. G., & Edwards, G. (1968). Hypnosis and desensitization for phobias: A controlled prospective trial. *British Journal of Psychiatry, 114,* 1263-1274.

Mather, M. D., & Degun, G. S. (1975). A comparative study of hypnosis and relaxation. *British Journal of Medical Psychology, 48,* 55-63.

Mavissakalian, M., & Barlow, D. H. (1981). Phobia: An overview. In M. Mavissakalian & D. H. Barlow (Eds.), *Phobia: Psychological and pharmacological treatment.* New York: Guildford Press.

McConkey, K. M., & Sheehan, P. W. (1982). Effort and experience on the Creative Imagination Scale. *International Journal of Clinical and Experimental Hypnosis, 30,* 280-288.

Miller, M. M. (1979). *Therapeutic hypnosis.* New York: Human Science Press.

Mott, T. (1982). The role of hypnosis in psychotherapy. *American Journal of Clinical Hypnosis, 24,* 241-248.

O'Brien, R. M., Cooley, L. E., Ciotti, J., & Henninger, K. M. (1981). Augmentation of systematic desensitization of snake phobia through post-hypnotic dream suggestion. *American Journal of Clinical Hypnosis, 19,* 231-238.

O'Donnell, J. M. (1978). Implosive therapy with hypnosis in the treatment of cancer phobia: A case report. *Psychotherapy: Theory, Research, and Practice, 15,* 8-12.

Paul, G. L. (1969). Physiological effects of relaxation training and hypnotic suggestion. *Journal of Abnormal Psychology, 74,* 425-437.

Pavlov, I. P. (1960). *Conditioned reflexes: An investigation of the physiological activity of the cerebral cortex.* (G. V. Anrep, Trans.) New York: Dover Publications (Original work published, 1927).

Ritow, J. K. (1979). Brief treatment of vomiting phobia. *American Journal of Clinical Hypnosis, 21,* 293–296.

Salter, A. (1961). *Conditioned reflex therapy: The direct approach to the reconstruction of personality.* New York: Capricorn.

Schneck, J. M. (1975). Prehypnotic suggestion in psychotherapy. *American Journal of Clinical Hypnosis, 17,* 158–159.

Schubot, E. D. (1967). The influence of hypnotic and muscular relaxation in systematic desensitization. *Dissertation Abstracts, 27,* 3681-3682.

Scott, D. L. (1970). Treatment of a severe phobia for birds by hypnosis. *American Journal of Clinical Hypnosis, 12,* 146–149.

Scrignor, C. B. (1981). Rapid treatment of contamination phobia with a handwashing compulsion by flooding with hypnosis. *American Journal of Clinical Hypnosis, 23,* 252–257.

Seif, B. (1982). Hypnosis in a man with fear of voiding in public facilities. *American Journal of Clinical Hypnosis, 24,* 288–289.

Sheehan, P. W. (1978). Hypnosis and the processes of imagination. In E. Fromm & R. E. Shor (Eds.), *Hypnosis: Developments in research and new perspectives.* (Rev. 2nd ed.). New York: Aldine Press.

Spanos, N. P., Valois, R., Ham, M. W., & Ham, W. L. (1973). Suggestibility and vividness and control of imagery. *International Journal of Clinical and Experimental Hypnosis, 21,* 305-311.

Speigel, D., Frischolz, E. J. Maruffi, B., & Speigel, H. (1981). Hypnotic responsivity and the treatment of flying phobia. *American Journal of Clinical Hypnosis, 23,* 239–247.

Surman, O. S. (1979). Postnoxious desensitization: Some clinical notes on the combined use of hypnosis and systematic desensitization. *American Journal of Clinical Hypnosis, 22,* 54–60.

T'Hoen, P. (1978). Effects of hypnotizability and visualizing ability on omagery-mediated learning. *International Journal of Clinical and Experimental Hypnosis, 26,* 45–54.

Todd, F. J., & Kelley, R. J. (1970). The use of hypnosis to facilitate conditoned relaxation responses: A report of three cases. *Journal of Behavior Therapy and Experimental Psychiatry, 1,* 295–299.

Ullman, L. P., & Krasner, L. (1975). *A psychological approach to abnormal behavior* (2nd ed.). Englewood Cliffs, NJ: Prentice-Hall.

Van der Hart, O. (1981). Treatment of a phobia for dead birds: A case report. *American Journal of Clinical Hypnosis, 23,* 266–268.

Van Dyke, P., & Harris, R. B. (1982). Phobia: A case report. *American Journal of Clinical Hypnosis, 24,* 284–287.

Wolpe, J. (1958). *Psychotherapy by reciprocal inhibition.* Stanford, CA: Stanford University Press.

Wolpe, J. (1973). *The practice of behavior therapy* (2nd ed.). New York: Pergamon Press.

Wolpe, J. (1976). *Themes and variations: A behavior therapy casebook.* New York: Pergamon Press.

Woody, R. H. (1973). Clinical suggestions and systematic desensitization. *American Journal of Clinical Hypnosis, 15,* 250--257.

Wyensighe, B. (1974). A vomiting phobia overcome by one session of flooding with hypnosis. *Journal of Behavioral Therapy and Experimental Psychiatry, 5,* 169–170.

Yamauchi, K. T. (1981). Dental fear in a chronic schizophrenia: A case report. *American Journal of Clinical Hypnosis, 24,* 128–131.

PART III

PSYCHODYNAMIC INTERVENTIONS

Chapter 7

Catharsis and Uncovering Therapies

Cynthia Nigro
Nova University

Jeffrey Jon Vidic
University of South Carolina

THE HISTORY OF HYPNOSIS AS RELATED TO CATHARSIS

While altered psychic states akin to hypnosis have been recorded from earliest history and were probably utilized even then to enhance emotional catharsis, the relationship between hypnosis and catharsis began to become established through the work of Anton Mesmer in the 1700s. Mesmer believed that he could cure people through the use of animal magnetism which he believed emanated from himself. This magnetic force could be transmitted to whatever object Mesmer chose.

Mesmer's clinic became widely known for its miraculous cure of patients' suffering from various forms of "mental disease." According to a description by Nichols and Zax (1977), the clinic featured elaborate decorations and ethereal music, which enhanced patient's expectations that something dramatic and mysterious was about the happen. The central feature of the treatment room was the baquet, a large oaken tub filled with iron filings, water, and powdered glass, from which a number of iron rods protruded.

The baquet contained fluid which had been magnetized by Mesmer. Patients would gather around the baquet, linking hands and touching the iron rods. Eventually, Mesmer would enter the room and pass amongst the patients, waving a wand over them. The patients would gradually become restless and agitated, until a "crisis" occurred. One or several patients would begin to scream, sweat, and convulse. These symptoms would spread rapidly to the other patients, until all of them were seized by hysterical convulsions. After several minutes of this behavior, the tension and hysteria would gradually fade away, and the patients would experience a remission of their presenting symptoms.

Eventually, a Royal Commission of which Benjamin Franklin was a member, was appointed to investigate Mesmer's animal magnetism and his miraculous "cures." Unfortunately, the Commission was more interested in determining whether or not Mesmer had discovered a new physical fluid, rather than whether or not his methods produced curative effects. From their tests, the Commission concluded that Mesmer's fluid was nothing out of the ordinary, and had nothing to do with the removal of the patients' symptoms. The final judgment of the Commission was that the cures were the result of suggestion and imagination, and Mesmer quickly fell into disrepute. However, his "cathartic method" of treatment spread rapidly throughout France and into Europe by the 1800s.

Jean Martin Charcot, an eminent French neurologist, was the first person to undertake scientific experiments using hypnosis. His were the earliest studies to deal with the hypothesis that forgotten memories could be retrieved under hypnosis.

Pierre Janet, Charcot's pupil and successor, investigated the use of hypnosis and hypnotic recall to create a sense of emotional catharsis in patients. Joseph Breuer and Sigmund Freud were also investigating the cathartic uses of hypnosis at the same time. Janet hypothesized that traumatic memories played a major role in producing hysterical symptoms and neuotic behavior. He advocated the use of hypnosis to uncover these forgotten memories and to encourage discharge of the affect which accompanied them. This was strikingly similar to the conclusions of Breuer and Freud, who were also using hypnosis as the basis of their "cathartic therapy."

The cathartic method, also called hypnotic abreaction, enjoyed much success when used to treat soldiers who broke down in battle during World War I and World War II. While this technique of cathartic hypnotherapy is still used by some practitioners today, it is not always as successful as it was with cases of traumatic stress reations to battle. Hypnoanalysis and hypnotherapy as practiced today are generally longer-term methods of intervention in comparison to the earlier methods which focused mainly on cathartic abreactions.

A DEFINITION OF CATHARSIS

Catharsis may be generally defined as an expression of emotions that were previously repressed or restrained from being manifested at the time of a prior incident. This unleashing of emotions often results in a temporary reduction in tension and anxiety. Cathartic abreactions are composed of two separate but related components. The first component involves intellectual functioning, and has been labeled the "cognitive-emotional aspect" by Nichols and Zax (1977). The cognitive-emotional aspect involves the recall of forgotten material or of a traumatic event to which a person did not originally respond with sufficient amounts of affect.

Nichols and Zax (1977) have labeled the second component the "somatic-emotional aspect." This aspect consists of the discharge of emotions through expressive actions such as tears, laughter, screaming, sweating, and so on. Since these two components of catharsis generally occur together in psychotherapy, the distinction between them is often ignored. Furthermore, it has not yet been clearly established whether the existence of both components is necessary to produce a satisfactory level of emotional catharsis.

Clinical evidence suggests that, in some cases, simply vividly recalling and talking about a traumatic experience, in the absence of an overt motoric discharge, will afford the client great relief. Other therapists have found that a somatic release, such as crying or yelling about an event which is not directly related to the client's problem, will afford some relief. An example of this would be when people weep over trivial incidents, or show emotional overreactions to minor events. It is possible that an inappropriate affective expression in the present may be traced to a past event for which the affect present at that time was insufficiently expressed. Nichols and Zax (1977), in a review of the literature on catharsis, concluded that the evidence suggests that "catharsis is most effective when it consists of both the cognitive and somatic aspects." (p. 12)

THEORIES EXPLAINING THE CATHARTIC REACTION

One of the first therapists to look into the dynamics which underlie catharsis was Sigmund Freud. Freud was first introduced to cathartic therapy by Joseph Breuer, who had used the method to successfully treat his patient, Anna O. Breuer found that having Anna, who was suffering from many hysterical symptoms, reexperience under hypnosis the event during which each symptom had originally developed, would cause the symptoms to disappear.

Freud was very impressed by Breuer's success, and began to use his "cathartic method" of therapy with his own clients. Together, Freud and Breuer published *Studies on Hysteria* in 1895 in which they explained how they believed the cathartic technique to work. They believed that hysterics' symptoms were the result of past experiences which generated large amounts of affect that were not expressed. Furthermore, the memory of the experience is cut off from the person's consciousness. The hysterical symptoms are symbolic of the unresolved unconscious conflict. In order to uncover the memory, the client must be hypnotized and then directed by the therapist to abreact, or relieve the original experience. Breuer and Freud found that:

> Each individual hypsterical symptom immediately and permanently disappeared when we had succeeded in bringing clearly to light the memory of the event by which it was provoked and in arousing its accompanying affect, and when the patient had described that event in the greatest possible detail and had put the affect into words. Recollection without affect almost invaribly produces no result. (Breuer & Freud, 1957, p. 6)

Freud and Breuer's theory has been criticized by Macmillan (1977) on the grounds that most of the treatment effects were due to the clients' expectations. In fact, however, Freud and Breuer had considered this hypothesis themselves but rejected it. In some of his later writings, Freud explained the effectiveness of the cathartic technique in terms of his hydraulic model of personality. "When emotions are not discharged, he said, they reside in inner space, incrementally accumulating tension" (Nichols & Zax, 1977, p. 3).

Later in his career as a therapist, Freud abandoned the use of hypnotically-induced cathartic abreactions. Nichols and Zax (1977) cite several reasons why he did so. One reason was that he found that he was unable to hypnotize a good number of his clients. Another problem was that, in many cases, symptoms were the result of multiple causes, and each cathartic abreaction only dealt with the unexpressed affect associated with that particular event. Thus, in order to effect permanent symptom removal, it would be necessary to have the clients hypnotically abreact every significant event from their past. Finally, by focusing exclusively on cathartic abreactions, the clients were never given the chance to explore the intrapsychic dynamics which were acting to produce the maladjusted behavior patterns. In short, the clients were not able to gain insight into the underlying motivations of their neurotic behavior.

The mechanisms underlying catharsis can also be explained from a learning theory point of view. What occurs in hypnotically-induced cathartic abreactions is strikingly similar to what occurs in flooding and implosive therapy. In flooding, a client is exposed to a real life object or stimulus which causes irrational levels of anxiety and fear. In implosive therapy, an imagined stimulus is used in place of the actual feared object or situation.

Both flooding and implosive therapy have proven to be very effective in reducing unwarranted levels of anxiety in clients. Their effectiveness has been explained in terms of the principle of extinction. When the conditioned stimuli are presented (whether real or imagined), clients are unable to follow their normal behavior patterns of escaping from the situations. By remaining in the feared situations, the clients learn that the feared consequences do not in fact occur, and eventually the fear responses extinguish.

Given this hypothesis, it is unclear why behavior therapists so strongly reject hypnotic abreaction of past events as a valid method of treatment Stampfl and Levis (1967) found that extinction in animals occur most rapidly when the animal is in the original situation where the unpleasant consequences first occurred. These authors further state that "extinction of a learned emotional response proceeds with the greatest rapidity when the organism is exposed to stimulus conditions most closely approaching those which were originally associated with painful stimulation" (p. 498). If this is indeed the case, would not the use of hypnosis facilitate a more accurate recall of the original experience which would result in better extinction of the inappropriate fear response? Of course the answer rests with the determination as to whether hypnosis enhances recall or merely effects the recaller's confidence in his ability to recall.

IS CATHARTIC THERAPY ALONE AN EFFECTIVE TREATMENT?

Unfortunately, there have been no well-controlled experimental studies in which cathartic abreactions have been the exclusive focus of therapy. However, there are enthusiastic advocates of this method of therapeutic intervention. Lipshitz and Blair (1960) cite a 1954 article by Symonds in which he investigated 68 reported changes of behavior. According to Symonds, 59 of the 68 reported changes could be directly traced to the client's experiençing a cathartic abreaction, and he concluded that the basic factor which underlies behavior change in psychotherapy is cathartic abreaction.

Lipshitz and Blair (1960) performed an experiment to "test the hypothesis that abreactions result in the extinction of the affective responsivity recallable from a particular traumatic incident and that this extinction follows the laws of classical conditioning" (p. 248). A 23-year-old female was used as a naive subject. During the first session, she was hypnotized and regressed back to a nonspecific frightening experience and an abreaction was induced. In subsequent sessions, she was hypnotically regressed back to the same incident and induced to abreact. In each session, various physiological measures were recorded. Generally, there was a diminuation of affective and antonomic responses. On the the basis of these results, the authors felt that their hypothesis was supported. However, it is not certain that this is what occurs during cathartic therapy, and it is even more uncertain that these types of changes would necessarily lead to overt behavior change in the client.

There have been two controlled experimental studies published in which levels of emotional catharsis were quantified and related to therapeutic outcome. Nichols (1974) conducted an experiment in which volunteer subjects from a college mental health clinic were divided into two treatment groups, one receiving emotive psychotherapy, and the other insight-oriented analytic therapy. Various measures of outcome were employed. Analysis of therapy sessions indicated that the emotive therapy did produce significantly higher levels of emotional catharsis. However, on measures of therapy outcome, the emotive group showed greater improvement on only one measure, the Personal Satisfaction Form. It was also found that subjects in the emotive group who manifested the highest levels of emotional catharsis during the therapy sessions were the ones who improved the most on the therapy outcome measures. Nichols interpreted this finding to be at least partially supportive of the effectiveness of emotional catharsis in producing favorable therapy outcomes.

The use of cathartic abreactions has been hypothesized to be a helpful adjunct to therapy in a number of areas. Nichols and Zax (1977) and Weiner (1974) feel that abreactions may reduce unexpressed anger which underlies psychosomatic illness. Grayson (1970) feels that cathartic abreactions help clients through mourning experiences.

THE USES OF HYPNOSIS IN PSYCHOTHERAPY

As was mentioned earlier in the chapter, the history of psychology and pschotherapy is filled with evidence of the use of altered states of consciousness, including hypnosis, in removing symptomology from patients. Hypnosis and hypnotherapy are in widespread use today, and adherents of these procedures claim that they are effective means of producing behavior change in clients.

Hypnosis can be used as an adjunct procedure to help the therapist overcome a client's initial resistance to entering therapy. Wolberg (1964) often uses hypnosis to induce a state of relaxation in overly anxious clients who are resistant to therapy. He has found that for many clients the mere ability to actually achieve a relaxed state often serves as a tremendous incentive for the client to seek further therapy.

INDUCED ANXIETY

Sipprelle (1967) developed a technique he called induced anxiety that uses emotional catharsis as a major component. This procedure grew out of Sipprelle's experience with clients in long-term therapy who experienced emotional blocking which impeded the progress of therapy. Sipprelle hypothesized that the blocking was due to repressed emotions associated with traumatic past events.

Induced anxiety is accomplished through a series of steps. First, hypnosis is explained to the client and then the client is hypnotized or put in a relaxed state. Next, the client is instructed to turn his or her attention inward and become aware of a growing feeling. The therapist does not label the feeling but verbally reinforces all signs of the client's experiencing emotion and encourages the client to "let it all out." Responses typically include agitation, sobbing, irregular breathing, or even hysterical laughter. Intense fear or anger are the most common reactions. Simultaneous with or immediately after the physical experience of emotion, the client will often spontaneously discuss the emotion eliciting events in his or her life. If these associated events are not brought up spontaneously, the therapist asks the client to relate his or her thoughts. After this catharsis of feeling and thoughts the client is given suggestions to return to a relaxed state followed soon after by instructions to awaken refreshed and relaxed with full recall for what had transpired. Finally, the therapist discusses and interprets the material which had been elicited during the induced anxiety state giving support and encouragement to the clients' effort to tolerate and assimilate what had transpired.

Sipprelle reports that this procedure gets the therapy past a "stuck point" and progress frequently resumes smoothly afterward. He suggests that this procedure can also be used as a diagnostic device when a prospective client has problems expressing feelings or shows blocking in attempting to specify problems while still in the assessment stage of therapy.

SHORT-TERM VS. LONG-TERM HYPNOTHERAPY

Hypnosis combined with age regression techniques has been shown to be a very effective tool in the treatment of acute behavioral reactions to traumatic incidents, such as those experienced during war time or during extreme disasters. What is hypothesized to have occurred is that the client, because of the situational demands which existed at the time, was unable to take action to relieve the tremendous anxiety that was felt. Another common emotion experienced by some patients is guilt over having survived an event while others were killed or injured. The person reacts to this inability to express anxiety or guilt by repressing his or her emotions. However, this repression is rarely complete, and emotions are usually manifested through some sort of symptom (e.g., hysterical paralysis of a limb, amnesia for the event, etc.)

During the First and Second World Wars, traumatic stress reactions to battle were often successfully treated using hypnotic regression to the traumatic event. Clients were then encouraged by the therapist to abreact the event and to allow emotions to be freely expressed. In cases where good premorbid personality adjustment was present, one or several sessions of hypnotic abreaction of the event were usually sufficient to remove pathological symptoms.

This short-term intervention, which focuses mainly on a specific traumatic incident, is very different in comparison to long-term hypnoanalysis. The main focus of such short-term therapy is the creation of a strong emotional abreaction of the event, which allows the client to experience emotional catharsis. The therapist does not need extensive training in psychoanalytic theory. The therapist also will tend to be much more directive in his interactions with the client in comparison to a therapist who is employing long-term hypnoanalysis with a client.

In order to practice long-term hypnoanalysis, the therapist must be well-grounded in analytic theory and must also be well-trained in the various techniques of hypnosis and hypnotic induction. An important point that is stressed by Wolberg (1964) is that in general, the hypnoanalyst will play a more active role in the therapy setting than the traditional "blank screen" psychoanalyst.

This higher level of activity on the part of such therapists, however, does not imply that they will be more directive in their interactions with clients. In order for hypnoanalytic procedures to be successful, Wolberg stresses that clients must play a very active role, even when in a hypnotized state. Clients who are hypnotized must remain free to accept or reject the analyst's interpretations, and must be able to actively verbalize their thoughts and emotions to the therapist.

HYPNOSIS AND ENHANCED EMOTIONAL CATHARSIS

In revewing the literature on the efficacy of hypnosis in producing a state of heightened emotional catharsis in therapy clients, the evidence seems to support the hypothesis that hypnotherapy produces more intense cathartic reactions than are usually seen during the course of normal psychoanalysis. This seems to be especially true in regard to the somatic-emotional component of the cathartic release. Wolberg (1964) states: "The mere induction of hypnosis may suddenly release a violent eruption of words and emotions that flood the treatment room, eventuating in emotional catharis and temporary symptom relief" (p. 11).

Hypnosis has been used successfully to facilitate the two basic processes which occur during psychoanalysis. The first process is that of free association, during which the client is encouraged to express whatever thoughts or feelings that may come to mind, no matter how trivial or unimportant they may seem. In a normal waking state, a client who has very well-developed defense mechanisms, such as repression or denial of problems, will avoid talking about issues which are ego-threatening. To talk about these threatening isues would cause the client to experience intense anxiety as a result of letting these significant thoughts and/or feelings into conscious awareness.

Wolberg (1964) points out that hypnosis is often a very useful tool which can be used by an experienced hypnoanalyst to remove this resistance to free association. He cites several reasons why hypnosis in the hands of a skilled analyst can overcome normal barriers to free association. First, superego controls are lowered when a person is placed in a hypnotic trance. Since it is mainly the superego that acts to repress threatening thoughts and feelings and keeps them from entering the clients conscious awareness, when these controls are lessened the client is more apt to express such material.

In order to deal with thoughts and feelings which provoke anxiety, the client must be operating from a position of adequate ego strength. Hypnosis seems to facilitate a fusing together of the egos of the client and the therapist, which results in the client gaining additional ego strength. If a client lacks sufficient ego strength, attempts to overcome resistance will usually meet with failure.

The hypnotic state also seems to enhance the client's ability to focus more intensely on inner thought processes and perceptions by deemphasizing awareness of the surrounding environment. Hypnosis seems to enhance imagery and fantasy in the client, allowing operation on a more primitive thought process level. Fromm, Oberlander, and Gruenwald (1970) and Levin and Harrison (1976) have provided experimental evidence supporting the existence of an increase in primary process thinking in hypnotically age-regressed adult subjects.

Several other factors may contribute to the client being more expressive of thoughts and feelings in the hypnotic state. The first deals with the inherent demand characteristics of the hypnotic relationship. By taking a more active role during hypnotherapy, the hypnoanalyst may convey certain expectations about how the client is supposed to respond. The client may focus on these cues and overrespond in order to please the therapist. This may be especially true in the case of emotional responding and the experiencing of cathartic abreactions.

Secondly, in American society there are social norms which prohibit or restrict direct expression of emotions. One would expect that under hypnosis, these norms are relaxed, especially when one considers the popular notions associated with stage hypnosis. It is common knowledge that a stage hypnotist is able to "make" hypnotized subjects engage in bizarre or silly behavior which violates certain normative standards. A client undergoing hypnoanalysis may therefore be excused for exhibiting emotional reactions which would normally be held in check, since such behavior was to some extent "beyond his control" while he was in the hypnotic state.

The second phase of both psychoanalysis and hypnoanalysis involves the development and interpretation of the transference relationship between the client and the therapist. During the transference phase, the client is encouraged to project hidden desires and impluses onto the therapist, who maintains an uncritical, accepting stance towards the client's inappropriate behavior. By carefully interpreting the thoughts and emotions which underlie the client's projections, the therapist attempts to help the client gain insight into the irrational motivations which potentiate such actions.

Hypnosis has been argued to be an effective tool in facilitating the development and interpretation of psychoanalytic transference relationships. Wolberg (1964) points out that the process of hypnotic induction itself is remarkably similar to the irrational positive transference that develops between the client and the analyst during regular psychoanalysis, in which the analyst is seen by the client as being the all-wise, all-knowing, all-caring healer. Kline (1955) states that hypnosis and transference both involve elements of recall, revivification, fantasy, affective feelings, displacement, dissociation, and amnesia. Because the underlying thought mechanisms are so similar, hypnosis used during psychoanalysis should produce a deeper and more insightful transference relationship.

Another reason that hypnosis may enhance transference relationships during therapy is that hypnosis tends to decrease superego controls. This decrease of superego control often allows a client to project thoughts and emotions onto the therapist that are so disgusting and threatening to the client that they could never be revealed in the normal waking state. Hypnosis also allows the transference relationship to develop at a more rapid pace than is usually seen in the course of regular psychoanalysis. Thus, the use of hypnosis as an adjunct to psychoanalysis can appreciably shorten the amount of time that a client must remain in therapy for lasting behavior change to occur.

It is very important that the analyst maintain an accepting, noncritical attitude towards the client's projections of negative thoughts and feelings. Such an attitude helps the client's ego from being overwhelmed by the anxiety that is associated with the expression of inappropriate thoughts and emotions. This leads to a strengthening of the client's ego, even when it occurs during the hypnotic state. This gradual strengthening of the ego through hypnotic association and projection of thoughts and feelings gradually lays the groundwork for the expression of this material in the waking state.

Wolberg (1964), Kline (1955), and other advocates of hypnoanalysis stress that, in order to achieve lasting behavior change, the material brought forth in the hypnotic state must later be recalled and worked through by the client in the waking state. Once this occurs, the analyst will give interpretations about what is going on to cause the client's behavior. This in turn allows the client to achieve insight into the motivating forces behind maladaptive behavior. The gaining of insight is the first step in the client's development of more adaptive behavior patterns to satisfy needs.

It is important to point out that allowing the client to experience intense emotional catharsis during the therapy session, whether hypnotically induced or not, is merely the starting point for true behavior change. Wolberg (1964) and Kline (1955) are in agreement that intense cathartic abreactions experienced by a client will almost always result in only temporary symptom relief. Before lasting change can take place, however, the client must gain insight into what motivates these maladaptive behaviors, and must make a conscious effort, with the help of the analyst, to generate more adaptive and socially acceptable ways of meeting needs. Merely coming into the therapy setting and experiencing intense catharsis, whether hypnotically induced or not, is in and of itself not enough to create lasting behavior change.

The proper use of hypnoanalytic techniques allows the analyst to proceed almost directly to the conflict areas that the client is wrestling with. Hypnotic recall of past traumas and upsetting incidents seems to set in motion a process of erosion in the client's defense mechanisms, so that the client is able to recall the emotionally threatening material in the waking state in a much shorter period of time than is usually required during traditional psychoanalysis. One successful technique used by Wolberg (1964) involves giving the client a posthypnotic suggestion to dream about the material brought forth in the hypnotic state. This seems to also help the client's ego gradually build strength to the point where it can handle the threatening material when recalled in the waking state.

It is important to keep in mind that a person's present behavior patterns are motivated by current environmental forces which impinge on longstanding, well-developed personality traits and styles of interaction. The behavior that results serves a purpose, in that client gets some sort of payoff by satisfying certain needs. These needs are often childish and immature in nature, and the analyst must carefully point this out to the client without the client becoming overly defensive. Such interpretations are often more readily accepted by the client while in a hypnotic state.

Wolberg (1964) stresses that interpretations given during a hypnotic session should be repeated to the client at a later point in time while the client is in the waking state, to insure that the client is totally free to accept or reject them. In order for lasting behavior change to occur, the client must actively choose to give up childish, dependency-oriented ways of behaving and replace them with more adaptive, rational, adult-oriented ways of responding. This choosing can only be done when the client is in the waking state; otherwise, a danger exists that the client is simply responding to the demand characteristics of the hypnotic relationship by saying things the analyst wants to hear.

Adherents of hypnoanalysis and hypnotherapy see hypnosis as an indispensable tool in the therapeutic process. Hypnosis allows the therapist to overcome the client's defenses and resistances much more quickly than can be done during regular therapy. Hypnosis also enables the therapist and the client to build a strong relationship in a shorter amount of time than is necessary during more traditional forms of therapy.

Because hypnotherapy and hypnoanalysis tend to be shorter in duration, they are therefore much more cost effective in comparison to more traditional forms of psychotherapy.

CRITICISMS OF HYPNOANALYSIS

Critics of hypnoanalysis and hypnotherapy argue that the procedure places the client in an overly-dependent relationship with the therapist, who is cast in the role of the all-powerful authority figure. They contend that little or no real behavior change occurs during therapy because the client is reacting to the therapist in a neurotic, dependent fashion. In order to please the authority figure therapist, the client will show "improvement" by ridding himself of his presenting problems. However, the original problem behaviors will be replaced by other irrational, unproductive behaviors, since no change has occurred in the client's underlying motivations and patterns of thinking.

Wolberg (1964) agrees that with some clients, there exists a danger of an adverse reaction to hypnoanalytic procedures. Hypnoanalysis is contraindicated when a client presents a pattern of behavior associated with dependent personality disorders. Wolberg suggests carefully screening all potential clients with a complete psychological assessment battery prior to undertaking hypnoanalytic therapy.

Other psychotherapists argue directly against the use of hypnosis to create high levels of emotional catharsis early in the course of therapy. It was Freud who first suggested the necessity for a slower, less dramatic unfolding of feelings and events during psychoanalysis in order to allow the ego sufficient time to react to and assimilate the uncovered material. Wolberg (1964) argues that if a hypnoanalyst is well grounded in the processes of psychoanalysis, there is little danger that such a therapist would push a client to reveal material that the client's ego is not capable of handling.

REQUIREMENTS FOR SUCCESSFUL HYPNOANALYSIS

Wolberg (1964) proposed the following criteria which must be met before a client can undergo successful hypnoanalysis:

1. The client must be hypnotizable, and must be trained prior to hypnoanalysis to reach a deep state of hypnotic trance as possible. This training should be done by the analyst himself. Wolberg stresses that even if the client can only be trained to reach a light or medium trance state, hypnoanalysis will still produce satisfactory results.
2. The best results are obtained when the client is able to remain active and verbally productive during the hypnotic trance.
3. It is important that the client be able to perform at least a limited amount of age-regression while in the hypnotic state.
4. The client should be capable of developing posthypnotic amnesia, and should also be able to carry out posthypnotic suggestions.
5. As mentioned earlier, the analyst must carefully assess whether the client possess sufficient ego strength to deal with the anxiety which may be released when the client's defenses and resistances break down during therapy. This can easily be determined through the use of an assessment battery prior to the beginning of hypnoanalytic therapy.

HYPNOANALYSIS AND PSYCHOTIC CLIENTS

Hypnosis and hypnotherapy techniques have been used very cautiously when dealing with clients who have been diagnosed as psychotic. Many analysts feel that psychotic clients lack sufficient ego strength to confront their problems directly, and that doing so may cause them to decompose further due to the overwhelming anxiety experienced. This anxiety, if released, may overrun their already fragile defenses. Conn (1960) also feels that there is an increased danger that psychotics may view the hypnoanalytic relationship as one of domination by and dependency on the therapist.

Crasilneck and Hall (1975) feel that such caution may be unwarranted. Bowers (1961) and Bowers, Brecher-Marex, and Polatin (1961) have reported the successful use of hypnotic age regression techniques during therapy with paranoid schizophrenics. Erickson (1970) was able to use hypnosis to produce positive therapeutic results with a schizophrenic client and three manic-depressive psychotics. Abrams (1963, 1965), Moore (1975), and Volgyesi (1959) all have reported improvements in attitude change and increased insight when using hypnotherapy with schizophrenic clients.

Wolberg (1948) and Scagnelli (1975) both feel that hypnosis and hypnotically-induced relaxation can be helpful adjunct procedures when doing therapy with schizophrenics. However, both authors caution that deep analytic probing should be avoided during hypnotic states, and that direct suggestions involving cathartic abreactions should also be avoided.

Crasilneck and Hall (1975) conclude that the use of hypnosis and hypnotherapy techniques with psychotic clients is, at best, an unsettled issue. One guideline they suggest is that a therapist should not use hypnotherapy on any client that the therapist would not feel competent to treat by more conventional methods. Readers interested in a more thorough review of the use of hypnotherapy and hypnotic techniques with psychotic clients should consult a review of the area by Abrams (1964).

REFERENCES

Abrams, S. (1964). The use of hypnotic techniques with psychotics: A critical review. *American Journal of Psychotherapy, 18,* 79-94.

Abrams, S. (1963). Short term therapy of a schizophrenic patient. *American Journal of Clinical Hypnosis, 5,* 237-247.

Abrams, S. (1965). The effects of motivation upon the intellectual performance of schizophrenic patients. *American Journal of Clinical Hypnosis, 8,* 37-43.

Bowers, M.K. (1964). Theoretical considerations in the use of hypnosis in the treatment of schizophrenia. *International Journal of Clinical and Experimental Hypnosis, 9,* 39-46.

Bowers, M. K., Brecher-Marer, S., & Polatin, A.H. (1961). Hypnosis in the study and treatment of schizophrenia: A case report. *International Journal of Clinical and Experimental Hypnosis, 9,* 119-138.

Breuer, J., & Freud, S. (1957). *Studies of Hysteria.* New York: Basic Books.

Conn, J.H. 1960). The psychodynamics of recovery under hypnosis. *International Journal of Clinical and Experimental Hypnosis, 8,* 3-16.

Crasilneck, H., & Hall, J.A. (1975). *Clinical hypnosis: Principles and applications.* New York: Grune & Stratton.

Erickson, M.H. (1970). Hypnosis: Its renaissance as a treatment modality. *American Journal of Clincal Hypnosis, 13,* 71-89.

Fromm, E., Oberlander, M., & Gruenwald, D. (1970) Perceptual and cognitive processes in different states of consciousness; The waking state of hypnosis. *Journal of Projective and Technical Personality Assessment, 34,* 375-387.

Grayson, H. (1970). Grief reactions to relinquishing of unfulfilled wishes. *American Journal of Psychotherapy, 24,* 287-295.

Kline, M. (1955). Hypnodynamic psychology. New York: The Julian Press.

Levine, R., & Harrison, R. (1976). Hypnosis and regression in the service of the ego. *International Journal of Clinical and Experimental Hypnosis, 24,* 400–418.

Lipshitz, K., & Blair, J. H. (1960). The polygraphic recording of a repeated hypnotic abreaction with comments on abreactive psychotherapy. *Journal of Nervous and Mental Diseases, 130,* 246-252.

Macmillan, M. B. (1977). The cathartic method and the expectancies of Breuer and Anna O. *The International Journal of Clinical and Experimental Hypnosis, 25, 106-118.*

Moore, M. R. (1975). *Treatment of psychosis with hypnosis: Report of a case.* Paper presented at the annual meeting of the American Society of Clinical and Experimental Hypnosis, Seattle, WA.

Nichols, M. P. (1974). Outcome of brief cathartic psychotherapy. *Journal of Consulting and Clinical Psychology, 42,* 403–410.

Nichols, M. P., & Zax. M. (1977). *Catharsis in psychotherapy.* New York: Gardner Press.

Scagnelli, J. (1975). Hypnotherapy with schizophrenic and borderline patients. Paper presented at the annual meeting os the American Society of Clinical and Experimental Hypnosis, Seattle, WA.

Sipprelle, C. N. (1967). Induced anxiety. *Psychotherapy: Therapy Research and Practice, 4,* 36–40.

Stampfl, T.G., & Levs, D. J. (1967). Essentials of implosive therapy: A learning-theory-based psychodynamic behavioral therapy. *Journal of Abnormal Psychology, 72,* 496-503.

Volgyesi, F. A. (1959). Schezophrenis, schezoide psychopathein und derun hypnosethreapie. *Acta Psychother Psychosom Orthopaedag, 7,* 37-52.

Weiner, H. (1974). Toward a body therapy. *The Psychoanalytic Review, 61,* 45-52.

Wolberg, L. R. (1948). *Hypnosis: Is it for you?* New York: Harcourt Brace Javanovich.

Wolberg, L. R. (1964). *Hypnoanalysis.* New York: Grune & Stratton.

Chapter 8

Hypnosis in the Treatment of Psychosomatic Disorders

Herman C. Salzberg
University of South Carolina

Mary Ann Hudgins
Nova University

The focus of this chapter is to summarize the review done by DePiano and Salzberg (1979) which covered the literature from 1967 to 1977 and to examine research that has been conducted since that time in terms of outcomes and methodology and in their relevance to and role in establishing hypnosis as a viable treatment procedure. DePiano and Salzberg found the greatest amount of hypnosis research focused on three psychosomatic disorders: the treatment of skin disorders, headaches, and asthma. This chapter is limited, as was this review, to these three disorders.

DePiano and Salzberg accepted the definition of psychosomatic disorders as those problems that are etiologically related to or exacerbated by psychological factors, even though physical symptoms are present and medical intervention is often necessary. It is further helpful to view psychosomatic disorders as those affected parts of the body innervated by the automatic nervous system whereas hysterical symptoms most often are manifested in parts of the body which the individual has control of and which are innervated by the central nervous system. Skin temperature, blood flow, and muscle tension in the head and the lungs are all controlled by the autonomic nervous system. Thus, skin disorders, headaches, and asthma would qualify as pyschosomatic disorders, using this definition.

When considered from a broader, holistic perspective all disorders have psychological antecedents or are maintained by psychological as well as other factors. Some of the diseases which have been linked with psychological antecedents and maintainers are heart disease, hypertension, gastric and duodenal ulcers, cancer, asthma, rheumatoid arthritis, headaches, and all sorts of allergic reactions. It has been repeatedly demonstrated that psychologically-produced stress reactions interfere with bodily functioning and it is commonly accepted that the individual, under frequent extreme psychologically-produced stress, will be more vulnerable to disease.

According to Bowers and Kelly (1979), hypnosis is considered as one of the major psychological interventions in the treatment of psychosomatic disorders. It has been used as a technique to control specific responses to stress, as an adjunct to other therapies in order to facilitate insight, and to increase an individual's coping in the face of stressful events.

According to Wadden and Anderton (1982) the principle way of using hypnosis in the treatment of psychosomatic disorders is to attempt to modify an ongoing experience. The basic strategies employed are geared towards a direct change in specific physiological functions, control enhancement, and explorative uncovering.

DePiano and Salzberg saw three ways in which hypnosis might be used as interventions in the treatment of psychosomatic disorders. One would be to get the individual to gain control of autonomic functions through suggestion, and thus change those physiological responses responsible, in some measure, for the symptoms of the disorder. A second would be by helping patients to understand the psychological factors that are creating and/or helping to maintain their symptoms. The third method involves changing the individual's perception of the consequences or his or her symptoms.

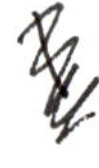

When hypnotic interventions are aimed at physiologic change there is an attempt to bring the nonvoluntary control systems under voluntary control. Direct suggestions are given to influence heart rate, blood flow, skin temperature, and other regulatory processes of the body. This is done in an attempt to alleviate the presenting symptoms. According to Spiegel (1975), control enhancement is utilized to increase an individual's sense of control by increasing and employing varied options in dealing with distressing symptoms. He delineated two methods of control enhancement: symptom alteration and attitude alteration. This procedure is similar to DePiano and Salzberg's third type of intervention where hypnosis is used to alter the way a patient perceives his or her disorder.

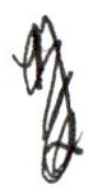

Treatment with this focus "veers the patient's attention away from his symptoms and concomitantly reminds him that more resourceful and effective means are available for his use in coping with problems of adaptation" (Spiegel, 1975, p. 1848). By altering attitudes held by the patient new, more adaptive, views can be adopted. DePiano and Salzberg (1979) indicate two salubrious effects of successful altered perceptions. Individuals may be able to function more adaptively when the debilitating effects of their symptoms are reduced and when the emotional response to the symptoms, which often exacerbate them, can be reduced.

The importance of helping the client gain insight into the disorder through the use of hypnosis has been pointed out by Bowers and Kelley (1979) and DePiano and Salzberg (1979). Frequently, it has been reported-particularly in case studies—that symptoms disappear soon after a connection is made between the symptoms and a significant aspect of the patient's experience.

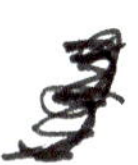

DePiano and Salzberg (1979) directed our attention to many of the methodological shortcomings of this type of research. The major problem has been the high number of case studies and multiple case studies and the few studies examining group data. Very few studies used a comparison group. Additional problems pointed out were vagueness in description of procedures, unreliable measuring devices, lack of control for experimenter bias, and placebo effects. With these limitations in mind let us look at the research on headaches, skin disorders, and asthma.

HEADACHES

Both migraine and tension headaches are common. Psychological factors often play a major role in their development and maintenance. Migraine headaches, an often debilitating problem, are precipitated by the vasoconstriction of cerebral blood vessels followed by an overcompensatory vasodilation. In addition to symptoms of severe pain, migraine may be accompanied by nausea and vomiting, chills, and other sensations which are mediated by the autonomic nervous system (Adams, Feuerstein & Fowler, 1980). Tension headaches are caused by prolonged muscle contraction about the face, scalp, and neck. In addition to pain, they are experienced as sensations of tightness, pressure, or constriction which vary widely in intensity, frequency, and duration.

In their review of hypnotic interventions employed in the treatment of headaches, DePiano and Salzberg (1979) examined nine studies. Seven of these studies attempted to change a specific physiological function by means of suggestions directed toward changing blood flow or directly suggesting the reduction or elimination of pain. Only one study focused on engendering insight, and the last study was an attempt to alter patients' perceptions. Five of the nine studies were case studies and suffered from many methodological shortcomings. However, DePiano and Salzberg concluded that, in spite of the methodological problems, hypnosis showed some promise as a treatment adjunct for headaches.

DePiano and Salzberg found the fewest studies using hypnosis in the treatment of headaches. There have been a surprisingly large number of studies applying hypnosis to the management of headache pain since the DePiano and Salzberg (1979) review. In fact, of the three disorders reviewed, most of the recent research in hypnosis has been in the treatment of headaches. A case study by Stambaugh and House (1977) use four treatment procedures with four reversals. The subject, a 51-year-old migraine sufferer, had a 23-year history of headaches which seemed to be exacerbated by stress. The first treatment procedure consisted of taped relaxation training with home practice. Then the therapist hypnotized the patient using a neutral hypnotic program initially, and later adding hypnotic glove anesthesia with transfer. The third procedure employed autohypnosis with heat transfer, and the fourth involved autohypnosis oriented towards posthypnotic analgesia. Headache duration, frequency and intensity were measured along with a tabulation of all consumption of analgesics. Both headache frequency and analgesic consumption showed an appreicable decrease only after the autohypnotic procedure was introduced. After the introduction of the first hypnotic treatment by the therapist, headache severity decreased 76 percent from baseline. The relaxation treatment did not lead to a decrement on any of the measures. Autohypnosis, therefore, was found to be the most effective treatment for dispelling pain in this one subject study. This finding would have to be replicated in a number of subjects before much credence could be given to it.

Another case study (Daniels, 1977) employed deep muscular and cue-controlled relaxation, hypnosis with handwarming, and cognitive behavior therapy in the treatment of severe migraine. The subject was a 38-year-old female with a 19-year history of migraines which had increased in severity during the last six years prior to treatment. After a reported six weeks of treatment, the subject was said to be symptom-free at a 12-month follow-up. No specific data was presented making it impossible to determine which intervention or combination of interventions was responsible for the treatment effect.

The role of hypnotizability or hypnotic susceptibility as it relates to treatment effectiveness has also been studied in a dissertation by Ubribe-de-Fazzano (1980) and in a study conducted by Friedman and Taub (1982). The latter looked at the interrelationship between hypnotic susceptibility, finger temperature elevation, and symptom relief. Twenty-three female subjects were divided into two groups in accordance with their hypnotic susceptibility. The highly hypnotizable group were each hypnotized and instructed to use visual imagery to increase their finger temperatures. The low susceptible subjects were given the same instructions, and were asked to simulate hypnosis. Both groups were instructed to engage in home practice using autohypnosis with the low susceptible subjects asked to go through the autohypnotic procedure in the same way as the highly susceptible group. Results indicated significant improvement in both groups on all measures. This improvement was maintained for at least six months. No difference was found between the high and low susceptible groups, suggesting that migraine pain reduction can be effected through hypnotic procedures with subjects of varied susceptibility.

In a 1980 dissertation by Uribe-de-Fazzano 26 subjects were matched in age, sex, and hypnotic susceptibility. Hypnotic treatment was compared to no treatment. No significant differences between the two groups were found, but both improved significantly in terms of the frequency, duration, and intensity of headache pain. However, a relationship was found between frequency of migraines and hypnotizability with the highly susceptible subjects reporting fewer headaches.

Bernal's (1978) dissertation compared hypnosis and biofeedback as to their effectiveness in treating tension headaches. He measured hypnotic susceptibility beforehand and assigned subjects of high, medium, and low susceptibility to each of four groups. One group received biofeedback, another hypnotic suggestion, a third group received alternating sessions of hypnosis and biofeedback, and the fourth group received pseudobiofeedback. Four self-report measures were administered during baseline, treatment, and follow-up. Level of muscle tension was also measured during the treatment phase. Results showed all three treatment groups were significantly more improved on two of the four self-report measures than the pseudobiofeedback control group. There were also significant measured decreases in frontalis tension in the three treatment groups but not for the control group. Two of the self-report measures showed no change. This highlights the need to use several measures for assessing change. This well-controlled study confirmed the usefulness of hypnosis as a treatment adjunct for tension headaches, and the quality of the research design was a great improvement over the bulk of the previous research in this area. This work was carried out at a "pain clinic" in the medical school of a major university illustrating how respectable hypnosis treatment has become.

Another two dissertations (Whalen, 1980; Schlutter, 1979) compared the efficiency of biofeedback and hypnosis in the treatment of tension headaches. Whalen (1980) found no relationship between hypnotizability and improvement, but supported Bernal's findings in that Whalen found biofeedback, hypnosis, and a combination of the two to be equally effective in controlling headache pain. Schlutter (1979) compared biofeedback, hypnosis, and progressive relaxation and found all treatments effective, corroborating the results of the other two studies. Apparently, all three dissertations were in progress at about the same time in different parts of the country on different populations and all came to similar independent conclusions.

In 1980, Schlutter, Golden, and Blume did another study comparing the effectiveness of hypnotic analgesia, frontalis biofeedback, and progressive relaxation with similar results. The researchers hypothesized that since significant improvement was documented in all treatment groups, relaxation was probably the significant variable responsible for the improvement. This study reported age as another significant variable as younger patients reported greater decrease in headache hours per week. Although Schlutter et al. posit relaxation as the common variable responsible for change, there is another possibility. All of these techniques also require focused concentration. Perhaps this type of concentration itself or in combination with other factors effected the change. More research is necessary to tease out the subtleties of these effects. However, hypnosis has certainly been recently shown to have great promise in the treatment of tension headaches.

There is still some justifiable criticism of hypnosis research in this area, even though the quality of research has shown great improvement recently. Case reports are still being published along with the well-controlled studies. The outcome data in this area is almost exclusively based on self-report which is practically inevitable in trying to assess headaches pain. Measurement has become more precise in the several recent well-executed studies on tension headaches. Standardizing hypnotic techniques used across studies and formulating a uniform definition of headache would be helpful in eventually finding appropriate and precise dependent measures. Whereas clinical case studies can have heuristic value early in the study of a phenomenon, it is heartening to see an increase in the proportion of well-executed controlled experimentation and particularly to see the good studies finding positive effects. DePiano and Salzberg (1979) reported, in looking at this research, that there was a relationship between less adequate research and more positive effects. This no longer appears to be the case.

SKIN DISORDERS

It has been stated "as the organ system most visible to inspection, the skin serves as a mirror of emotional states" (Engels and Wittkower, 1975, p. 1685). Disorders of the skin are often considered to have a psychological basis. Because the skin is richly supplied by small blood vessels, the autonomic nervous system is closely involved in its regulation. This close connection with the autonomic nervous system involves the skin in defensive reactions of the body such as the skin's development of allergic reactions and possibly of warts. When the natural immunological defensive reactions are exaggerated, disorders can arise (Bowers and Kelley, 1979).

DePiano and Salzberg reviewed 14 studies applying hypnotic interventions to the treatment of skin disorders. Nine of these focused on effecting direct physiological change, three were aimed at increasing subjects insight, and two were geared toward altering subjects' perceptions of their symptoms. The major and almost exclusive method of measuring effects of treatment was the observation of physical changes in the condition of the skin. Mediating physiological changes such as blood flow and skin temperature were generally not monitored. Only three of the studies used a treatment group and the two studies with a control group yielded negative results. It was surprising that hypnosis in the treatment of skin disorders yielded the poorest results as there had been many earlier published clinical reports of astonishing success using hypnosis to treat warts (Sulzberger and Wolf, 1934; Dunbar, 1954). Apparently there are high baseline rates of spontaneous remission of warts which must be controlled for in investigating treatments using hypnosis.

Unfortunately the research completed since the DePiano and Salzberg review continues to be uncontrolled case reports except for the Johnson and Barber (1978) investigation of the treatment of warts.

A case study is reported where hypnosis was applied to the treatment of psychogenic pupura (characterized by recurrent, painful echymoses) in a 27-year-old woman whose symptoms, prior to the hypnotic procedures, were unremitting. Suggestions of trance depth, relaxation, and positive change led to marked symptom improvement (Roden, 1979).

Although a viral etiology has been implicated in the development of some types of warts, Gravitz (1981) and Sheehan (1978) emphasize the importance of psychological factors in their appearance and remission. Sheehan presented two case studies employing hypnosis in the effective treatment of warts. In the first case Sheehan reports a 14-year-old girl's warts disappearing after, through the use of a hypnotic induction and autohypnosis, she recognized the underlying "meaning" of her warts. Treatment description was very vague.

In the second case, Sheehan (1978), the focus of the hypnotic intervention was on direct suggestions for physiological change. It was suggested that the patient visualize his wart melting away. Vascular changes surrounding the wart were noted immediately following the suggestion, and these changes lasted for fifteeen minutes. The wart disappeared in a week. It is impossible to determine if the "vascular changes" or spontaneous remisssion explained the disappearance of the wart.

Barber (1978) has postulated that hypnotic inductions in the treatment of skin disorders such as dermatitis and warts are superfluous. He has maintained that suggestion with a hypnotic induction would have the same effects. He postulated that "believed-in suggestions which are incorporated into ongoing conditions, affect blood supply in localized areas" (p. 25). Johnson and Barber (1978) randomly assigned 22 subjects to one or two groups. The hypnotic treatment group were given a standard 10-minute induction relying on suggestions for relaxation, drowsiness, and sleep. The comparison group received a treatment labeled "focused contemplation" which had all the elements of the hypnotic treatment, but they were not exposed to the standard hypnotic induction. Both groups were told to imagine tingling in the warts targeted for remission.

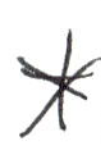

Only three of the 22 subjects showed remission of their warts; all were in the hypnotic group. Johnson and Barber attributed the remission of the warts in the three subjects to either spontaneous remission or the subjects "believed-in efficacy" of the hypnosis treatment and not to the effects of hypnosis. They argued that the focused contemplation group did not command the same set of expectancies. Barber and his colleagues have consistently argued against the effect of hypnosis, per se, in changing behavior, so it is not surprising that they did not attribute the wart remission to hypnosis in this study. Nevertheless, the data suggests that hypnosis, and not expectancies, accounted for the change.

The evidence for the effectiveness of hypnosis in treating skin disorders remains equivocal. More controlled clinical studies are needed, particularly those using autonomic measures in addition to observation of external skin changes. Altered blood flow as a mediator of change in skin disorders is an interesting area for further research. Much of the treatment of skin disorders in the past has involved the use of numerous useless salves, balms, and lotions and sometimes rather drastic attempts at alleviating symptoms such as X-ray radiation and acid. The expectations of the client has frequently been the major factor in cure. The controlled research in the use of hypnosis as a treatment can serve as a model for research using other treatment methods.

ASTHMA

It was believed earlier that allergic, infective, and psychological factors interacted in the etiology of asthma and that the importance of each factor varied with the age of the individual. Up until the age of 16, infective factors predominate, but psychological factors play an increasing role. Psychological factors progressively decrease in importance until middle age where psychological factors again became consequential (Rees, 1964). Coleman, Butcher, and Carson (1984) cite research by Alexander which casts doubt on the idea that the broncheolar constriction characteristic of asthma is brought on by emotional conflict. Coleman, et al. state "in many—perhaps most—cases of asthma there may be some type of innate vulnerability to interference with the autonomic regulation of breathing. Support for this position is provided by the fact that asthma attacks sometimes occur at times when the individual is not under stress" (p. 28). They do acknowledge that emotional factors may trigger an attack in some individuals and that some asthmatics learn to use their symptoms to control other people.

In spite of the fact that current thinking has emphasized physical factors over psychological factors in the etiology of asthma, DePiano and Salzberg (1979) found a great deal of good research investigating the use of hypnosis in the treatment of asthma. Of the three disorders, the greatest number of controlled studies on the largest number of subjects had been conducted on the use of hypnosis to treat asthma with improvement found especially when self-report was the dependent variable. Physiological measures of change were less promising. At the very least, asthma appeared to be the most fruitful area of research at the time of the DePiano and Salzberg review with the most applicability to clinical practice. Hypnosis was found to be effective when attempting to reduce symptoms by suggestions focusing on physiological change and by attempting to get patients to change the way in which they perceived their asthma.

In view of the relative success found using hypnosis to treat asthma, it was disappointing to find so few subsequent publications in this area. Only two case studies were found since the DePiano and Salzberg review. This drop in interest in research in this area may coincide with the change in current thinking about the importance of psychological factors in the etiology of asthma.

Lazar and Jedliczka (1979) reported the successful use of hypnosis with a moderately retarded 11-year-old boy. Neinstein and Dash (1982) reported hypnosis to have been a beneficial adjunct in the treatment of a 17-year-old male suffering from moderately severe asthmatic attacks. Four hypnotic sessions produced reported improvement which was maintained at a one-year follow-up. Unfortunately, these two cases studies add little to our knowledge or to our sophistication of research methodology in this promising area of research.

CONCLUSIONS

DePiano and Salzberg, in concluding their review of 38 studies of these three disorders, found asthma to be the best researched and most promising area for clinical application. Subsequent research appears to have emphasized asthma least, and the most and best research has been done in the treatment of headaches. Several carefully controlled studies in treating tension headaches found hypnosis effective in reducing several indices of headache symtomatology. DePiano and Salzberg suggested that future investigators should use measures of vasoconstriction and muscular tension along with the usual self-report measures. Bernal (1978) did indeed find a measured decrease in frontalis muscular tension in his hypnosis treatment group and not in his control group.

Except for some further speculation about vascular changes associated with wart remission, little theoretical sophistication has been added to the research on the use of hypnosis in treating skin disorders since the DePiano and Salzberg review. The precise role of mediating physiological mechanisms has yet to be systematically assessed.

DePiano and Salzberg called for several improvements in research methodology; control for spontaneous remission of symptoms, placebo effects, and assessment of hypnotic susceptibility using a standard research scale. Recent studies on skin disorders and asthma did not include these methodological improvements. Again, only the headache research incorporated many of these research design improvements.

Much work is yet to be accomplished in these areas, especially because hypnosis continues to be widely used clinically in the treatment of these disorders either as the sole treatment modality or as an adjunct to other treatments.

Scientific progress is helped by the efficiency with which scientists can communicate their results to one another. Because of the varied perspectives and lack of controls in hypnosis research, this communication has been difficult to achieve. Future research needs more clearly specified treatment procedures and dependent variables. Standard measures of hypnotizability and hypnotic induction procedures would help in the evaluation of treatment effectiveness across studies.

REFERENCES

Adams, H., Feuerstein, M., & Fowler, J. (1980). Migraine headache: Review of parameters, etiology, and intervention. *Psychological Bulletin, 87* (2), 217-238.

Barber, T. (1978). Hypnosis, suggestions, and psychosomatic phenomena: A new look from the standpoint of recent experimental studies. *The American Journal of Clinical Hypnosis, 21* (1), 13-27.

Bernal, G. (1978). *A study of the differential effectiveness of biofeedback and hypnosis for the treatment of tension headaches.* Unpublished doctoral dissertation. University of South Carolina, Columbia.

Bowers, A., & Kelly, P. (1979). Stress disease and hypnosis. *Journal of Abnormal Psychology, 88* (5), 490-505.

Coleman, J. C., Butcher, J. N., & Carson, R. C. (1984). *Abnormal psychology and modern life* (7th ed.) Glenview, IL: Scott Foresman.

Daniels, L. (1977). Treatment of migraine headache by hypnosis and behavior therapy: A case study. *American Journal of Clinical Hypnosis, 19* (4), 241-244.

DePiano, F., & Salzberg, H. (1979). Clinical applications of hypnosis to three psychosomatic disorders. *Psychological Bulletin, 86* (6), 1223-1235.

Dunbar, F. (1954). *Emotions and bodily changes* (4th ed.) New York: Columbia University Press.

Engels, D., & Wittkower, E. (1975). Psychophysiological allergic and skin disorders. In A. Freedman, H. Kaplan, & B. Sadock (Eds.), *Comprehensive Textbook of Psychiatry* (Vol. 1, 2nd ed.) Baltimore: Williams & Wilkins.

Friedman, H. & Taub, H., (1982). An evaluation of hypnotic susceptibility and peripheral temperature elevation in the treatment of migraine. *American Journal of Clinical Hypnosis, 24* (3), 172-182.

Gravitz, M. (1981). The production of warts by suggestion as a cultural phenomenon. *American Journal of Clinical Hypnosis, 23* (4), 281-283.

Johnson, R., & Barber, T. (1978). Hypnosis, suggestions, and warts: An experimental investigation implicating the importance of "believed-in efficacy". *American Journal of Clinical Hypnosis, 20* (30), 165-174.

Lazar, B., & Jedliczka, Z. (1979). Utilization of manipulative behavior in a retarded asthmatic child. *American Journal of Clinical Hypnosis, 21,* (4) 287-292.

Neinstein, L. & Dash, J. (1982). Hypnosis as an adjunct therapy for asthma: Case report. *Journal of Adolescent Health Care, 3* (1), 45-48 (Abstract)

Rees, L. (1964). The importance of psychological, allergic, and infective factors in childhood asthma, *Journal of Psychosomatic Research* 7, 253-262.

Roden, R. (1979). Psychoanalytically oriented hypnotic treatment of autoerythrocytic sensitization and blindness. *American Journal of Clinical Hypnosis, 21* (4) 278-281.

Schlutter, L. (1979). A comparison of treatments for prefrontal muscle contraction headache. *Dissertation Abstracts International,* 39, 5086B. (University Microfilm No. 79-04, 890)

Schlutter, L., Golden, G., & Blume, H. (1980). A comparison of treatments for prefrontal muscle contraction headache. *British Journal of Medical Psychology, 53,* 47-52.

Sheehan, D. (1978). Influence of psychosocial factors on wart remission. *American Journal of Clinical Hypnosis, 20,* 160-164.

Spiegel, H. (1975). Hypnosis: An adjunct to psychotherapy. In A. Freedman, H. Kaplan, & B. Sadock (Eds.), *Comprehensive Textbook of Psychiatry,* (Vol. 1, 2nd ed.). Baltimore: Williams & Wilkins.

Stambaugh, E., & House, A. (1977). Multimodality treatment of migraine headache: A case study utilizing biofeedback, relaxation, autogenic and hypnotic treatments. *American Journal of Clinical Hypnosis, 19* (4), 235-240.

Sulzberger, M. B., & Wolf, J. (1934). The treatment of warts by suggestion. *Medical Record of New York,* 140, 552-556.

Uribe-de-Fazzano, C. (1980). Effectiveness of hypnosis in the treatment of migraine: The role of hypnotizability. *Dissertation Abstracts International, 41,* 703B. (University Microfilm No. 80-18, 169)

Wadden, T., & Anderton, C. (1982). The clinical use of hypnosis. *Psychological Bulletin, 91* (2), 215-243.

Whalen, S. (1980). The use of EMG biofeedback and hypnosis in treatment of tension headaches. *Dissertation Abstracts International, 40,* 4014B. (University Microfilm No. 80-03, 139)

PART IV

Hypnosis and Enhanced Performances

Chapter 9

Effects of Hypnosis on Physical and Athletic Performance

Sharon Jacobs
University of South Carolina

Cheryl Gotthelf
Nova University

Studies in physical and athletic performance have been of interest to hypnosis investigators for the past ninety years. Experimental work in this area dates back to 1889 when Moll (1889/1958) claimed that the hypnotized subject "may exert a degree of strength which is quite impossible under normal conditions." Since that time, a considerable number of research studies have evaluated the relationship between hypnosis and physical performance, but results are contradictory.

This chapter will critically examine the studies which have been published in the literature including significant early research that led to the more recent investigations. The three major areas discussed include muscular strength and endurance, motor performance, and athletic performance.

OVERVIEW OF PRE-1972 LITERATURE

Early reviews of the literature on hypnosis and physical performance by Hull (1933), Gorton (1949), Crasilneck and Hall (1959), Johnson (1961b), and Weitzenhoffer (1963) basically concluded that in some situations hypnosis enhances physical performance. However, the conditions under which this occurs are ambiguous. Comparisons between these earlier studies are difficult to perform because of the variations in procedures, depths of trances, and content and style of suggestions (Johnson, 1961b; Weitzenhoffer, 1963). However, these early studies indicate that hypnotic suggestions to decrease performance are more likely to be effective.

Barber (1966) examined the experimental studies on hypnosis and performance and reported that (1) the research fails to demonstrate that hypnosis (without direct suggestion for improved performance) has any significant effect on muscular strength and endurance and (2) motivational suggestions are as effective in enhancing performance when given to subjects in the waking state as in the hypnotic state. He cautions, however, that the evidence is equivocal due to methodological inadequacies which include a lack of random assignment to groups and failure to counterbalance the experimental treatments or to control for experimenter bias.

More recently, Morgan (1972) reviewed the research related to hypnosis and and its effect on muscular strength and endurance, physiological variables, psychomotor behavior, and athletic performance. He concluded that efforts to decrease physical performance by means of hypnotic suggestions are generally effective but recognized that one would also intuitively expect similar results when testing subjects in the waking state. In fact, Morgan (1972) identified the confounding of suggestion and state as one of the most serious methodological problems in the experimental research. A comprehensive analysis of methodological problems may be found in Sheehen and Perry (1976).

MUSCULAR STRENGTH AND ENDURANCE

In 1949, Mead and Roush made a significant contribution to the hypnosis research literature because the results of their study highlighted the importance of task specificity when examining the relationship of hypnosis to muscular performances. The investigators did not confound treatment with suggestions, reported the reliability of the assessment instruments, and used a larger number of subjects than previous studies (Morgan, 1972). They examined the effects of hypnosis on an arm dynamometer (a measure of elbow flexion), and a hanging by hands task (a measure of endurance) with 11 highly susceptible female subjects. Standardized instructions that suggested increased strength and an ability to do well were read to subjects while they were being tested in both the control and waking states. Subjects performed significantly better under hypnosis on the arm dynamometer test, but there were no significant differences on the grip dynamometer of endurance test. Watkins (1949) stated that "one of the limiting factors in muscular work, particularly maximum efforts of short duration, is pain or discomfort or apprehension" (p. 705) and hypothesized that the arm dynamometer test produces less discomfort than other tests. Since suggestions were given only to increase strength, Watkins (1949) proposed that the discomfort factor led to the differences in performance for the various tasks.

Roush (1951) replicated the Mead and Roush study but changed the standardized instructions to include suggestions of painlessness and numbness throughout the tests. Additional changes included testing subjects under three conditions–waking, hypnotic, and posthypnotic–and counterbalancing the order of testing. Five male and 10 females capable of amnesic somnabulism participated in this study. Results indicated that the performance on the endurance test was not significantly different under the various conditions. Performance on the hand and arm dynamometer indicated that subjects demonstrated increased strength in the hypnotic and posthypnotic state than in the waking state. Performances in the hypnotic and posthypnotic states were not significantly different. Roush (1951) suggested that instructions to disregard pain leads to enhanced performance under hypnosis and that this is the result of the inhibition of those factors which usually limit maximum performance in the waking state. Subjects were also given the same instructions in the waking state, however, so it appears unlikely that these instructions, per se, account for the increased performances under the hypnotic condition. One limitation of this study is that some of the subjects participated in the previous study so it is difficult to assess if the effects are due to their previous experience or to the effect of the experimental treatment.

Johnson and Kramer (1961) report a dramatic example of a "superhuman feat" performed under hypnosis. The subject, a professional athlete, initially demonstrated an exceptional performance under the waking control condition on the supine press of a 47-pound barbell (endurance task). He almost doubled his performance under the three hypnotic trials. When retested later without hypnosis or suggestions, his performance was more than 2½ times greater than his initial performance. Subsequent age regression by the investigators indicated that the subject accepted the suggestions of increased strength and endurance as unquestionable truths. Nevertheless, it is difficult to explain why some subjects accept hypnotic suggestions so vividly and unquestionably and how this interacts with other variables to enable some individuals to perform with exceptional strength and endurance. Methodologically, this study may be easily criticized as there was an inaccurate measure of baseline performance; however, if one accepts it validity, the possibility of replications with other individuals and other tasks is a factor that contributes to the spurring interest in understanding the relationship between hypnosis and muscular strength and endurance.

Johnson and his colleagues (Johnson & Kramer, 1960; Johnson & Kramer, 1961, and Johnson, Massey & Kramer, 1960) conducted a series of additional investigations in the early 1960s with highly susceptible male subjects who were athletes or physical education majors in excellent physical condition. In the first study, Johnson et al. (1960) evaluated the effects of posthypnotic suggestions on a maximal effort of short duration of 100 revolutions of a bicycle ergometer with 26.8 pounds of resistance. The 10 subjects were hypnotized and the experimental treatment included suggestions to increase strength and feel free from fatigue. Testing was performed after subjects were awakened from the hypnotic trance. Posthypnotic suggestions of improved ability did not facilitate performance, however, Johnson et al. (1960) pointed out that the subjects previous athletic experiences "had already accustomed them, more or less to the discomfort of acute fatigue symptoms–with the results that posthypnotic suggestions to ignore such discomfort might not be as effective with them as with nonathletic subjects" (p. 145). Johnson and Kramer (1960) assessed the effect of various types of hypnotic suggestions on a supine press of a 47-pound barbell to exaustion. Ten subjects participated in four counterbalanced treatments: (1) stereotyped suggestions (deliberate, quiet, and authoritative) of improved performance while in a hypnotic state; (2) pep talk suggestions (urgent, excited) appealing to subjects' egos given in a hypnotic state; (3) posthypnotic suggestions of improved performance given in a hypnotic state but acted upon after awakening; and (4) posthypnotic failure suggestions of decreased performance given in the hypnotic state but acted upon the waking state. Subjects' performance under stereotyped, pep-talk and posthypnotic suggestions did not differ significantly; however, performances under posthypnotic suggestions for failure was significantly lower than the other three conditions. In a third study, Johnson and Kramer (1961) assessed the effects of various types of nonhypnotic, hypnotic, and posthypnotic suggestions on strength as measured by hand dynamometer, power, as measured by a jump and reach test, and endurance which was measured by supine press of 47 pound barbell to exaustion. The 11 subjects, some of whom had participated in previous studies, underwent four counterbalanced treatments: (1) waking control; (2) deep hypnotic trance; (3) deep hypnotic trance with performance tested upon awakening; and (4) light hypnotic trance with posthypnotic testing. The light trance consisted of instructions to remain completely awake and aware of the environment (with the exception of visual cues) and be able to recall hypnotic suggestions. Standardized suggestions of improved performance were given under each experimental condition. Statistical significance was found only in the endurance task when deep and light hypnotic trance suggestions with posthypnotic performance were compared with suggestions given in the waking state.

The studies evaluated thus far lend support to the view that enhancement of performance through hypnosis is task specific. The extent to which the susceptibility of subjects, their level of physical training, and subjects' sex interact with treatment effects remain unclear. The following group of reports evaluate the effects of various types of suggestions on motor performance.

London and Fuhrer (1961) evaluated the performances of 16 highly susceptible female subjects and 16 unsusceptible female subjects on a hand dynamometer, weight holding, and tremor task, under balanced hypnotic and waking conditions. Subjects received exhortation instructions (motivational suggestions designed to convince subjects of their ability to overcome their previous performance limits and to reinterpret feelings of fatigue and discomfort as signals to continue rather than to stop), and were retested under both experimental conditions. Results indicated that (1) low susceptible subjects consistently performed better than high susceptible subjects, (2) hypnosis with no suggestions for improved performance had no effect on strength or endurance, and (3) exhortation instructions are equally effective in the hypnotic and waking state. In a complementary study, Barber and Calverly (1964) assessed the strength of grip and weight holding endurance of 60 female subjects. Subjects were then randomly assigned to one of the four following treatment groups: (1) task motivating instructions which consist of instructions suggesting to subjects that they are capable of producing and are expected to produce excellent performances; (2) hypnotic induction; (3) hypnotic induction and task motivating instructions; and (4) control. The strength of grip was not significantly influenced by any of the experimental treatments whereas weight-holding endurance was negatively affected by the hypnotic induction. However, significant results were demonstrated by subjects on the weight-holding task when they received motivational instructions with or without hypnosis, suggesting that motivational instructions may be the significant variable in efforts to improve motor performance.

Additional studies concerning the influence of exhortation instructions have been pursued by Slotnik and his colleagues (Slotnik, Liebert & Hilgard, 1965; Slotnik & London, 1965). In 1965, Slotnik and London assigned 50 female subjects who were either high or low hypnotizables to one of three experimental groups or a control group. With the exception of the control group (which always performed in the waking state), groups were tested under both hypnotic and waking conditions on hand dynamometer, weight endurance, and tremor tasks. The groups differed in that they received either base rate instructions, analgesic instructions, exhortative instructions, or a combination of the latter two. The design allowed the experimenters to assess combined and separate effects of analgesic and exhortation instructions, waking and hypnotic states, and the susceptibility of subjects. Results indicated that special instructions are effective in improving performance of the grip dynamometer and muscular endurance tasks, but only under hypnotic treatment. This contradicts earlier research but may be partially explained by the investigators failure to counterbalance experimental treatments; therefore, order effects and demand characteristics may influence results. Another interesting finding is that exhortative instructions appear to be more effective than analgesic instructions. The results of this study suggest that hypnosis may interact with instructions to produce task specific effects on performance.

In a related study, Slotnik et al. (1965) investigated the effects of exhortation instructions and exhortation plus involving instructions, which are statements repeated by the subjects themselves on a muscular endurance task. Twelve high susceptible females who were pretested in a hypnotic state following exhortation instructions were matched according to their pretest performances and assigned to a group in which they received exhortation and involving instructions in either waking or hypnotic state. Both groups improved with combined instructions, however, the hypnotic group improved significantly more than the waking group.

A recent study by Albert and Williams (1975) assessed the effects of posthypnotic suggestions on maximal endurance capacity, subjective ratings of perceived exertion, and heart rate. Twenty highly susceptible subjects were tested on a bicycle ergometer and after being matched on pretest scores, were assigned to posthypnotic or waking suggestion groups. Suggestions to facilitate performance, retard performance, and neutral suggestions were given in randomized order to all subjects. Endurance time was not significantly different between groups with facilitative suggestions. Suggestions to retard performance led to a significant decrease in endurance time only for those in the hypnotic group. Neutral suggestions had no effect on performance. The perceived rates of exertion were in the predicted direction, but the posthypnotic suggestions had the strongest effect. Heart rate was not significantly different across groups. One interesting finding of this study was the nonoccurrence of a significant decrement in performance in waking control subjects following suggestions designed to inhibit their performance. In a similar study, Jackson, Gass, and Camp (1979) assessed the relationship between endurance on a treadmill task and posthypnotic suggestions. Fifty-five male subjects who were able to reach maximum endurance performance were assigned to one of the following groups: (1) hypnosis alone; (2) motivating instructions alone; (3) low susceptibles with motivating instructions; (4) high susceptibles with motivating instructions; and (5) control. The highly susceptible subjects receiving hypnosis and motivational instructions and those receiving only motivational suggestions demonstrated significant improvement in performance on a treadmill task. Low susceptible subjects receiving task-motivating suggestions did not show improvement in performance. This study lends some support to Barber's (1966) conclusion that exhortation suggestions enhance performance whether given in the hypnotic or waking state, but also suggests that there is an interaction between response to these instructions and hypnotic susceptibility.

The studies investigating the effects of various suggestions on performance indicate that performance may be enhanced by means of task-motivating suggestions. Exhortation instructions are more effective than analgesic instructions and this effect may be enhanced with involving instructions; however, the research is equivocal as to whether or not these instructions are equally effective in the waking and hypnotic state. Several design inadequacies are apparent including failure to counterbalance treatment or control for demand characteristics, experimenter bias, or subject expectancies. In more methodologically rigid studies, results indicate that these suggestions are equally effective under hypnotic or waking conditions (Barber & Calvery, 1964; Jackson, et al., 1979).

Evans and Orne (1965) and Slater (1967) have conducted important studies that have highlighted the influence of order effects and subject expectancy on muscular performance. In a well--designed study, Evans and Orne (1965) tested 36 males and 24 females for hypnotic susceptibility, hand dynamometer, weight-holding endurance, and tremor task. Testing was counterbalanced with one-half of the subjects tested under hypnosis first and the other half tested in the waking state. Baseline measures of endurance were significantly higher when subjects were tested in the waking condition first and the only difference between baseline and hypnotic endurance trials was under this condition. Performance on the hand dynamometer also indicated a similar trend; however, there were no significant differences found for level of susceptibility or the experimental treatment. Although subjects reported that the suggestions of drowsiness and deep relaxation had a negative effect on their performance, Evans and Orne (1965) hypothesized that the subjects performances decreased from the hypnotic to the waking state because of their expectations that performance should be higher under hypnosis. The authors recommend that these expectations and other demand characteristics of the experimental situation be carefully assessed in future studies. Slater (1967) assessed the strength of grip of 72 male subjects and then asked them if they expected hypnosis to improve their performance. Subjects were stratified according to expectancy and randomly assigned to hypnotic and waking conditions. Both groups were retested following task-motivational instructions. There was no significant effect on performance due to hypnosis or expectancy alone, but the interaction of the two variables was significant. Therefore, if subjects expect hypnosis to improve performance, it is more likely to do so.

The results of studies investigating the effects of hypnosis and suggestions on muscular performance have been evaluated. The specific tasks involved include performance on hand dynamometer, weight holding, supine barbell press, treadmill, bicycle ergometer, and/or tremor task. Results indicate, (1) hypnosis alone does not have a significant effect on performance; (2) motivational instructions appear to be equally effective whether given in the hypnotic or waking state, however, this finding needs additional systematic investigation; (3) posthypnotic suggestions to inhibit performance produce significant changes in the predicted direction, however, similar suggestions given to waking subjects did not produce similar results and needs replication; and (4) order effects subject expectancies, and other subject characteristics (i.e., susceptibility, physical fitness) may interact in a unique way to influence muscular performance.

MOTOR PERFORMANCE

Recently, investigators have been interested in the relationship between hypnosis and motor performance. In contrast to studies regarding muscular performance, most of these studies focus on the influence of hypnotic suggestions on reaction time and motor learning.

Edmonston and Marks (1967) studied the effects of hypnosis with task motivating instruction instructions on learning a complex motor sequence task. Subjects were tested for kinesthetic learning rather than physical endurance or coordination. Twenty-four male subjects, matched for susceptibility, were assigned to one of the following groups: (1) hypnosis with task-motivating instructions: (2) hypnosis with task-motivating instructions and deepening suggestions; (3) task-motivating instructions alone; and (4) control group. Experimental treatments did not facilitate performance. Edmonston and Marks (1967) acknowledge that these results are contradictory with literature that demonstrated a facilitative effect of task motivating instructions on muscular performance; however, these results are consistent with those of other investigations reviewed in the previous section that found no significant influence of instructions on the performance of a tremor task. The choice point stylus maze task used in the Edmonston and Marks (1967) study is similar to the tremor task in that it is dependent on skill rather than exertion. Arnold (1971) investigated the effect of hypnosis and involving suggestions on learning two novel skills, mirror tracing (fine motor) and ball bouncing (gross motor). Forty-five highly susceptible male subjects either received positive and involving suggestions in the waking state as posthypnotic suggestions, or served as controls. Fifteen unsusceptible male subjects received positive involving suggestions in the waking state. The experimental treatments had no effect on learning for either susceptible or unsusceptible subjects. The results of these studies indicate that positive involving, or exhortative instructions with or without hypnosis, are not effective in enhancing performance on a skilled task.

A number of investigations have evaluated the relationship of hypnosis and suggestions to performance on reaction time tasks. Graham, Olsen, Parrish, and Leibowitz (1968) assessed 10 subjects on a stimulus response task under prehypnotic conditions with the hypnotic states counterbalanced across subjects to control for order effects. There was a significant performance decrement under the hypnotic condition which increased when fatigue suggestions were added. Rader (1972) randomly assigned sixty male subjects to one of four conditions; hypnosis with exhortation instruction; hypnosis; exhortation instructions in the waking state; and control. Groups that received motivating instructions performed significantly better than the control group. Hypnosis alone signifigantly decreased reaction time. Rader (1972) concluded that the motivating instructions (1) accounted for the faster reaction time and (2) undermined the relaxation effects of a traditional hypnotic induction. Ham and Edmonston (1971) assigned 30 highly susceptible male subjects to a relaxation induction, alert induction, or relaxation control group. The mean reaction time on a simple visual task was significantly faster for the alert induction group. The relaxation group and the traditional induction group did not differ in performance. The investigators concluded that it is the suggestions of relaxation and not the altered state that produces retardation in reaction time and they recommend the use of alert inductions when attempting to enhance motor performance or learning.

These studies indicate hypnosis alone retards performance on a reaction time task; however, this effect was removed by motivational instructions and alert induction techniques which suggests that relaxation may be the critical variable inhibiting performance.

Fehr and Stern (1967) examined the effect of hypnosis on the reaction time of 24 female subjects. Subjects performed a simple vigilance task in either the hypnotic or waking condition and an extraneous auditory stimulus was repeatedly presented throughout the task. Hypnotized subjects responded slower than control subjects and were less responsive to extraneous stimulation. In a similar study, Blum and Porter (1974) compared the performance of three highly susceptible hypnotic subjects with three unselected nonhypnotic controls. Hypnotic subjects were given posthypnotic suggestions for deafness to an irrelevant tone for half the experimental trials; control subjects were given similar waking suggestions to ignore the tone. Only the posthypnotic suggestions were effective in attenuating the alerting effect of the tone and slowing down reaction time. Their reports indicate that hypnotic subjects are less responsive to external cues and support Hilgard's (1965) contention that hypnosis results in a narrowing of attention.

In a case study with a highly susceptible female subject, Blum and Wohl (1971) investigated the effects of monetary, intrinsic, and hypnotically-induced affective states as incentive conditions for a reaction time task. The incentive conditions did not elicit significantly different reaction times; however, without baseline assessments, the results of this study may indicate superior performance across the three incentive conditions.

In order to assess the relationship between psychomotor speed in the normal and waking state, Kratochvil and Shubat (1971) assessed the speed of finger-tapping and circle-drawing for 12 highly susceptible subjects under hypnotic and waking conditions. There was no difference in maximal speed for either task in the hypnotic or waking state. The authors concluded that psychomotor speed in the hypnotic state is partly a function of psychomotor speed in the waking state.

Other studies regarding the relationship of hypnosis to motor performance concern the effects of suggestions to slow down or speed up the subjective experience of time. Zimbardo and his collagues (Zimbardo, Maslach, & Marshal, 1972; Zimbardo, Marshal, White & Maslach, 1973) compared the performance of highly susceptible subjects on a key-tapping task after receiving suggestions for time distortion under hypnotic, hypnotic simulation, or a waking non hypnotized control condition. Subjects were taught to press a key at different rates in order to illuminate various target lights. The order in which instructions for time distortion were given were counterbalanced across subjects and did not significantly effect task behavior. The two studies differed in that Zimbardo et al. (1973) provided objective feedback for half the subjects during both experimental trials. Only the hypnotic subjects in both experiments were able to significantly alter their sense of personal time. Performance was in direction that paralleled the suggestions. Although external feedback improved all subjects' performance, it was the most effective for the simulation and waking group which suggests that they were responding primarily to the task rather than to an internalized altered sense of time. These studies lend further support to the view that hypnosis involves a narrowing of attention and suggests that this focus is toward the inner, subjective reality of the individual.

Two recent experiments by Baer (1979; 1980) assessed the effects of time-slowing suggestions on performance. Baer (1979) trained five highly susceptible females to maintain an operant response on a variable interval schedule of reinforcement. Subjects were than given posthypnotic suggestions for time-slowing and performance was assessed using a within-subjects withdrawl design. Subjects received continuous feedback about the correctness of their responses and were led to believe that their speed of responding would determine the number of tokens they earned. During the time distortion, four of the five subjects showed noticeable decreases in their mean response rate as compared to their preceding baseline performance. In a postexperiment inquiry, the fifth subject reported that she was not sure she was hypnotized and the author hypnothesized that she was not suggestible to time slowing suggestions and/or the brief presentation of these suggestions was not adequate for her to acquire the skill. Baer (1980) assessed the effects of time-slowing suggestions on performance accuracy in a perceptual motor task. Three highly susceptible subjects participated in playing a video sports game. Suggestions for time slowing were presented and included imagery regarding the ball bouncing slowly across the screen. Control was established by using hypnotic induction with time-normal suggestions for each subject. Three sessions took place. Results showed that time slowing suggestions led to performance decreases in the first session; however, the second and third phase of time distortion suggestions resulted in significantly longer volleys than during the control periods. These studies are important because they provide an objective assessment of the behavioral effects of time-slowing suggestions. The small sample size and lack of appropriate waking control comparisons limit generalization of results.

In sum, the results of 12 recent studies that assessed the relationship of hypnosis and suggestions to motor performance suggest: (1) Exhortation and involving suggestions have no effect on learning a motor task: (2) traditional hypnotic inductions inhibit reaction time but this effect may be eliminated with task-motivational instructions or alert inductions; (3) hypnosis involves a narrowing of attention and increases the individual's responsiveness to internal cues; (4) hypnotic suggestions to slow down the experience of time may facilitate learning a visual motor task. These conclusions can only be tentative presently since additional replications in well-designed studies with rigorous methodological controls are yet to be done.

ATHLETIC PERFORMANCE

This last section focuses specifically on the application of hypnosis to athletic performance. The emphasis is on complex motor behavior whereas the previous section dealt with relatively simple motor responses. Unfortunately, at this point in time the literature consists primarily of anecdotal reports and case studies.

The following reports are primarily concerned with alleviating psychological problems that interfere with sports performance. For example, Naruse (1965) discusses performance anxiety in terms of "stage fright." This acute and intense psychological stress may occur at the time of competition. or days and weeks in advance. The author utilized progressive relaxation, direct hypnotic suggestions, and posthypnotic suggestions to induce autohypnosis in order to train several champion and amateur athletes in self-hypnosis. The individual's personality characteristics and experience of stage fright would then determine which additional hypnotic techniques were used. These include: physiological relaxation by means of autogenic training; dissociation from reality by detatching one's self from sports or everyday life in order to relax; catharsis and self-understanding in order to help the individual become aware of the psychological problems that interfere with performance; mental rehearsal by imagining performing in the actual situation in order to gain practice or desensitize fears; and mental warming up or creating a mental set to increase concentration and competitiveness. Naruse (1965) presents anecdotal evidence of the effects of these techniques on the performances of athletes involved in a variety of sports. McCord (1970) hypnotized a professional athlete who was concerned about his performance. After receiving posthypnotic suggestions of improved performance, the athlete reported lifting weights that were 25 pounds heavier than he had ever lifted previously.

The above reports indicate that hypnosis aimed at increasing relaxation and alleviating psychological anxiety may have positive and enhancing effects on the performance of athletes. Unfortunately, since the studies reviewed are limited to case studies, the results are only suggestive.

Johnson (1961b) presented a unique study involving a baseball player who was having difficulty batting. The subject was unable to identify the problems with his performance in a waking state. In a hypnotic state, however, he was able to identify a multitude of problems in timing, coordination, and position. Although the pretreatment batting average was not reported. Johnson indicated that the subject finished the season with a .400 average. Johnson suggested that it was the hypnotic state that enabled the individual to possess "extensive body movement awareness which is apparently not ordinarily accessible to conscious verbal representation" (p.263). It would be interesting to see if other techniques such as relaxation or imagery training would achieve the same effects.

Ryde (1964) has used a somewhat different application of hypnosis to athletic performance. Although he does not attempt to facilitate athletic performance directly, he uses hypnotic techniques to alleviate the minor ailments of athletes (i.e., tennis elbow, shin splints) that interfere with performance.

The use of hypnosis in facilitating athletic performance does not appear to be very common. A recent survey of sports psychologists (Ogilvie, 1979) indicated that relaxation training, motor visual rehearsal, and autogenic training are the preferred techniques. Nevertheless, the literature that was reviewed suggests that hypnosis may successfully alleviate certain psychological, behavioral, or physical problems that interfere with athletic performance. Whether or not the effects of hypnosis would produce clinically significant improvements in sports performances is debatable. Carefully controlled, systematic research in this area is needed. Additionally, comparative studies are needed to rule out the likely possibility that other techniques are equally effective in achieving these goals.

CONCLUSIONS

Although well-controlled outcome studies generally have provided equivocal support for hypnosis as facilitating athletic or motor performances, case reports indicate positive results. This section will address an explanation for the discrepancies in results, and suggests the possibility that there may be conditions under which hypnosis may facilitate performance. Finally, some tentative ideas will be discussed regarding treatment considerations and methodology.

A weakness found in much of the hypnosis literature is that a multidimensenional approach to increase performance has not been considered. There may not be sufficient incentive for a subject participating in a study to improve performance because the tasks are generally not interesting enough to promote a subject to put forth an all-out effort. Subjects who are the focus of a case report are generally goal-oriented with regard to their performance. In other words, there is sufficient motivation to increase performance, such that it becomes important enough to these subjects to improve. Personality factors also may need to be considered in studies of performance and hypnosis. Muscular tension and/or high levels of anxiety are known to decrease performance. Anxiety is the most commonly cited reason for seeking hypnosis treatment to improve performance. Concentration and attention factors are important components of athletic and motor performance. Practice effect contributes to the acquisition of skills; however, the cognitive set with which one enters a situation may influence outcome.

Given that individual differences exist among people, there may be a combination of factors under which an increase in performance could be seen. A population with specific characteristics may benefit more than others. For example, subjects who score high on hypnotic susceptibility scales have been known to accept suggestions more readily than those who score low (Jackson, Gass, & Camp, 1979). Another variable may be the physical ability one has regarding a physical activity. A basic understanding or competence in an activity must be present before it can be improved upon. Another consideration is how suggestions are given. Direct suggestions for improving specific motor movements have been found to be more effective than general non-task specific suggestions (Barber, 1966). Evans and Orne (1965) have found that demand characteristics in the context of expectancy can also influence performance. Following this line of reasoning it may well be possible that subjects who are told to expect performance improvements may benefit. Additionally, time-slowing suggestions have been shown to be effective in achieving a narrowed focus of attention and concentration which may facilitate visual acuity and motor movement (Baer, 1979, 1980; Zimbardo et al 1973). Finally, relaxation training with imagery and autohypnosis skills may assist subjects to decrease anxiety, thereby increasing performance.

There has been a lack of consistency between the results of hypnosis and performance studies done in the laboratory and those presented as case reports. Some of the variables that need to be examined include motivation, incentive to improve performance, personality variables, and basic ability to perform the task in question. Additionally, the literature has outlined some conditions under which a subject could improve or increase performance. It appears that if the following conditions were combined, performance could be enhanced. (1) high hypnotic susceptibility, (2) direct suggestions to improve performance, (3) waking suggestions for improved performance to set up expectancy, and (4) relaxation training.

Many sports psychologists who employ hypnosis as a means to improve performance have suggested several treatment approaches. In general, it appears that most athletes benefit from some type of relaxation training (Naruse, 1965). Initially, the training should focus on teaching the athlete to discriminate between tension and relaxation. This can be accomplished by contrast exercise in which the student tightly contracts a muscle group such as the forearm (by making a tight fist), then releases. The difference between tension and relaxation is pointed out with each successive muscle group to make the student aware of subtle differences. When discrimination training has been completed, a progressive relaxation or another comparable method should be taught to condition a relaxed response. Since this is a learned conditioning model, the athlete needs to practice this technique daily. This can be accomplished initially be means of an audio tape recording or autohypnosis instructions. When this skill has been conditioned sufficiently to elicit a relaxation response, hypnotic inductions can be easily achieved and direct suggestions can be implemented. These may include appropriate imagery scenarios to decrease performance anxiety. For example, one type of imagery might include suggestions for optimal performance in a nonthreatening setting. Imagery might also be used to pinpoint a subtle change that needs to be made in the execution of a movement to increase performance. Time-slowing or slow motion suggestions may be facilitative in changing a cognition regarding a motor movement. This method often permits close scrutiny of a performance. An example of when this would be particularly applicable is in a situation where speed is emphasized as in swimming competition. Generally, the input from a coach or trainer may be helpful in structuring suggestions. Other suggestions include ego strengthening, positive self-statements, and concentration and attention on the task which can help to block out environmental cues that distract from performance.

Many practitioners report that hypnotic treatment to improve athletic performance can be accomplished in a four to six week period if the student is motivated to practice by means of audio tape recordings or autohypnosis conditioning techniques. The ultimate goal in general is to provide the athlete with the proper conditioned learning skills to elicit the desired response, thereby increasing performance and decreasing dependency on the hypnotist.

SUMMARY

This chapter has presented a review of those reports on the effects of hypnosis on muscular strength and endurance, motor performance, and athletic performance. Some of the conclusions reached at this point are that hypnosis. (1) does not improve simple motor performance; (2) does not augment the effect of task-motivating suggestions; and (3) does not inhibit performance except on reaction time tasks; however, this decrease in performance appears to be the result of the effects of relaxation. Hypnotic suggestions to drecrease performance have a significant effect in the predicted direction. One hypothesis is that this effect is due to the asymptopic level of performance in these tasks which only allows for limited improvement. In contrast, there is greater room for variability in behavior following suggestions designed to inhibit performance.

New and promising areas of investigation concering the effects of time distortion lend insight into the characteristics of the hypnotic state and suggest applications regarding the use of hypnosis in enhancing performance. For example, suggestions to slow down the experience of time may improve critical evaluations of performance difficulties (see Johnson, 1961b). Suggestions to speed up the experience of time might improve reaction time on certain tasks (see Baer, 1979). Competing alternative explanations such as the effects of relaxation or experimental demand characteristics accounting for the observed effects need to be ruled out with additional studies and well-controlled replications.

REFERENCES

Albert, I., & Williams, M. H. (1975). Effects of posthypnotic suggestions on muscular endurance. Perceptual and Motor Skills 40, 131-139.

Arnold, J. (1971). Effects of hypnosis on the learning of two motor skills. *Research Quarterly, 42,* 1-6.

Baer, L. (1979). Effect of time-slowing suggestions on rate of emission of an operant response. *Psychological Record, 29,* 389-400.

Baer, L. (1980). Effect of a time-slowing suggestion on performance accuracy on a perceptual motor task. *Perceptual and Motor Skills, 51,* 167-176.

Barber, T.X. (1966). The effects of 'hypnosis' and motivational suggestions on strength and endurance. A critical review of research studies. *British Journal of Social Clinical Psychology, 5,* 42-50.

Barber, T.X., & Calvery, D. S. (1964). Toward a theory of hypnotic behavior. Enhancement of strength and endurance. *Canadian Journal of Psychology, 18* (2), 156-167.

Blum, G. S., & Porter, M. L. (1974). Effects of the restriction of conscious awareness in a reaction time task. *The International Journal of Clinical and Experimental Hypnosis, 22,* 335-345.

Blum, G. S., & Wohl, B. M. (1971). Monetary, affective, and intrinsic incentives in choice reaction time. *Psychonomic Science, 22,* 69-70.

Crasilneck, H. B., & Hall, J. A. (1959). Physiological changes associated with hypnosis: A review of the literature since 1948. *Journal of Clinical and Experimental Hypnosis, 7,* 9-50.

Edmonston, W. E., & Marks, H. E. (1967). The effects of hypnosis and motivational instructions on kinesthetic learning. *The American Journal of Clinical Hypnosis, 9,* 252-255.

Evans, F. J., & Orne M. T. (1965). Motivation, performance, and hypnosis. *The International Journal of Clinical and Experimental Hypnosis, 13* (2), 103-116.

Fehr, F. S., & Stern, J. A. (1967). The effect of hypnosis on attention to relevant and irrelevant stimuli. *The International Journal of Clinical and Experimental Hypnosis, 15,* 134-143.

Gorton, B. E., (1949). The physiology of hypnosis. *Psychiatric Quarterly, 23,* 457-485.

Graham, C., Olsen, R. A., Parrish, M., & Leibowitz, H. W. (1968). The effect of hypnotically induced fatigue on reaction time. *Psychonomic Science, 10,* 223—224.

Ham, M. W., & Edmonston, W. E., Jr. (1971) Hypnosis, relaxation, and motor retardation. *Journal of Abnormal Psychology, 77,* 329-331.

Hilgard, E. R. (1965). Hypnosis. *Annual Review of Psychology, 16,* 157-180.

Hull, C. L. (1933). *Hypnosis and suggestibility.* New York: Appleton-Century Co.

Jackson, J. A., Gass, G. C., & Camp, E. M. (1979) The relationship between posthypnotic suggestion and endurance in physically trained subjects. *The international Journal of Clinical and Experimental Hypnosis, 27* (3), 278-293.

Johnson, W. R. (1961). Body movement awareness in the nonhypnotic and hypnotic states. *Research Quarterly, 32* (2), 264-265. (a)

Johnson, W. R. (1961). Hypnosis and muscular performance. *Journal of Sports Medicine and Physical Fitness, 1,* 71-79 (b)

Johnson, W. R., & Kramer, G. F. (1960). Effects of different types of hypnotic suggestions upon physical performance. *Research Quarterly, 31,* 469-473.

Johnson, W. R., & Kramer, G. F. (1961) Effects of stereotyped nonhypnotic, hypnotic, and posthypnotic suggestions upon strength, power, and endurance. *Research Quarterly, 32,* 522-529.

Johnson, W. R., Massey, B. H. & Kramer, G. F. (1960). Effects of post-hypnotic suggestions on all-out effort of short duration. *Research Quarterly, 1960, 31,* 142-146.

Kratochvil, S, & Shubat (1971). Activity-passivity in hypnosis and in the normal state. *The International Journal of Clinical and Experimental Hypnosis, 19,* 140-146.

London, P., & Fuhrer, M. (1966) Hypnosis, motivation and performance. *Journal of Personality, 34,* 71-79.

McCord, H. (1970). Measuring hypnotic effects by the pound. *Journal of the American Society of Psychosomatic Dentistry and Medicine, 17,* 69-70.

Mead, S., & Roush, E. S. (1949). A study of the effect of hypnotic suggestion on physiologic performance. *Archives of Physical Medicine, 30,* 700-705.

Moll, A. (1958). *A study of hypnosis: Historical, clinical and experimental research in the techniques of hypnotic induction.* New York: Julian Press, (Original Publication, 1889).

Morgan, W. P. (1972). Hypnosis and muscular performance. In W. P. Morgan (Ed.), *Ergogenic aids and muscular performance.* New York: Academic Press.

Nicholson, N. C. (1920). Notes on muscular work during hypnosis. *John Hopkins Hospital Bulletin, 31,* 89-91.

Ogilvie, B. C. (1979). Clinical issues in the application of clinical psychology in the sport setting. *International Journal of Sport Psychology, 10* (3), 178-183.

Rader, C. M. (1972), Influence of motivational instructions on hypnotic and nonhypnotic reaction time performance. *The American Journal of Clinical Hypnosis, 15,* 98-101.

Roush, E. S. (1951) Strength and endurance in the waking and hypnotic states. *Journal of Applied Physiology, 3,* 404-410.

Ryde, D. (1964). A personal study of some uses of hypnosis in sport and sports injuries. *Journal of Sports Medicine and Physical Fitness,* 4, 241-246.

Sheehen, P. W., & Perry C. (1976). *Methodologies of hypnosis: A critical appraisal of contemporary paradigms of hypnosis.* Hillsdale N. J. Erlbaum.

Slater, C. (1967). Expentancy and hypnotic performance. Doctoral dissertation, Washington State University, Pullman.

Slotnick, R. S., & Liebert, R. M., & Hilgard, E. R. (1965). The enhancement of muscular performance in hypnosis through exhortation and involving instructions. *Journal of Personality, 33,* 37-45.

Slotnick, R. S., & London, P. (1965). Influence of instructions on hypnotic and nonhypnotic performance. *Journal of Abnormal Psychology 70*, 38–46.

Naruse, G. (1965). The hypnotic treatment of stage fright in champion athletes. *The International Journal of Clinical and Experimental Hypnosis, 13* (2), 63–70.

Watkins, D. A. (1949). Discussion: A study of the effect of hypnotic suggestion on physiologic performance. *Archives of Physical Medicine, 30*, 705–706.

Weitzenhoffer, A. M. (1963) *Hypnotism: An objective study in suggestibility.* New York: John Wiley & Sons.

Zimbardo, P. G., Marshall, G., White, G., & Maslach, C. (1973). Objective assessment of hypnotically induced time distortion. *Science, 181*, 282–284.

Zimbardo, P., Maslach, C., & Marshal, G. (1972). Hypnosis and the psychology of cognitive and behavioral control. In E. Fromm & R. E. Shor (Eds.), *Hypnosis: Research developments and perspectives.* Chicago: Aldine Atherton.

Chapter 10

Hypnosis: Enhancement of Cognitive Capacity

Wendy Blumenthal
Jean Heaton
Nova University

The quest for knowledge began thousands of years ago. According to Aristotle, "All men wonder why things are" (Aristotle in Watson, 1978). The discovery of new methods of learning has been the goal of educators and educational researchers for hundreds of years. Since hypnosis was reported by clinicians to be useful in facilitating their client's memories of previously forgotten material, researchers have examined hypnosis as a possible facilitator of, and/or an aid to memory and learning.

Learning will be defined as the acquisition of new responses or the enhanced execution of old ones while recall is concerned with the persistence of previously acquired responses or the enhancement of the responses. Both recall and learning are a function of memory; learning has to do with the storage of material in memory and recall has to do with the retrieval of that material stored in memory. Hull (1933) defined hypnosis as a state of consciousness characterized by a heightened responsiveness to direct suggestion. Treloar (1967) operationally defined hypnosis as a state of consciousness which is produced by exposure to a hypnotic production procedure. If the operational definition conforms to Hull's definition, hypnosis could enhance memory and recall through suggestions to focus attention, increase motivation, and promote greater effort, which are known to be important variables in recall of material stored in memory.

Numerous investigations, dating as far back as 1924 (Hadfield, 1924), have focused on the effects of hypnosis on cognitive performance. The findings of these studies often conflicted, their results were mixed. Therefore, the utilization of hypnosis to increase cognitive capacity has been a controversial treatment modality and no clear-cut answer to the question of whether or not hypnosis can enhance cognitive capacity has as yet been found.

To further compound the controversy in the area, research on the effects of hypnosis on learning has been plagued with methodological flaws. In the 1960's, many articles appeared criticizing the methodologies used by early investigators in the area. Studies were criticized for lack or inappropriate use of control, experimental procedures, and statistical analysis (Parker & Barber, 1964; Barber, 1966; Treloar, 1967; Cole, 1979). Furthermore, as with most investigative areas in the field of hypnosis, depending upon the orientation of the evaluator, studies have been criticized for either (1) incorporating too much control causing an alteration in the hypnotic "state" or (2) not having enough control making it difficult to determine the variables responsible for the results obtained (Shor, 1979). Those researchers who advocate more stringent controls have identified the following as possible confounding variables: expectancy, susceptibility, demand characteristics, and motivation. These and other methodological difficulties have led to what Salzberg and DePiano (1980) described as a moratorium on studies which examine the effects of hypnosis in learning. Since 1975, less than a dozen studies, including unpublished doctoral dissertations, could be found in the area (Illovsky & Friedman, 1976; Johnson, 1976; Garver, 1977; Bowers, Montiero, & Gilligan, 1978; Cole, 1979; Ingram, Saccuzzo, McNeill & McDonald, 1979; Salzberg & DePiano, 1980; Saccuzzo, Safran, Anderson & McNeill, 1982; Stein, 1982). Most of these recent studies utilized acceptable research methodologies, however, the results are still mixed. Therefore, no definitive conclusions may be reached regarding the efficacy of hypnosis on enhancing cognitive capacity.

At this point questions arise concerning the availability of information pertaining to hypnosis and learning, and/or whether, even though empirical findings have been mixed, any of this information can be utilized by the practicing clinician, educational consultant, or interested researcher. The purpose of this chapter is to review the major issues and findings on the effects of hypnosis on cognitive performance. In addition, an attempt will be made to ferret out the useful clinical applications of hypnosis on cognitive performance and identify the areas in the field which still remain virtually unexplored by experimental studies.

ALERT VS. TRADITIONAL INDUCTION

Some investigators in the field posit that it is possible to create essentially different kinds of "trance states" within hypnosis. The concept of an active or alert hypnotic "state" is not a recent phenomena, but was noted as far back as de Puysegur's time. De Puysegur demonstrated at least two phases of mesmerism in his most famous case, Victor Race. The first phase was a general arousal of the nervous system induced by the type of induction used with the subject (the hysteria of Mesmer's patients). The second phase of hypnotic alertness occurred during the hypnotic trance, and allowed the patient to carry out extremely difficult suggestions which would be impossible to perform if the patient was in a traditional trance. "Initially Race was passive, in a sleep-appearing condition (which led to de Puysegur's credit for the passivity and relaxation that is hypnosis), but upon instruction, during mesmerism, Race became alert, carrying out various suggestions, and, in fact, taking on personality characteristics that seemed most unlike him" (Edmonston, 1981, p. 195). Although White (1967) was not the first to distinguish between an active and passive hypnotic "state," he clearly differentiated between the two states. "The active subject behaves as if he were in a completely submissive state. He seems to fall in eagerly with the hypnotist's assertion(s). The passive subject seems bent on immobility. He can be made to move, or to wake, only by urgent efforts on the part of the hypnotist." (White, as cited in Edmonston, 1981). The concept of alert hypnotic conditions has led to a hypothesis that different suggestions or induction procedures may also produce different hypnotic "states." This hypothesis has led to investigations which compare the effects of alert hypnotic suggestions or inductions, to traditional (relaxation) ones, on cognitive performance.

The majority of hypnotic subjects experience an overall feeling of relaxation, however, a hypnotic trance can be produced without suggestions of relaxation (Hilgard, 1977). Alert hypnotic suggestions and alert inductions differ procedurally. Alert or involving suggestions occur after the subject is already hypnotized in a traditional (relaxation) manner. Alert inductions, on the other hand, avoid suggestions of relaxation and sleep during the hypnotic induction.

The studies on alert hypnosis and those comparing alert hypnosis with the more traditional hypnosis are limited. Oetting (1964) presented and discussed a study investigating alert hypnosis, however, this study did not compare an alert induction with a more traditional relaxation induction. Although Oetting gave instructions to enable a subject to concentrate and remain alert while studying, he presented no data to support his claims that the alert induction has advantages over a traditional induction.

In 1965 Liebert, Rubin, and Hilgard conducted a study comparing the effects of alert and traditional hypnotic inductions on learning. They used 15 undergraduate students who had obtained high scores (upper quartile) on the Stanford Hypnotic Susceptibility Scales, form A or form C. Each subject served as his/her own control in a paired associate learning task (16 word-number pairs). Waking baseline scores were obtained for each subject before beginning one of three treatments (waking repeat, traditional hypnosis, and "alert hypnosis"). During the treatment condition, subjects were remeasured on an equivalent list of word number pairs. The traditional hypnosis induction was from the Stanford Susceptibility Scale, Form A (SHSS:A); the alert induction was essentially the same except instructions were modified to eliminate all references to sleep or relaxation. The results indicated that the alert induction significantly enhanced learning over the traditional induction. Subjects under alert hypnosis produced fewer errors in learning than those in the traditional induction group. There were no significant differences in learning found between waking and alert induction conditions.

In contrast, Vingoe (1968) urges subjects to relax both muscularly and physically but to remain mentally alert in the Group Alert Trance Scale (GAT). Vingoe mixes suggestions for relaxation of the body with alertness of the mind in the same hypnotic induction. The author claims this combination induction is advantageous for education and experimental studies. A study by Ham and Edmonston (1971) compared alerting instructions, a traditional induction, and non-hypnotic relaxation. When the experimenters measured simple reaction times, they found no difference between the traditional induction group and the non-hypnotic relaxation group, however a difference was found between the alerted group and the other two groups. The other groups' reaction times were longer than the alert group and the reaction increased over time.

A study conducted by Swiercinsky and Coe (1971) examined the effects of "alert" hypnosis and hypnotic responsiveness on reading comprehension. The ability to increase reading comprehension was compared in three antecedent conditions. The three conditions were: (1) "alert" hypnosis followed by a posthypnotic suggestion of enhanced recall, (2) talk motivating instructions to subjects to imagine and concentrate as much as possible, and (3) no special instructions (control). No significant differences were found among any of the three conditions.

Thurman, in a 1974 unpublished doctoral dissertation, investigated the effect of hypnosis on learning meaningful material. Although specific induction strategies were not discussed in the abstract, Thurman reported that subjects who were given "alert" instructions did not perform any better than subjects who were given "relaxation" instructions on questions pertaining to brief passages from the Davis Reading Test.

The final study was conducted by Salzberg and DePiano (1980) in which they attempted to ferret out the separate effects of hypnotic susceptibility, task motivating suggestions, and the hypnotic trance state on performance on three cognitive tasks. Three treatment conditions were utilized: (1) a traditional hypnotic induction procedure (Salzberg, 1960); (2) an alert induction procedure; and (3) a short interview format, control group. Their findings did not support the hypotheses that alert induction procedures would counteract the inhibiting effects of traditional hypnosis (drowsiness and sleepiness) on cognitive tasks. In fact, there were no significant differences in performances between subjects in alert, traditional or control conditions (Salzberg & DePiano, 1980).

Although it would not be appropriate to make any definitive conclusions from these studies, two tentative formulations could be hypothesized First, alert hypnotic inductions as compared to traditional (relaxation) inductions are at least as effective (Thurman, 1974; Salzberg & DePiano, 1980) and may be more effective (Liebart et al., 1965) in producing learning. Second, alert hypnotic inductions do not appear to be any more effective than awake states in producing learning of new material (Swiercinsky & Coe, 1971; Salzberg & DePiano, 1980).

HYPNOTIZABILITY

Hypnotizability refers to an individual's level of suggestibility during a hypnotic induction. In general, research subjects are grouped according to high or low hypnotic suggestibility. This is based on the hypothesis that hypnosis may have differential effects on subjects' learning depending upon their abilities to respond to hypnotic suggestions. Concern surrounding the matter of hypnotizability came to the forefront after Barber (1965a, 1965b) criticized Salzberg's (1960) design for confounding experimental treatment with preexisting differences among subjects with regard to hypnotizability or suggestibility. Since then, investigators have focused upon, as well as controlled for, possible differences in learning during hypnosis which could be explained by different levels of hypnotizability.

Parker and Barber (1964) attempted a replication of Salzberg's (1960) study with several modifications to determine if Salzberg's results, which indicated that hypnotic and posthypnotic task motivating suggestions were effective in significantly enhancing performance on three cognitive tasks, could be repeated if appropriate experimental controls were utilized. They used tasks similar to Salzberg's (1960) (digit symbol substitution, memory for words, and abstract reasoning), however, the experimental treatments were somewhat altered. Parker and Barber (1964) used four experimental groups. Suggestible subjects were randomly assigned to one of three experimental treatments: task motivating instructions, hypnotic induction procedure with task motivating instructions, and control group. Nonsuggestible subjects were given task motivating instructions without a hypnotic induction procedure. Parker and Barber (1964) did not find any significant differences among experimental groups on the memory or abstract reasoning tasks, but on the digit symbol substitution task they found that suggestible subjects who did not receive task motivating instructions performed significantly worse than subjects in the three groups who received motivating instructions.

Other studies since Parker and Barber's (1964) have appeared to confirm the hypothesis that high and low susceptible subjects perform essentially equivocally when both are given task motivating instructions. In 1970, Swiercinsky and Coe attempted to isolate the effects of hypnotic induction on recall of meaningful material. They found no significant differences between conditions (group hypnotic induction followed by posthypnotic suggestions of enhanced concentration and recall ability, task motivating instructions, and control group). The authors reported that there were essentially no differences in the performances of high and low susceptible subjects (Swiercinsky & Coe, 1970). Cooper and London (1973) also reported finding no significant effect on the ability to recall meaningful material based on levels of hypnotic suggestibility. In 1980 Salzberg with DePiano made another attempt to determine the effects of hypnotic susceptibility on cognitive performance. In terms of hypnotic susceptibility, they did not find any significant differences except between simulating and real subjects on a digit symbol task which the authors held reflected the simulating subjects' superior baseline performance on this task (Salzberg & DePiano, 1980).

Many investigators have also hypothesized about the existence of a relationship between hypnotizability and the ability to selectively attend and/or visual information processing. Bowers (1976) hypnothezied that highly suggestible as compared to low-suggestible people may be better at processing and appraising information. Two recent experiments investigated this hypothesis. In the first study, Ingram, Saccuzzo, McNeill, and McDonald (1979) employed a backward masking paradigm to evaluate the relationship between hypnotic susceptibility and information processing. Backward masking is a procedure which can be used to evaluate group differences at various stages of information processing. The results of this procedure indicated that highly susceptible subjects process information significantly faster than low-susceptible subjects (Ingram et al., 1979). The results of the second investigation were not as clear-cut. In an attempt to extend and replicate the first study Saccuzzo, Safran, Anderson, and McNeill (1982) used a masking paradigm utilizing both forward and backward informational masking. The results supported those of Ingram et al. (1979) and thus, provide additional evidence for the hypothesis that there may be an inherent attentional or informational processing capability difference among high and low hypnotizable subjects; however, the differences between high and low suggestible subjects, although significant, were small and subtle, only occurring during one of two experimental phases. Therefore, caution should be used when interpreting the results of these two studies.

In summary, based on the limited amount of literature it would appear that hypnosis does not have differential effects on learning as a result of high or low levels of hypnotizability. Hypnotizability appears to be related to attentional and/or informational processing capabilities, however, further evidence is needed before any definitive relationships can be delineated.

MOTIVATION AND HYPNOSIS

After reviewing the results of studies pertaining to the effects of hypnosis on learning and recall, including the Salzberg (1960) studies discussed in the last section, Barber (1965a) concluded that,

> (1) Hypnosis by itself, without suggestions for high performance, does not significantly enhance either learning or recall.
> (2) Task motivating suggestions or suggestions for improved performance are at times effective with hypnotic Ss and are also at times effective with nonhypnotic Ss in facilitating acquisition and recall. (p. 24)

This statement challenged investigators in the area of hypnosis and learning. If nonhypnotic variables could yield effects equivalent to those produced by hypnotic induction, this would provide a more parsimonious alternative explanation, motivating instructions, for the effects of hypnosis on learning.

Some early investigators hypothesized that motivational differences among subjects may even exist during baseline measures before any treatment is initiated. Specifically, London and Fuhrer (1961) and Rosenhan and London (1963a; 1963b) reported that waking baseline performance of subjects not susceptible to hypnosis was significantly higher than that of subjects highly susceptible to hypnosis. Evans and Orne (1966) replicated these earlier studies but did not find any differences between performances of high and low susceptible subjects on any of four experimental measures. Therefore, since Evans and Orne's (1966) findings, pretreatment motivation has either been deemed manipulable by experimental treatments or controlled for by interactional designs which include hypnotic susceptibility and motivation factors.

Three types of motivational instructions have been used by investigators in the area - task motivating, exhortation, and involving instructions (Roeder, 1978). Task motivating instructions were developed by Barber and Calverly (1962; 1963a, 1963b) to include all the elements found in standard inductions which could be considered nonhypnotic such as verbal suggestions of increased memory, attention, and concentration (Barber, 1969). Exhortation instructions developed by London and Fuhrer (1961), contain content which encourages subjects by (1) explaining that most people underestimate their own capabilities, (2) urging them not to give up because of fatigue as discomfort, and to reinterpret these feelings as cues to continue rather than stop, and (3) telling them the experiment cannot be successful without their maximal efforts. Involving instructions were introduced by Slotnick et al. (1965) to be used in addition to exhortation instructions. They stress commitment and involvement and require the subjects to verbally state their desires to do well. Although these procedures are somewhat different and each technique varies somewhat depending on the nature of the experiment, for the purposes of this review all three procedures will be viewed as equivocal in elliciting subjects' optimal performance.

Every study reviewed in the literature since 1964 reported that when motivation was experimentally controlled no significant differences in learning could be found between hypnotic and nonhypnotic conditions (Parker & Barber, 1964; Lenox, 1970; Swiercinsky & Coe, 1970; 1971; Arnold, 1971; Gilbert & Barber, 1972; Willis, 1972; Thurman, 1974; Zamansky, 1977; Cole, 1979; Salzberg & DePiano, 1980). In general, Barber's conclusions in 1965 were supported. Swiercinsky and Coe (1970; 1971) found that motivated subjects in both hypnotic and waking conditions performed equally on tasks of reading recall (1970) and comprehension (1971). In a 1971 study, Arnold found no significant differences in the learning of two motor tasks between subjects given suggestions of a positively involving nature either post-hypnotically or without hypnosis (Arnold, 1971). Willis' (1972) results from a study on the effect of self-hypnosis on reading rate and comprehension indicated that reading and motivating suggestions, but not hypnosis, facilitate reading rate. In another study examining the effects of hypnosis on reading, Thurman (1974) found no significant differences between the experimental groups of standard hypnosis, self-hypnosis, task motivating instructions and a control group. Finally, in 1980, after finding task motivating suggestions were effective in enhancing performance for all three experimental groups on the digit symbol and abstract reasoning tasks, but not on a memory task, Salzberg and DePiano (1980) concluded that when the experimental design of a study controls for motivating suggestions, hypnosis does not facilitate cognitive performance. In summary, it would appear that hypnosis does not enhance performance differently from nonhypnotic comparison groups when appropriate experimental controls are utilized.

OTHER RELATED AREAS

Sleep Learning

The Soviet countries have reported widespread success of hypnopadea sleep learning, for many years (Hoskovec, 1967). Interest in laboratory investigations of sleep learning was also widespread in America during the 1940s and 1950s. However, since Simon and Emmons (1956) carefully controlled EEG studies research in the area has waned. Simon and Emmons (1956) reported that subjects could not recall stimuli presented during sleep unless alpha activity occurred simultaneously with the stimulus material. They concluded that since alpha activity indicates arousal during sleep, than any learning displayed occurred during the awake state and not during sleep. Generally, in earlier sleep learning studies lack of retention upon awakening was considered as evidence that registration and acquisition did not occur during sleep. However, two recent studies have shown that retention can and does occur during sleep, demonstrating that registration and acquisition has occurred during sleep. The first study was done by Cooper and Hoskovec in 1972. In this cleverly designed study, the experimenters first taught the eleven subjects ten simple Russian-English word pairs upon awakening on an adaption night as a learning within subjects control. Prior to going to sleep on the experimental night, the subjects were hypnotized, and given suggestions to perceive and remember the word pairs presented while asleep. During Stage I REM sleep, a second set of English-Russian word pairs was presented. Cooper and Hoskovec (1972) found waking learning and recall to be superior to hypnotic sleep learning and recall, recall of the learned material averaged 90 percent and 30 percent, respectively. It should be noted though that material learned during sleep was still three times more than what would be anticipated by chance alone. The second investigation was an unpublished study reported by Evans (1979). Although the design differed from the one used by Cooper and Hoskevec (1972), the results were quite similar. Evans (1979) reported that the average recall of material during Stage I sleep, was 28 percent which he pointed out exceeded chance recall. The findings of these two studies combined with the reportedly widespread practice and success of sleep learning in Soviet countries (Hoskovec, 1967), suggest that under optimal conditions in the laboratory sleep learning is possible with subsequent waking recall, but it may not be practical (i.e., 30 percent of the material is learned as compared to 90 percent under the same instructions when awake).

Hypnotic Time Distortion

In the hypnotic distortion of time, hypnosis is used to modify the perception of nominal time. "This involves both the estimation of the rate at which events are (or should be) occurring and affective reactions to different rates of stimulus impact" (Maslach, Zimbardo, & Marshall, 1979, p. 664). This causes an alteration in the amount of effective time available to subjects to learn and/or perform tasks. Investigators have hypnothesized that this alteration in perceived affective learning time may give rise to an increased learning rate. Although a couple of investigators have reported increased learning rates based on perceived time passage (Krauss, Krauss, & Kratzell, 1974; Cooper & Erickson in Maslach et al., 1979), most of the studies that have measured performance increment have generally yielded negative results (Johnson, 1976; Maslach et al., 1979). However, since all but two of the studies found in the literature were conducted before 1968, it is probably premature to conclude with any confidence whether or not hypnotic time distortion techniques are capable of enhancing learning proficiency.

Recall vs. Recognition

Recall and recognition involve different memory processes. In recognition the target information is provided and the individual must evaluate its familiarity in a specified context, however, in recall tasks the individual must provide the memory with fewer cues. Anderson and Bower (1972) present a two-stage theory of recall and recognition. This theory states that new experiences are integrated into an existing network of associated ideas and memories. According to this theory, remembering begins with a search through the existing network for associated ideas, this search generates several possible alternative memories; one of these alternative memories is chosen as the most probable choice. Recall utilizes both the search and decision processes, while recognition does not involve the search process because the presentation of a target item eliminates the need to search for that item; therefore, recognition only necessitates a decision as to whether a specific target item meets a criterion.

The episodic ecophory theory (Tulving & Thompson, 1973) and the levels of processing theory (Craik & Lockhart (1972) differ in their theory as to the relationship between perception and memory. Tulving states that the memory trace of an event is encoded in memory as a set of features representing the event and the experiential context in which it took place. Successful retrieval involves a match between the encoded features and those that are contained in the memory code. Craik and Lockhart's levels of processing theory proposes that memory is the result of perceptual activity; the ease with which an event can be remembered depends on (1) the number of perceptual-cognitive operations performed at the time the event occurred, (2) the degree to which the event is elaborated within any level of processing, (3) the extent to which the event matches its context, and (4) the uniqueness of the fit between the trace and the memory probe. The two theories tend to agree that recall and recognition do not involve processes different in quality, and that one is not a subset of the other. Both theories propose that remembering requires a sufficient overlap between information associated with memory trace and corresponding information in the memory probe. However, the two theories differ in their conception of the relationship between the memory trace and memory probe. According to Tulvig, all that is required for the trace to enter consciousness as a remembered event is a successful match between the memory trace and the memory probe, whereas Craik and Lockhart (1970) assert that sufficient early contact between probe and trace will encourage continued reconstructive activity until a memory is formed. Both theories hold that the processes involved in recognition and recall are essentially the same, except that less information is provided by the probe in recall than is provided in the memory probe in recognition.

Williamsen, Johnson, and Eriksen (1965) investigated the supposition that a comparison of recall and recognition memory would lead to a more detailed account of the processes of posthypnotic amnesia. In Experiment I, subjects who were deeply hypnotized learned a list of six common words and then received a suggestion for posthypnotic amnesia. The subjects exhibited a virtually complete inability to remember the critical material in an initial recall test. After they performed other tasks related to learning, the subjects were shown a list containing the original six common words and six distracters. On this recognition task, they showed improvement in memory compared to their initial recall performance. However, the recall performance of the hypnotized group was still inferior to that of the waking control group. In Experiment II, recall and recognition testing took place in close succession; no difference was found between the outcome of the recall and recognitions tasks. This outcome suggests that the difference found in Experiment I was due to the interference in remembering learning tasks performed due to the interval between tests, not a function of the difference between recall and recognition memory.

Kihlstrom and Shor (1978) conducted two complementary studies investigating hypothesized differences in recall and recognition. Experiment I was a normative study which controlled for time of recognition and recall while Experiment II assessed the generalizability of Experiment I. The outcome of the two experiments indicated that recognition testing produces a break in posthypnotic amnesia. The finding of relative rather than a significant superiority of recognition to recall is explained by all three theories of memory: (1) two-stage theory, (2) episodic ecphory, and (3) levels of processing.

Hypnotic Amnesia

Much research has been done in the area of hypnotic amnesia. At one time it was used as a criteria to determine whether or not a person was in a hypnotic state. If the "forgetting" associated with hypnotic amnesia can be explained, perhaps the forgetting associated with recall can be understood as both types of forgetting seem to be a process of attentional focus.

"Hypnotic amnesia is a temporary, suggestion induced deficit in recall. The temporary nature of the deficit is shown by its reversibility." (Spanos, Radtke, and Dubreuil, 1982). Hilgard (1965) listed different kinds of hypnotic amnesia: (1) source amnesia is when material learned under hypnosis is remembered, but the fact that it was learned under hypnosis is forgotten, (2) posthypnotic recall amnesia is amnesia for the events within the hypnotic session, and (3) posthypnotic partial amnesia, in which the subject is told he will forget some but not all of the the material learned within the hypnotic session. In general, hypnotic amnesia can be viewed as temporary forgetting that is associated with the hypnotic process.

Kihlstrom, Evans, Orne, and Orne, (1980) reported that a suggestion for posthypnotic amnesia produced deficits in episodic (learned word lists) but not semantic (word association) memory tasks. A more recent study (Spanos et al., 1982) confirmed Kihlstrom's results. In addition, Spanos et al. supported the cued inattention hypothesis. This hypothesis does not deny that the hypnotic subject temporarily forgets the target material but states that through hypnotic suggestion the Ss (subjects) attention is diverted away from the material by suggestions from the hypnotist. Evans and Kihlstrom (1973) postulated that posthypnotic amnesia involves disrupted retrieval in memory organization. Support for this hypothesis comes from a more recent study that investigates the restricted use of success cues during posthypnotic amnesia (Pettinati, Evans, Orne, & Orne, 1981). A study that investigated the selective recall of successful experiences (Pettinati & Evans, 1978) controlled for potential bias in the scoring procedure by modifying the selective recall index to account for the differences in the recall pools available to hypnotizable and unhypnotizable subjects. This study found no significant difference between highly hypnotizable Ss and low hypnotizable Ss, however, the highly hypnotizable Ss were less likely to selectively recall successful experiences.

Numerous studies have been conducted to investigate hypnotic amnesia and many hypotheses explaining this phenomena have come out of these studies, for example: proactive interference and ablation of memory, (Wickens & Grittis, 1974); disrupted retrieval, (Evans & Kihlstrom, 1973); selective recall, (Pettinati & Evans, 1978); dissociative process, (Coe, Basden, Basden, & Graham, 1976); disorganized recall, (Nace, Orne, & Hammer, 1974; Spanos & Radtke-Bodorik, 1980). However, many of these hypotheses have been discomfirmed: disrupted search, (St. Jean & Coe. 1981); proactive interference and the ablation of memory, (Dillon & Spanos, 1983); and disorganized recall, (Spanos, Radtke, Bertrand, Addie, & Drummond, 1982). In addition studies have investigated the recovery of memory after posthypnotic amnesia (Kihlstrom & Evans, 1976); attempts to breach posthypnotic amnesia (Kihlstrom, Evans, Orne & Orne, 1980); a comparison of spontaneous recovery of memory during posthypnotic amnesia and recovery of memory by hypnotic suggestion (Kihlstrom, Easton, & Shor, 1983); and residual effects of posthypnotic amnesia among hypnotizable subjects (Kihlstrom & Evans, 1977).

Meaningfulness of Material

Many of the studies previously reviewed made a point of investigating the effects of hypnosis on learning meaningful material. Obviously, it would not be worthwhile to learn meaningless material. However, nonsense material has been a vehicle in experiments on learning since Ebbinghaus' revolutionary work with nonsense syllables (Ebbinghaus in Watson, 1978). In its conception, Ebbinghaus hypothesized that learning could most objectively be examined when the material learned has no associative value. Still, hypnotic material is best learned if it is meaningful. Furthermore, the literature suggests that the hypnotic learning increment is a monotonicly increasing function by the "degree of meaningfulness" (Weitzenhoffer, 1963). Again, as in previous areas discussed in the review, investigators found no significant differences in learning material, nonsensical or meaningful, between waking and hypnotic conditions (Edmonstron & Stanek, 1966; Lenox, 1970; Swiercinsky & Coe, 1970; Thurman, 1974; Stein, 1982).

Memory and Recall

Hypnosis has been used by clinicians to facilitate recall of forgotten or repressed material for years. However, there is no strong experimental support for the use of hypnosis to enhance recall. Barber and Calvery (1966) proposed that hypnosis has never improved recall in a controlled study. Dhanens and Lundy (1975) conducted a study to examine the various factors in hypnosis as they relate to enhanced recall. Two variables (high and low susceptible subjects) and six treatments (hypnosis plus motivating suggestions, motivating instructions without hypnosis, hypnosis with regression suggestions, regression suggestions without hypnosis, relaxation suggestions alone, and a no treatment control group) were used. The learning tasks were a taped biographical sketch of Nicholas Butler and a list of 13 nonsense syllables. There was a significant improvement in recall for highly susceptible Ss with a combination of hypnosis and motivating suggestions using contexual material.

A large number of case studies have been reported (Smith, 1983) in which hypnosis has been used to solve a crime. Because of these case studies police departments and other investigative agencies have developed a belief that hypnosis can be used to recall memories. The results of some laboratory studies do not support this belief. However, a 1981 study by DePiano and Salzberg investigated the effectiveness of hypnosis in enhancing the recall of meaningful and incidentally learned material, presented under three types of arousal. The researchers used film induced arousal: traumatic arousal (typical of crime situations), sexual arousal (high arousal not typical of a crime situation), and low arousal (a calming effect on Ss). The information was meaningful, learned incidentally, and was part of a contexual sequence. The Ss were 108 students from an undergraduate class. The arousal level was monitored through the use of a Basal Skin Resistance Monitor and a Cardio-Tachometer ECG. A self report arousal rating form was used to obtain a self report of arousal. The Ss were randomly assigned to three groups, each group was shown a different film: high arousal film, low arousal film, and a sexual arousal film. The Ss were then randomly assigned to either a hypnosis group or a nonhypnotic group. The hypnosis group was then given a standard hypnotic induction. Both groups were played recorded task motivating instructions and were tested verbally for recall. The results of this study indicate that hypnosis with task motivating instructions enhanced recall more than motivating instructions alone. However, the arousal level did not tend to influence recall of material presented during or after the arousal film.

A study investigating the relationship between mood and memory (Bower, Monteiro, & Gilligan, 1978) found that recall of a given target was enhanced when the mood state during learning was the same as the mood state during the recall of the list. The authors had hypnotized subjects learn two word lists, one list while feeling "happy" and the other while feeling "sad". They found a mood-dependent retention effect, recall was best when the mood-state during recall was the same as during learning (Bower et al., 1978). Thus, mood cue may provide a helpful retrieval cue for material learned while hypnotized.

It has been hypothesized that the relationship between the hypnotist and subject may have an effect on recall and memory. Shubat (1969) used four experimental conditions: (1) no hypnotic state and minimal relationships between experimenters and subjects, (2) hypnotic state and minimal relationship between experimenter and subjects, (3) hypnotic state and maximal relationship between experimenter and subjects, and (4) no hypnotic state and maximal relationship between experimenter and subjects. The findings of this study indicated that the relationship between experimenter and subjects was the significant factor in enchancing recall.

Hypnosis in Academic Settings

The method of success imagery (Porter, 1978) has been reported to be clinically useful for problems of concentration, attention span, recall, test anxiety, and performance fear. This procedure is effective for adults returning to school as well as for children already in an academic setting. Suggestions are given while the individual is in a hypnotic trance. These suggestions should be adapted for the individuals level of understanding and emotional state. The individual adaptations of the following suggestions are used:

1. Work efficiently without being fatigued by the sheer effort of study, it will come naturally and easily. . . .
2. Enjoy the learning process, find it easy and natural to study and to learn. . . .
3. Ability to learn and recall information, to integrate new information with what you already know, and answer appropriately any oral or written questions. . . .
4. Spend adequate time to ensure success. Take sufficient rest pauses to remain alert and efficient. . . .
5. Have increasing belief in your own abilities and certainty that you will succeed. . . .

6. Gain ability to switch on the internal success mechanism within the mind, instead of the failure mechanism . . . until very soon you forget even how to switch on the failure mechanism. . . .
7. Treat failures as merely pointers to a new path to success. . . .
8. Have general confidence in your ability to do not only what you have to do but what you want to do. . . .
9. Maintain a pleasant balance between work and pleasure while remianing always on an overall path to success. . . .
10. As belief in your own abilities increases, you will see potential as unlimited. . . .
11. Given the opportunity to learn and the ability, you can do anything if you have the desire. . . .
12. Do the necessary practice and the determination to bring success, but you will be able to do this without having to strive unduly. . . . The entire process will be enjoyable and pleasant and you will have the overall conviction that you can be a success. . . .
13. Have an increasing sense of achievement and accomplishment. (Porter, 1978).

The literature on the effects of hypnosis on academic performance portrayed mixed and inconclusive results. As with other areas of study on hypnosis, even though many of the findings are provactive, research and clinical reports contain pervasive methodological flaws which prevent the formation of definitive conclusions. In 1966, Krippner tailored individual inductions for nine children, with an average age of eleven years, nine months, enrolled in a 5-week remedial reading program. Hypnotic suggestions pertained to reading focused on three areas: reducing tension and anxiety, enhancing motivation to recall, and increasing concentration and attention span (Krippner, 1966). Using alternate forms of the California Reading Test, he compared the reading improvements of the nine children who received hypnosis to those of the forty other children who attended the remedial program who did not receive hypnosis. Krippner (1966) found that children who received hypnotic remediation improved significantly more than children in the control group, however, the actual amount of improvement (six months versus five months) was too small to be of much practical value. In a reading comprehension study, Mutke (1967) reported that this hypnotic suggestion group reached a peak reading rate faster than controls, however, he confounded hypnosis, image rehearsal, susceptibility, and therapy which he reported providing to some experimental subjects. Donk, Knudson, Washburn, Goldstein, and Vingoe (1968) also looked at the effects of using specific suggestions to increase reading efficiently. He found suggestions which included content to eliminate specific reading problems, increase reading speed, and maintain and/or increase comprehension resulted in significant increase in subjects reading speed while their comprehension levels remained stable. However, in a 1970 replication study using alert and traditional hypnotic inductions, Donk et al. did not find significant results (Donk, Virgoe, Hall, & Doty ., 1970), causing the results of both studies (Donk et al., 1968; 1970) to be unreliable and subject to speculation.

Anxiety tends to interfere with a person's attentional focus during test taking. A 1983 study by Boutin and Tosi examined the effects of four treatment modalities on the modification of irrational ideas and test anxiety in 48 female nursing students. The treatments used were as follows: (1) Rational Stage Directed Hypnotherapy (*RSDH*), (2) a hypnosis only treatment, (3) a placebo group, and (4) a no treatment control group. Significant treatment effects were found for both *RSDH,* and hypnosis, however, hypnosis alone was not as effective as *RSDH.* There were also significant results when the grade point average was measured before and after treatment with *RSDH* and hypnosis only. *RSDH* as a combination of hypnosis and cognitive restructuring seems to be an effective treatment for reducing test anxiety.

The only case studies relating hypnotic suggestions to academic performance were presented by Krippner (1971). Krippner described six cases in which he used a clinical approach on students referred to him for academic counseling. Suggestions were chosen to treat the specific academic problem(s) of each child. Krippner (1971) sees hypnosis as a potentially helpful aide for the improvement of study habits and test taking skills and the enhancement of academic motivation. Although he did not use any statistical analysis, he concluded that hypnosis is not a panacea but can be used to motivate and reinforce student's skills to enable attainment of their maximal performance capabilities (Krippner, 1971).

In a direct response to Krippner's work and others who hypothesize that hypnosis can be used to remediate some academic problems, Cole (1979) conducted a study on the effects of hypnosis on academic and test taking skills. The hypnotic treatment was administered by prerecorded cassette tapes over a four week period during college class time. The tapes consisted of hypnotic and waking suggestions related to course content and general academic skills. Cole's (1979) results indicated that hypnotic and waking suggestions did not facilitate academic skill learning significantly more than regular classroom curriculum alone.

Finally, the effects of hypnosis on children with learning disabilities has also been investigated by a couple of researchers. In the first, Jampolsky (Jampolsky in Gardner & Olness, 1981) used hypnotherapy to overcome the negative reinforcement to which a small group of third- and fourth-grade reading disabled children had been repeatedly subjected. Jampolsky combined group hypnotic inductions with suggestions which utilized imagery techniques to reduce negative associations and formulate new positive images (for specific suggestions see

Jampolsky, 1975). Over a one month period, the experimental group averaged an increase in reading skills of 1½ years as compared to the control group's average of only one month. Furthermore, parents and teachers reported marked increases in the experimental subject's self esteem (Jampolsky in Gardner & Olness, 1981). The second study investigated the effectiveness of hypotherapy with 48 out of 180 children referred to a clinic for behavior and learning problems in school (Illovsky & Friedman, 1976). In general, the children selected by the authors manifested short attention span, acting-out behavior, and distractibility. Taped hypnotic inducions were utilized and hypnotic suggestions focused on improved learning and increased ability to cope with emotional problems. Teachers reported improved self-confidence in the children exposed to hypnotherapy. Unfortunately, teacher bias, lack of an experimental control group, and no available statistical analyses make the data almost impossible to interpret objectively.

In summary, the results of studies on the effectiveness of hypnosis on academic problems are mixed. Therefore, no conclusions concerning its usefulness with academic problems can be made. Based on the results of the two studies presently available, hypnotherapy appears to be a promising new remedial approach for children with learning problems, however, clinicians should use it cautiously until such findings are replicated.

CONCLUSIONS AND CLINICAL IMPLICATIONS

The results of much of the research on the effects of hypnosis on learning are mixed, however, some trends do appear in the currently available data. These tentative conclusions are: (1) There does not appear to be a significant difference in the amount of learning which occurs during hypnotic and waking states. Learning does not appear to be enhanced by hypnosis. The results of early studies, which found hypnosis enchanced learning, were probably confounded by uncontrolled variables and, in particular, by motivating suggestions. When task-motivating instructions are appropriately controlled, no differences in learning and/or cognitive performance have been found. (2) Although the differential effects on learning of alert and traditional inductions are still debatable, neither is any more effective than learning while awake. Most studies have reported equivocal performances among subjects in experimental conditions of traditional induction procedures, awake induction procedures, and awake controls. (3) Learning under hypnosis is not differentially effected by subject's levels of hypnotic suggestibility/susceptibility. Hypnotic subjects of both high and low levels of hypnotic responsiveness perform similarly on learning tasks. However, highly susceptible hypnotic subjects may process information differently than low susceptible subjects. (4) Hypnotic sleep learning may be possible, but does not appear to be practical. Learning under such conditions appears to be occurring as performance is greater than that predicted by chance. (5) There is no difference in learning nonsense or meaningful material between hypnotized and awake subjects, both groups perform essentially the same when appropriate controls are utilized. (6) Hypnosis does not appear to be effective in enhancing reading rate or comprehension. Hypnotherapy may or may not, be effective in remediating other academic areas. The results reported by clinical studies indicate that hypnosis may be effective in remediating some problems associated with difficulties in learning and learning disabilities. No conclusions about the effects of hypnotic time distortion on learning can be made at this time. It is stressed, that these conclusions are at best tentative. More research is needed, in almost all of these areas, to substantiate and expound upon the currently available data.

Future research needs to focus on other variables as well. Many investigators have hypothsized that the length of hypnotic inductions may effect hypnotic learning. Gilbert and Barber (1972) found extended hypnotic inductions tended to produce higher scores on a visual-motor coordination task than a shorter induction and control group. This finding is very provocative, however, no other studies on the length of hypnotic induction were found in the literature. Another area which has been speculated upon and suggested by clinical observations is the consequences of long-term hypnotic training on enhancing meaningful learning (Swiercinsky & Coe, 1971). Many studies have been criticized for not verifying whether or not hypnosis had actually been achieved by experimental subjects, long-term training in hypnosis could control for this as well as being utilized as an experimental variable itself. Also, Garver (1977) found hypnosis to be useful in cognitive rehearsal of athletic performance, perhaps it could be useful in rehearsing other learned skills as well. The potential list of related research areas is limitless. Although this area is very complex and acknowledgably difficult to investigate, the state of the art is still relatively primitive. More well designed research is needed to ascertain how hypnosis can effect cognitive capacity.

Based on the current research methodologies, experimental studies do not find that hypnosis facilitates either memory or recall of learned material, while clinical studies report success in enhancing cognitive capacities. The difference in the two types of studies is that experimental studies use controls while clinical studies are primarily case studies. Should clinicians discontinue the utilization of hypnosis as a treatment modality and wait for positive results from experimental studies or should the clinician continue to use hypnosis with selected patients for which his/her clinical judgement (based on experience) indicates that hypnosis is the treatment of choice?

Barber's apparent doubts about the existence of the hypnotic trance have motivated him to perform numerous studies in attempts to confirm his doubts. Erickson is on the opposite side of the controversy surrounding hypnosis. He compares experimental researchers with the seven blind men describing an elephant and this analogy may hold some truisms today. The experimental scientist insists that when we conduct hypnotic studies we must control for the following variables: (1) relationship between experimenter and subject, (2) motivation, (3) expectations of both subject and experimenter, (4) susceptibility, (5) suggestibility, and (6) whether the subjects eyes are open or closed. All of these variables, with the exception of number six, are a significant part of any therapy; yet these stringent controls are not used in experimental studies of other treatment modalities. If a study investigating the efficacy of cognitive restructuring was conducted and the findings indicated that the cognitive restructuring group showed significant improvement, but the control group had a lower motivation level than the treatment group, would we have to report that high motivation, not cognitive restructuring, was responsible for the improvement? Would we even doubt the existence of cognitive restructuring? We think not. The conclusion which must be reached is that the clinician should continue to use hypnosis in his or her clinical practice when it is the treatment of choice for selected patients. Hypnotherapy may be helpful in increasing motivation, reducing test anxiety, improving studying and test taking skills, and with learning disabled children's secondary problems (i.e. poor self concepts and overcoming negative reinforcement). Hypnotherapy may also aide cognitive rehearsal. In general, when used with the proper caution, hypnotherapy may be a viable treatment for some learning problems.

REFERENCES

Anderson, J. R., & Bower, G. H. (1972). Recognition and retrieval processes in free recall *Psychological Review, 79,* 97-123.

Arnold, J. (1971). Effects of hypnosis on learning of two motor-skills. *Research Quarterly, 42,* 1-6.

Barber, T. X. (1965a). The effects of "hypnosis" on learning and recall: A methodological critique. *Journal of Clinical Psychology, 21,* 19-25.

Barber, T. X. 1965b). Experimental analysis of "hypnotic" behavior: A review of recent empirical findings. *Journal of Abnormal Psychology, 70,* 132-154.

Barber, T. X. (1966). The effects of "hypnosis" and motivational suggestions on strength and endurance: A critical review of research studies. *British Journal of Social and Clinical Psychology, 5,* 42-50.

Barber, T. X. (1966). *Hypnosis: A scienfific approach.* New York: Van Nostrand and Reinhold.

Barber, T. X. & Calvery, D. S. (1963a). The relative effectiveness of task motivating instructions and trance induction procedures in theproduction of "hypnotic like" behaviors. *Journal of Nervous and Mental Diseas, 137,* 107–116. (a).

Barber, T. X., & Calvery, D. S. (1963b). Toward a theory of hypnotic behavior: Effects on suggestibility of task motivating instructions and attitude toward hypnosis. *Journal of Abnormal and Social Psychology, 67,* 557-565.

Barber, T.X., & Calverley, D. S. (1966). Effects on recall of hypnotic induction, motivational suggestions, and suggested regression: A methodological and experimental analysis. *Journal of Abnormal Psychology, 71,* 169-180.

Bootin, G. E., & Tosi, D. J. (1983). Modification of irrational ideas and test anxiety through Rational Stage Directed Hypnotherapy (RSDH). *Journal of Clinical Psychology, 39,* 382-391.

Bowers, G. H., Montiero, K. P., & Gilligan, S. G. (1978). Emotional mood as context for learning and recall. *Journal of Verbal Learning and Verbal Behavior, 17,* 573–585.

Bowers, K. S. (1976). *Hypnosis for the seriously curious.* Montery, CA: Brooks-Cole.

Coe, W. C., Basden, B., Basden, D., & Graham, C. (1976). Posthypnotic amnesia: Suggestions of an active process in dissociative phenomena. *Journal of Abnormal Psychology. 85,* 455-458.

Cole, R. D. (1979). The use of hypnosis in a course to increase academic and test-taking skills. *International Journal of Clinical and Experimental Hypnosis, 27,* 21-28.

Cooper, L. M., & Hoskovec, J. (1972). Hypnotic suggestions for learning during stage I REM sleep. *American Journal of Clinical Hypnosis, 15,* 102-111.

Cooper, L. M. & London, P. (1973). Reactivation of memory by hypnosis and suggestion. *International Journal of Clinical and Experimental Hypnosis, 21,* 312–323.

Craik, F.I.M., & Lockhart, R.S. (1972). Levels of processing: A framework for memory research. *Journal of Verbal Learning and Verbal Behavior, 11,* 671-684.

DePiano, F.A., & Salzberg, H.C. (1981). Hypnosis as an aid to recall of meaningful information presented under three types of arousal. *International Journal of Clinical and Experimental Hypnosis, 29,* 383-400.

Dhanens, T.P., & Lundy, R.M. (1975). Hypnotic and waking suggestions and recall. *International Journal of Clincal and Experimental Hypnosis, 23,* 68-79.

Dillon, R. F., & Spanos, N. P. (1983a). Levels of processing: A framework for memory research. *Journal of Verbal Learning and Verbal Behavior, 11,* 671-684.

Dillon, R. F., & Spanos, N. P. (1983b). Proactive interference and the functional ablation hypothesis: More disconfirmatory data. *International Journal of Clinical and Experimental Hypnosis. 31,* 47-56.

Donk, L. J., Knudson, R.G., Washburn, R.W., Goldstein, A.D., & Vingoe, F.J. (1968). Toward an increase in reading efficiency utilizing specific suggestions: A preliminary approach. *International Journal of Clinical and Experimental Hypnosis, 16,* 101-110.

Donk, L. J., Vingoe, F. J., Hall, R. A., & Doty, R. (1970). The comparison of three suggestion techniques for increasing leading efficiency utilizing a counter-balanced research paradigm. *International Journal of Clinical and Experimental Hypnosis, 18,* 126-133.

Edmonston, W. E., Jr. (1981). *Hypnosis and relaxation: Modern verification of an old education.* New York: Wiley.

Edmonston, W. E., Jr., & Stanek, F. J. (1966). The effects of hypnosis and meaningfulness on material on verbal learning. *American Journal of Clinical Hypnosis, 8,* 257–260.

Evans, F. J., & Kihlstom, J. F. (1973). Posthypnotic amnesia as disrupted retrieval. *Journal of Abnormal Psychology, 82,* 317-323.

Evans, F. J. (1979). Hypnosis and sleep: Techniques for exploring cognitive activity during sleep. In E. Fromm & R. E. Shor (Eds.), *Hypnosis: Developments in research and new perspectives.* (pp. 15–44). New York: Alpine.

Evans, F. J., & Orne, M. T. (1966). Motivation, performance, and hypnosis. *International Journal of Clinical and Experimental Hypnosis, 13,* 103-116.

Gardner, G. G., & Olness, K. (1981). *Hypnosis and hypnotherapy with children.* New York: Grune & Stratton.

Garver, R. B. (1977). The enhancement of human performance through neuromotor facilitation and control of arousal level. *American Journal of Clinical Hypnosis, 19,* 177-181.

Gilbert, J. A., & Barber, T. X. (1972). Effects of hypnotic induction, motivational instructions, and level of suggestibility on cognitive performance. *International Journal of Clinical and Experimental Hypnosis, 20,* 156-168.

Goldstein, M. S., & Sipprelle, C. N. (1970). Hypnotically induced amnesia versus ablation of memory. *International Journal of Clinical and Experimental Hypnosis. 18,* 211-216.

Hadfield, J. A. (1924). *The psychology of power.* London: Macmillan.

Ham, M. W., & Edmonston, W.E., Jr. (1971). Hypnosis, relaxation, and motor retardation. *Journal of Abnormal Psychology, 77,* 329–331.

Hilgard, E. R. (1977). *Divided Consciousness: Multiple Controls in Human Thought and Action.* New York: Wiley.

Hilgard, E. R. (1965). *Hypnotic susceptibility.* New York: Harcourt Brace & World.

Hoskevec, J. (1967). A review of some major works in Soviet hypnotherapy. *International Journal of Clinical and Experimental Hypnosis, 15,* 1-10.

Hull, C. L. (1933). *Hypnosis and suggestibility: An experimental approach.* New York: Appleton-Century-Crofts.

Illovsky, J., & Friedman, N. (1976). Group suggestion in learning disabilities of primary grade children: A feasibility study. *International Journal of Clinical and Experimental Hypnosis, 24,* 87-97.

Ingram, R. E., Saccuzzo, D. P., McNeill, B. W., & McDonald, R. (1979). Speed of information processing in high and low susceptible subjects: A preliminary study. *International Journal of Clinical and Experimental Hypnosis, 27* (1), 42-47.

Jampolsky, G. G. (1975). *Hypnosis in the treatment of learning problems.* Paper presented at the 17th annual scientific meeting of the Society for Clinical and Experimental Hypnosis, Chicago.

Johnson, R. F. (1976). Hypnotic time distortion and the enhancement of learning: New data pertinent to the Krauss–Katzell–Krass experiment. *American Journal of Clinical Hypnosis, 19,* 98-102.

Kihlstrom, J. F., Easton, R. D., & Shor, R. E. (1983). Spontaneous recovery of memory during posthypnotic amnesia. *International Journal of Clinical and Experimental Hypnosis, 31,* 309-323.

Kihlstrom, J. F., & Evans, F. J. (1976). Recovery of memory after posthypnotic amnesia. *Journal of Abnormal Psychology, 85,* 564-569.

Kihlstrom, J. F., & Evans, F. J. (1977). Residual effect of suggestions for posthypnotic amnesia: A reexamination. *Journal of Abnormal Psychology, 86,* 327-333.

Kihlstrom, J. F., Evans, F. J., Orne, E. E., & Orne, M. T. (1980). Attempting to breach posthypnotic amnesia. *Journal of Abnormal Psychology, 89,* 603-616.

Kihlstrom, J. F., & Shor, R. E. (1978). Recall and recognition during posthypnotic amnesia. *International Journal of Clinical and Experimental Hypnosis, 26,* 330-349.

Krippner, S. (1966). The use of hypnosis with elementary and secondary school children in a summer reading clinic. *American Journal of Clinical Hypnosis, 18,* 261-266.

Krippner, S. (1971). Hypnosis as verbal programming in educational therapy. *Academic Therapy, 7,* 5-12.

Lenox, J. R. (1970). A failure of hypnotic state to effect numerical task performance. *Dissertation Abstracts International, 31,* 2186.

Liebart, R. M., Rubin, N., & Hilgard, E. R. (1965). The effects of suggestions of alertness in hypnosis on paired-associate learning. *Hypnosis and Learning,* 605-612.

London, P., & Fuhrer, M. (1961). Hypnosis, motivation, and performance. *Journal of Personality, 29,* 321-333.

Maslach, C., Zimbardo, P., & Marshall, G. (1979). Hypnosis as a means of studying cognitive and behavioral control. In E. Fromm & R. E. Shor (Eds.), *Hypnosis: Developments in research and new perspectives* (pp. 649-686). New York: Aldine.

Mutke, P. H. C. (1967). Increased reading comprehension through hypnosis. *American Journal of Clinical Hypnosis, 9,* 262-266.

Nace, E. P., Orne, M. T., & Hammer, A. G. (1974). Posthypnotic amnesia as an active psychic process: The reversibility of amnesia. *Archives of General Psychiatry, 31,* 257-260.

Oetting, E. R. (1964). Hypnosis and concentration in study. *American Journal of Clinical Hypnosis, 7,* 148-151.

Parker, P. D., & Barber, T. X. (1964). Hypnosis, task-motivating instructions, and learning performance. *Journal of Abnormal and Social Psychology, 69,* 499-504.

Pettinati, H. M., & Evans, F. J. (1978). Posthypnotic amnesia: Evaluation of selective recall of successful experiences. *International Journal of Clinical and Experimental Hypnosis, 36,* 317-329.

Pettinati, H. M., Evans, F. J., Orne, E. C., & Orne, M. T. (1981). Restricted use of success cues in retrieval during posthypnotic amnesia. *Journal of Abnormal Psychology,* 345-353.

Porter, J. (1978). Suggestions and success imagery for study problems *International Journal of Clinical and Experimental Hypnosis, 26,* 63-75.

Roeder, G. D. (1978). *Hypnosis and performance: A critical review of the recent literature.* Paper submitted to the University of South Carolina.

Rosenhan, D., & London, P. (1963a). Hypnosis: Expectation, susceptibility, and performance. *Journal of Abnormal and Social Psychology, 66,* 77-81.

Rosenhan, D., & London, P. (1963b). Hypnosis in the unhypnotizable: A study in rote learning. *Journal of Experimental Psychology, 65,* 30-34.

Saccuzzo, D. P., Safran, D., Anderson, V., & McNeill, B. (1982). Visual information processing in high and low susceptible subjects. *International Journal of Clinical and Experimental Hypnosis, 8,* 251-258

Salzberg, H. C. (1960). The effects of hypnotic, post-hypnotic and waking suggestion on performance using tasks varied in complexity. *International Journal of Clinical and Experimental Hypnosis, 8,* 251-258.

Salzberg, H. C., & DePiano, F. A. (1980). Hypnotizability and task motivating suggestions: A further look at how the affect performance. *International Journal of Clinical and Experimental Hypnosis, 28,* 261-271.

Shor, R. E. (1979). The fundamental problem in hypnosis research as viewed from historic perspectives. In E. Fromm & R. E. Shor (Eds.), *Hypnosis: Developments in research and new perspectives* (p. 15-44). New York: Aldine.

Shubat, N. L. (1969). The influence of state and relationship on the hypnotic recall of previously presented material: A test of hypnotic hypernesia. *Dissertation Abstracts International, 30,* 69-11, 980 (Abstract)

Simon, C. W., & Emmons, W. H. (1956). EEG consciousness and sleep. *Science, 124,* 1066-1069.

Smith, M. C. (1983). hypnotic memory enhancement of witnesses: Does it work? *Psychological Bulletin, 94,* 387-407.

Spanos, N. P., & Radtke-Bodorik, H. L. (1980). Integrating hypnotic phenomena with cognitive psychology: An illusion using suggested amnesia. *Bulletin of British Society of Experimental and Clinical Psychology, 3,* 4-7.

Spanos, N. P., Radtke, H. L., Bertran, L. D., Addie, D. L., & Drummond, J. (1982). Disorganized recall, hypnotic amnesia and subject's faking. *Journal of Clinical and Experimental Hypnosis, 28,* 261–271.

Spanos, N. P., Radtke, H. L., & Dubreuil, D. L. (1982). Episodic and semantic memory in posthypnotic amnesia: A reevaluation. *Journal of Personality and Social Psychology, 43,* 565-573.

St. Jean, R., & Coe, W. C. (1981). Recall and recognition memory during posthypnotic amnesia: A failure to confirm the disrupted-search hypothesis and the memory disorganization hypothesis. *Journal of Abnormal Psychology, 90,* 231-241.

Stein, V. T. (1982). The effect of traditional hypnosis, alert hypnosis and task motivation suggestions on recall of contextual material by college students. *Dissertation Abstracts International, 42,* 4176.

Stotnick, R. S., Liebart, R. M., & Hilgard, E. R. (1965). The enhancement of muscular performance in hypnosis through exhortation and involving instructions. *Journal of Personality, 33,* 37-45.

Swiercinsky, D., & Coe, W. C. (1970). Hypnosis, hypnotic responsiveness, and learning meaningful material. *International Journal of Clinical and Experimental Hypnosis, 18,* 217-222.

Swiercinsky, D., & Coe, W. C. (1971). The effect of "alert" hypnosis and hypnotic responsiveness on reading comprehension. *International Journal of Clinical and Experimental Hypnosis, 19,* 146-153.

Thurman, C., Jr. (1974). The effect of hypnosison learning meaningful material. *Dissertation Abstracts International, 34,* 6253B.

Treloar, W. W. (1967). Review of recent research on hypnotic learning. *Psychological reports, 20,* 723-732.

Tulving, E. (1972). Episodic and semantic memory. In E. Tulving & W. Donaldson (Eds.), *Organization of Memory.* New York: Academic Press.

Tulving, E., & Thompson, D. M. (1973). Encoding specificity and retrieval process in episodic memory. *Psychological Review, 80,* 352–373.

Vingoe, F. J. (1968). The development of a group alert-trance scale. *International Journal of Clinical and Experimental Hypnosis, 16,* 120-132.

Vingoe, F. J. (1969). Introversion-extroversion, attitudes toward hypnosis, and susceptibility to the alert trance. *Proceedings of 77th Annual Convention of APA* (pp. 903-904).

Vingoe, F. J. (1973). Comparison of the Harvard Group Scale of Hypnotic Susceptibility, Form A and the group alert trance in a university population. *International Journal of Clinical and Experimental Hypnosis, 21,* 169–179.

Watson, R. I. (1978) *The Great Psychologists.* (4th ed.). New York: Lippincott.

Weitzenhoffer, A. M. (1963). The influence of hypnosis on the learning process some theoretical considerations: II. Recall of meaningful material. In M. Kline (Ed.), *Clinical correlations of experimental hypnosis* (pp. 185–209). Illinois: Thomas Books.

White, R. W. (1967). Two types of hypnotic trance and their personal correlates. *Journal of Psychology, 4,* 279-289.

Wickens, D. D., & Gittis, M. M. (1974). The temporal course of recovery from interference and degree of learning in the Brown-Peterson paradigm. *Journal of Experimental Psychology, 102,* 1021-1026.

Williamsen, J. A., Johnson, H. J., & Eriksen, C. W. (1965). Some characteristics of posthypnotic amesia. *Journal of Abnormal Psychology, 70,* 123-131.

Willis, D. C. (1972). The effect of self-hypnosis on reading rate and comprehension. *American Journal of Clinical Hypnosis, 14,* 249-255.

Zamansky, H. S. (1977). Suggestion and countersuggestion in hypnotic behavior. *Journal of Abnormal Psychology, 86,* 346–351.

Chapter 11

The Forensic Use of Hypnosis

Charles H. Anderton, J. D., Ph.D.
University of South Carolina

During the past decade interest in using hypnosis in forensic arenas has greatly increased. In federal and state court systems, both civil litigation and criminal prosecutions rely heavily on witnesses' and victims' memories of events. Numerous reports have described the effectiveness of hypnosis in aiding memory in the following contexts: assisting recall of witnesses or victims of crime in order to enhance pretrial investigation or provide in-court testimony, confirming which of an uncertain witness' statements is true, obtaining exculpatory evidence from amnesic criminal defendants, or evaluating a defendant's state of mind at the time of the crime (Reiser and Neilson, 1980; Warner, 1979; Worthington, 1979). Cases have been reported, for example, in which a victim who reported little memory of an event underwent hypnosis and produced a lead which was later verified by incontrovertible fingerprint evidence, resulting in conviction (Schafer and Rubio, 1978). Considering these reports, one may be led to believe forensic hypnosis is a tool that should be used in almost all circumstances.

Several questions arise, however, which temper such a conclusion. Are statements made by a witness during or after hypnosis reliable? Are such statements accurate memories, distortions, confabulations, or a combination of all three? Does the use of hypnosis unduly sway juries? Does enhanced self-confidence in a hypnotized witness deprive the opposing party of the right to examine the original "witness" to the events? What hypnotic techniques are effective? Who is qualified to serve as a hypnotist? Finally, what, if any, procedural safeguards are necessary?

The purpose of this chapter is to acquaint the reader with the following: (1) facets of hypnosis which affect its forensic use; (2) research concerning the use of hypnotic techniques to enhance memory, and concerning the alteration of memory in nonhypnotic (waking) and hypnotic subjects; (3) forensic uses of hypnosis; (4) selected cases in which hypnosis has been used; (5) legal decisions

*The author wishes to thank Thomas A. Wadden, Ph.D., for his review of this chapter and valuable comments.

regarding forensic hypnosis; (6) procedural safeguards for forensic use of hypnosis; and (7) suggestions for future research. The chapter will draw upon an excellent recent review by Orne, Soskis, Dinges, and Orne (in press).

FACETS OF HYPNOSIS WHICH AFFECT ITS FORENSIC USE

It will be helpful first to describe what generally transpires during a forensic hypnosis session. The therapist or hypnotist first provides a rationale for the use of hypnosis and briefly explains what hypnosis is. After answering any questions the subject has and establishing adequate rapport, the hypnotist conducts an induction, which usually consists of suggestions for relaxation, sleepiness, focused attention, or related trancelike experiences (Barber, Spanos, and Chaves, 1974). Following the induction, direct suggestions are given for enhanced recall of the events in question, often by asking the subject to reexperience them visually in imagination. A posthypnotic suggestion may be given suggesting that the subject will recall everything that happend during the session, including reliving the events in question and new recollections about those events.

Hilgard (1965) conceptualizes hypnosis as an altered state of consciousness in which a subject experiences increased susceptibility to suggestions. He believes that a subject loses willingness to act independently, develops readiness to engage in fantasy, tolerates some degree of reality distortion, and experiences redirection of attention and changes in perception based on the hypnotist's demands. Others have similarly described hypnosis in terms of augmented amenability to suggestions (Barber et al., 1974; Hull, 1933). Theorists such as Orne (1977) have emphasized the unique, subjective experience which hypnotized subjects undergo, consisting of changes in memory, perception, and cognition. Regardless of how hypnosis occurs, Orne believes that the key characteristic of hypnosis is that the subject experiences it as real, believes in it, and is not merely acting as if he did. Further, individuals with hypnotic ability are more likely to experience dissociative states and perceptual alterations which cannot be accounted for by nonhypnotic events such as relaxation, task-motivational instructions, or placebo effects (McGlashan, Evans, and Orne, 1969).

Hypnotizability (the capacity of a subject to respond to suggestions) varies from person to person but is regarded as a stable characteristic of an individual (Hilgard, 1965). It can be assessed using standardized instruments such as the Barber Suggestibility Scale (Barber, 1976), the Harvard Group Scale of Hypnotic Susceptibility (Shor and Orne, 1962), or the Stanford Hypnotic Susceptibility Scales, Forms A and B (Wietzenhoffer and Hilgard, 1959) and Form C (Weitzenhoffer and Hilgard, 1962). The increased capacity and willingness of a hypnotic subject to accept suggestions requires that the subject temporarily suspend critical judgment. Hypnotic subjects appear to be able to do so for several reasons (Orne et al., in press). First, the subject is normally highly motivated to please the hypnotist because of the therapist-subject interpersonal relationship, in which the therapist either explicitly or implicitly shares his belief that hypnosis involves compliance (Orne, 1981a). Second, subjects' expectations and beliefs about the power of hypnosis tend to be positive. Subjects frequently have been influenced by media and literature to believe that hypnosis is unique and powerful in improving memory. A recent survey found, for example, that 96 percent of college students surveyed expressed this belief (Orne , et al., in press). As a result, the hypnotic subject may believe beforehand that his hypnotic recollections, regardless of content, will be accurate. This belief, in turn, can significantly increase a subject's feeling of confidence in the accuracy of his memories.

Third, it is likely that a hypnotic subject who closes his eyes and enters a state of relaxation places faith in the hypnotist to take responsibility for the subject's well-being during the session. As a result, the subject is often susceptible to subtle contingency reinforcement given by the expert in the form of cues and suggestions. These cues, in the form of verbal responses ("good" or "uh-huh") or silence can reinforce or extinguish, respectively, a subject's efforts to explore an area of inquiry. These cues can produce greater quantities of information than could have been produced without hypnosis, and they may have more to do with the subject's performance than the subject's critical faculties.

Two other facets of hypnosis deserve note. They are the belief that subjects can perform behaviors under hypnosis which they are not capable of displaying in a waking state and the belief that no one can fake hypnosis. First, research has not shown that hypnosis can persuade people to do what they ordinarily would not do. For example, hypnotic subjects cannot be induced to commit antisocial acts (Erickson, 1939). In addition, clinical research has shown that hypnosis does not generally enable people to eliminate undesired behavior, such as excessive eating, smoking, or drinking (Wadden and Anderton, 1982).

Second, research has shown that individuals can feign hypnosis (Orne, 1979). Experienced hypnotists can be deceived by subjects instructed to simulate hypnosis and act as they think the hypnotist wants them to act (Hilgard, 1977; Sheehan, 1972). It has also been shown that deeply hypnotizable subjects can purposely lie (Orne, 1961). Purposeful lying would not generally occur in a clinical setting in which a hypnotic subject is presumably seeking help for a problem. However, the possibility of lying or faking is high in a forensic setting, in which potential consequences of litigation are great for both victims of crimes (imprisonment of criminal so victim can be safe from reoccurrence) and criminal defendants (liberty or imprisonment).

In summary, during hypnosis a subject experiences focused attention and heightened susceptibility to suggestions by the therapist. Changes in memory, perception, and cognition make a subject less willing to act independently and more willing to act in accordance with the hypnotist's direct and subtle demands. Subjects often have high expectations that hypnosis will produce accurate memories and are often highly motivated to conform to the hypnotist's expectations. Research has shown that hypnosis cannot make a subject do what he ordinarily would not do and that hypnosis can indeed be feigned. These two findings are of particular importance in the forensic setting, in which great faith is often placed in the results of hypnosis and in which motivation to dissimulate may be great.

Several other issues must be addressed, however, before one can decide whether hypnosis should be used in forensic settings. These include the examination of hypnotic techniques to enhance memory, alteration of memory in waking and hypnotic subjects, and interrogation techniques.

RESEARCH REGARDING (a) ENHANCEMENT AND ALTERATION OF MEMORY AND INTERROGATION TECHNIQUES

Hypnotic Techniques to Enhance Memory

Several techniques are used in hypnotic recall. Each has potential benefits and risks. We will look at three of these techniques: hypnotic age regression, hypermnesia (increased recollection) suggestions, and removal of amnesia. The first, *hypnotic age regression,* was initially utilized by Freud to help adult patients reexperience traumatic childhood events causing unconscious emotional conflict and psychological symptoms (Breuer and Freud, 1895/1955). Freud was impressed by the ostensible accuracy and details of the patient's memory under hypnosis and by the fact that symptoms disappeared after the cathartic effect produced by this vivid recollection. Later Freud concluded that patients' memories were not totally accurate but included confabulation and fantasy. Nevertheless, whether hypnotic memories of past traumatic events were accurate was not important in Freud's psychoanalysis as it would be in the forensic setting. He believed that symptoms developed as long as the patient *thought* that the memoies were accurate and that remembered events actually occurred.

Modern research on hypnotic age regression, however, has focused on the issue of historical accuracy, that is, whether the subject actually returns in his mind to earlier life stages, as manifested by psychological and physiological responses. Studies have been conducted in which subjects have been age-regressed to six months of age in an effort to obtain the type of postive Babinski sign seen in infants (Gidro-Frank and Bowers-Buch, 1948). Anecdotal evidence also exists showing that age regression produces accurate memories of earlier events (Young, 1926). Later reviews (Barber, 1962), however, have found little evidence for the phenomenon.

In an early study by Orne (1951), for example, age-regressed subjects drew pictures from childhood memories, but an expert in children's drawings examined the drawings and concluded that they were not done by children and indicated "sophisticated oversimplification." O'Connell, Shor, and Orne (1970) attempted to replicate an earlier study supporting the accuracy of age regression memories (Reiff and Scheerer, 1959). They age-regressed both hypnotic and simulating subjects to ages 10, 7, and 4. No differences were found between real and simulating subjects with regard to accuracy of remembered events, such as specific days on which birthdays occurred. No evidence of hypermnesia was found among any subjects. Further, although subjects often gave vividly detailed reports of matters such as who sat next to them in the second grade, these ostensibly credible statements were found to be false by later investigation of school records.

Unfortunately, it is sometimes impossible to ascertain which memories are true and which have been caused by suggestive cues by the therapist or stimulation of unrelated memories of the subject. Only independent verification can determine the truth of material produced by hypnotic age regression. Richness of detail is hardly dispositive. Surprisingly, few studies have even attempted to verify specific memories through subsequent investigation (Yates, 1961).

The second technique consists of *suggestions for hypermnesia.* Research on this problem has usually compared recall under hypnosis with recall without hypnosis of events witnessed minutes, hours, or weeks earlier in a nonhypnotic state. A large part of the research , however, is not directly relevant to the questions surrounding forensic hypnosis because of three limitations. First, information recalled in laboratory research has often consisted of word lists, nonsense syllables, and other nonmeaningful information, whereas information sought in forensic contexts involves meaningful events. Second, laboratory subjects are rarely aroused or under stress, whereas victims or witnesses of crimes are almost always aroused when they observe the events in question. Third, laboratory subjects are often instructed to observe or remember events, whereas victims and witnesses of crimes observe events without instructions to remember events (DePiano and Salzberg, 1981).

Regarding the first limitation, that studies have utilized nonmeaningful material, most studies using contextually *nonmeaningful* material have found that hypnotic suggestions for hypermnesia do not enhance recall beyond that realized in nonhypnotic conditions (Barber and Calverly, 1966; Huse, 1930, Salzberg and DePiano, 1980). On the other hand, studies using contextually *meaningful* material, such as literature or pictures, have generally found that hypnosis enhances recall beyond that of nonhypnotic conditions (DePiano and Salzberg, 1981; Dhanens and Lundy, 1974; Stalnaker and Riddle, 1932; White, Fox, and Harris, 1940). Several researchers have reached contrary results, however. Augustynek (1978, 1979), for example, found that hypnosis enhanced recall of all material, regardless of its meaningfulness, and Shaul (1978) found that recall under hypnosis was not enhanced beyond that obtained with instructions seeking to increase subjects' motivation for the task.

Regarding the second limitation, that studies have not always manipulated state of arousal, Rosenthal (1944) found that recall in hypnotic subjects exceeded that in nonhypnotic subjects for stimuli observed in a state of arousal or anxiety. Other studies, however, have not replicated Rosenthal (Burch, 1974; DePiano and Salzberg, 1981; Helwig, 1978; Shaul, 1978).

Regarding the third limitation, that laboratory subjects observe events intentionally, several studies in the last five years have utilized simulated accidents and mock crimes to investigate hypnotic hypermnesia for unintentionally witnessed events. These studies are of great relevance to forensic hypnosis. Despite Griffin's (1980) finding that hypnosis significantly enhanced recall of witnessed mock crimes, numerous other studies found no enhanced recall with hypnosis regarding witnessed mock crimes (Sheehan and Tilden, 1983; Timm, 1981), witnessed accidents (Putnam, 1979; Zelig and Beidleman, 1981), and facial recognition (Wagstaff, Traverse, and Milner, 1982). Sheehan and Tilden (1983), for example, showed subjects slides of a street sequence in which a wallet was stolen from a woman's shoulder bag. Afterward, subjects were tested either under hypnosis or in the waking state for memory of events depicted in the slides. Results indicated that whether a subject had been hypnotized or not was unrelated to the number of correct responses a subject made.

The seminal study in this area of hypermnesia involved suggestions that subjects would remember prose committed to memory in elementary school (Stalnaker and Riddle, 1932). Hypnotic subjects' responses appeared to be more detailed and accurate than those of waking subjects. However, later investigation revealed that hypnotic subjects, despite their increase in quantity of accurate memories, exhibited an even greater increase in quantity of confabulated, inaccurate memories.

Orne (1979) describes confabulation as the filling in of memory gaps with plausible, inferred details. The hypnotized subject who receives the commonly utilized suggestion that on waking he will remember all details vividly, both those memories existing before and those obtained during hypnosis, may unconsciously confound hypnotic memories with waking, prehypnosis memories. This recall, as experienced in hypnosis, may become the authoritative version, and there may be no practical way to distinguish between accurate recall derived from the original experience and inaccurate recall derived elsewhere.[1]

[1] The extent to which confabulation can occur in hypnosis is also clear when a subject is given suggestions to experience a future event about which no memories yet exist. For example, in age progression, subjects are given the suggestion that it is the year 2000 and asked to describe the world (Kline and Guze, 1951). Subjects then provide specific, convinicing descriptions, presumably limited only by the subject's technical background and creativity.

Stalnaker and Riddle's (1932) research in hypermnesia was important in indicating that hypnotized subjects produced a greater number of responses and a resultant increase in accurate recollections, as compared to nonhypnotized subjects. Nevertheless, hypnotized subjects exhibited an even greater increase in *inaccurate* recollections. Orne et al. (in press) suggest that these increases may reflect reduced critical judgment and laxness in the subject's response criterion. Rather than memory being enhanced, the subject simply reports memories previously considered too uncertain to report, with some being accurate but more being inaccurate. Although recent hypermnesia research has monitored both accurate and inaccurate recollections, as well as total recollections, increases in productivity have not been adequately controlled for or investigated.

Only two research groups have attempted to control for increases in productivity by comparing increases from waking hypermnesia techniques with increases from hypnotic hypermnesia techniques (Dywan and Bowers, 1983; Stager and Lundy, in press; see also Stager, 1974). In a significant recent study Dywan and Bowers (1983) showed subjects a series of 60 black and white pictures and then assessed recall of the subjects in daily tests for a week using a form of forced recall. Most subjects correctly remembered about 30 of the pictures on the first forced recall. After one week, half of the subjects were hypnotized, and half were told to relax and focus attention on the pictures seen a week before (task-motivational instructions). Results indicated that hypnotic subjects recalled an average of five more pictures than they had recalled before hypnosis, twice as many new pictures as nonhypnotic, task-motivation subjects recalled. However, an average of four of the five new pictures recalled by hypnotic subjects were inaccurate, even though subjects reported that all five new memories were true. Therefore, despite an increase in accurate recall, hypnotic subjects experienced a threefold increase in inaccurate recall. Dywan and Bowers suggest that increased correct recall in hypnosis may not indicate enhanced memory as much as a shift in report criterion and decrease in caution in what subjects are willing to report as memories, resulting in a proportionally greater number of errors. They suggest social cues, demand characteristics, and expectations engendered by the hypnotic situation as possible sources for this shift.

Stager and Lundy (in press), however, used a probed recall technique to assess recollection of details from a film observed by highly hypnotizable subjects both with and without hypnosis. Consistent with prior research, results showed that highly hypnotizable subjects who were hypnotized exhibited an increase in accurate memories, while highly hypnotizable subjects who were not hypnotized and low hypnotizable subjects (with or without hypnosis) exhibited no such increase. In contrast to the results of Dywan and Bowers (1983), however, highly hypnotizable subjects who were hypnotized exhibited a *decrease* in inaccurate memories. Orne et al. (in press) suggest that these results may be explained on grounds that probed recall formats provided a highly structured response set, as well as detailed and accurate information regarding events about which the subject was asked. Such questions as the following were asked: "Immediately after the title of the film was shown, a young man carrying some books was shown walking along in front of several billboards. What was the color of his sports jacket?" (Stager, 1974, p. 94). Stager and Lundy's results are valuable in demonstrating the positive effect of hypnosis on memory when specific retrieval cues are used. Unfortunately, such cues are rarely available in nonresearch settings.

The final technique is *removal of amnesia* (Orne, 1979), which must be distinguished from previously mentioned therapeutic efforts to have a patient relive past traumatic events (Breuer and Freud, 1895/1955). In the latter, full reexperiencing and spontaneous expression of affect are encouraged for therapeutic reasons. In the former, however, no presumption of psychopathology exists, and memory is refreshed with suggestions that the subject will not experience strong affect. The memory is usually analogized to a large television where memories can be seen in a film which can be stopped, run forward, or run backward at the subject's request (Reiser, 1980). The suggestion is made that the subject will be a spectator of the film without participating or experiencing pain in any way.

Unfortunately, however, the human memory does not function like a tiny videotape recorder. Such a view, called the "exact copy" theory of memory, has not been accepted by memory theorists (Bourne, Dominowski, and Loftus, 1979; Crowder, 1976). Nor has such a view been supported by research described above indicating that hypnosis enhances recall of contextually meaning information but not nonmeaningful information. If the videotape model of memory were correct, there would be no effect for meaningfulness of information, and everything would be remembered equally. Rather, accepted theory holds that memory is constantly changing and involves reconstruction and alteration, as well as intact reproduction, of past events (Bartlett, 1932; Crowder, 1976). We will now review evidence regarding these processes of reconstruction and alteration of memory in both waking and hypnotic subjects.

Alteration of Memory in Waking (Nonhypnotic) Subjects

The processing of information in memory consists of three stages (Hilgard and Loftus, 1979, Loftus, 1979). First is acquisition, in which information is encoded and stored in memory. Second is retention, the period between acquisition and later recollection of material, during which time original stored information can remain the same or be merged with or supplanted by new information. Third is retrieval, discussed below, in which a person recalls stored information. Loftus has studied alteration of memory during the second stage, retention, by asking subjects to recall an event a second time, with the first recall considered an event during retention interval. For example, Loftus' (1975) subjects viewed eight men in a film and were then asked, "What were the *four* men wearing?" When asked later to recall the number of men, they tended to report six men. Loftus calls this "compromise memory" because people tend to compromise their own recollections to fit what seems expected.

Similarly, Loftus (1979) has effectively introduced nonexistent objects into memory during retention. A typical experiment involves showing subjects a film and later asking questions about the film which are intended to bias memory. For example, subjects viewed a film in which no barn existed and then were asked, "How fast was the car going as it went by the barn by the crossroads?" When subsequently asked whether they had seen a barn, subjects given the biased question tended to report that they had seen a barn more than subjects not given the biased question.

The third stage of memory processing, retrieval, is particularly important for forensic hypnosis. In this stage two major factors may undermine the reliability of hypnotic interrogation. They are wording of questions and type of retrieval. Regarding wording of questions, minute changes in wordings have been shown in the laboratory to evoke significantly different responses. In two revealing studies subjects observed films and were then questioned about events therein (Loftus and Palmer, 1974; Loftus and Zanni, 1975). Loftus and Palmer (1974) showed an automobile accident and then asked questions which were identical except for one word. Some subjects were asked, "How fast were the cars going when they *contacted* one another?" Others were asked, "How fast were the cars going when they *smashed* one another?" The former gave the lowest speed estimates; the latter, the highest. Similarly, Loftus and Zanni (1975) asked subjects about a nonexistent car. Half were asked, "Did you see *the* car?" The other half was asked, "Did you see *a* car?" Twenty percent of the "the" group reported seeing the nonexistent car, while only 6 percent of the "a" group reported seeing the car.

These studies reveal the power and dangers of subtle wording which can lead the person interrogated to a specific answer. Leading questions not only inquire but also give information. "Did you see the car?" implies that a car was present, while "Did you see a car?" involves no implication either way. Loftus (1979) has shown that by shrewdly suggestive questions witnesses can be convinced that a robber had a mustache when he did not and that a red light was green.

Regarding the second influence on retrieval, type of retrieval, there are two primary forms of questions: (1) free recall or open-ended, in which the subject recollects events in narrative form (e.g., "What did you see?"), and (2) closed, recognition-based questions, such as multiple choice or yes-no questions ("Was the robber heavy, thin, or average in build?"). Cady (1924) found that the free recall form of questions gives more accurate but less complete information, while closed questions give more complete but less accurate information Marquis, Marshall, and Oskamp (1972) similarly found that after showing subjects films, accuracy is highest and completeness lowest for free recall questions. As retrieval becomes more specifically detailed and structured, accuracy decreases while completeness increases. It appears that free recall questions followed by more specific questioning constitute the most effective method of interrogation.

If the aforementioned possibilities for alteration of memory exist for waking subjects, the potential for bias and alteration of memory may be even greater for hypnotized subjects due to increased suggestibility, increased compliance, and decreased response criterion in the latter.

Alteration of Memory in Hypnotic Subjects

Several memory studies have investigated the issue of whether hypnosis augments the biasing effects of various types of questions. Putnam (1979) had subjects observe a mock accident and then complete a questionnaire asking both nonleading questions and leading questions containing misinformation. Hypnotized and nonhypnotized subjects did not differ in the accuracy or inaccuracy of their responses to nonleading questions. However, hypnotized subjects made more inaccurate responses to leading questions (which referred to nonexistent items, e.g., "Did you see the passenger in the car?") than did nonhypnotic subjects. Putnam concluded that hypnotic subjects are more suggestible and easily influenced by leading questions than nonhypnotic subjects. These results were largely replicated by Zelig and Beidleman (1981).

Laurence and Perry (1983a) found similar biasing effects with hypnosis. Twenty-seven highly hypnotizable subjects were asked during hypnosis to choose one night from the previous week. Subjects were than ascertained to have had no specific memories of awakening at any time during that night. Through an age regression technique, subjects were then asked to reexperience that night and were asked whether they had heard some loud noises that had awakened them that night. Results revealed that nearly half of the subjects thereafter responded to the suggestion implicit in this leading question by reporting both during and after hypnosis that they had heard loud noises during the night. Some of these subjects maintained their belief that the noises occurred even after being told that the hypnotist had suggested the noises to them during hypnosis.

Contradictory results were obtained by Sheehan and Tilden (1983) and Sturm (1983). Both studies found that hypnotic subjects did not exhibit any more susceptibility to bias and inaccurate recall of information from leading questions than did nonhypnotic subjects.

Interrogation Techniques

Various metaphors are used in hypnotic interrogation. As mentioned above regarding removal of amnesia, a frequently utilized metaphor is the videotape recorder or television (Reiser, 1976). Reiser (1980) states that the hypnotist

> indicates that the subject in imagination will be watching a special documentary film on television from a safe, secure, and comfortable place. This special documentary can be speeded up, slowed down, stopped, reversed, with close-ups possible on any person, object, or thing in the film. The sound can be turned up high so that anything that is said, even a whisper, can be heard very clearly. This will be a documentary film of the incident in question and will depict accurately and vividly everything of significance and importance the subject perceived and experienced in relationship to that crime scene. And even though what occurred was very traumautic, the subject watching the TV documentary will be able to remain calm and relaxed, feeling detached from what is happening on the television set. The subject will be observing it as a reporter, covering an event to be written up accurately for a news story. (p. 159)

The metaphor is indeed alluring in terms of its ostensible potential for accurate recall of detailed facts. However, as a model of memory the metaphor is inadequate. It omits various stages of information processing and has not been accepted by memory theorists (Bourne, Dominowski, and Loftus, 1979; Crowder 1976). In addition, its potential for misuse is great. The model entails both an implicit suggestion that the facts are available to the subject somewhere in his memory and an explicit suggestion that facts remembered based on viewing the documentary are accurate. It is not hard to imagine how much more detailed a subject would be in testifying were he to believe he had visually reviewed the exact events in question. Indeed, the subject would not believe he was testifying from the documentary but from his own memory of the actual events. Separating testimony based on actual memories and testimory based on confabulated memories created during hypnosis would be extremely difficult.

Similarly, a subject's confidence in his recollections can be enhanced immeasurably if he believes hypnosis has helped him remember accurated details. Although the self-confidence of a witness is not a crucial factor when hypnosis is being used to obtain investigative leads which can later be corroborated by independent evidence, self-confidence is a key factor in in-court testimony. Self-confidence not only enhances a witness' ability to withstand hostile cross-examination but also allows a witness to appear credible to a jury when being directly examined by his own attorney. It has been shown that the greater certainty a witness feels in his memory, the greater will be his perceived credibility (Lindsay, Wells, and Rumpel, 1981; Wells and Leippe, 1981; Wells, Lindsay, and Ferguson, 1979). In addition, Loftus (1979) has shown that great weight is given to statements by a person claiming to be an eyewitness.

Sheehan and Tilden (1983) have shown that hypnotic subjects, especially highly hypnotizable subjects, experience greater certainty in the accuracy of their memory than waking subjects. Putnam (1979), although finding no significant difference between hypnotic and waking subjects' confidence ratings, found that hypnotic subjects speculated that they were more accurate with hypnosis than they would have been without hypnosis. Further, Timm (1982) found that hypnotizable subjects who remembered events during hypnosis were more confident that inaccurate memories were accurate than were unhypnotizable subjects who recalled without hypnosis. Hence, the danger of obtaining inaccurate memories during hypnosis is matched by an equally great danger that hypnosis can greatly enhance a subject's confidence in inaccurate memories obtained through hypnosis.

In summary, regarding *hypnotic techniques to enhance memory*, research has not generally shown *hypnotic age regression* to be effective in returning a subject to a prior life stage and in generating accurate memories of that stage. Research on *hypermnesia* has shown that hypnosis can enhance recall over that of nonhypnotic techniques if the information to be remembered is contextually meaningful. No such effect, however, appears to exist for hypnosis over waking techniques when the subject is in a state of arousal or when the events to be remembered were witnessed unintentionally. Hypnosis appears to lower subjects' response criterion and increase productivity of responses. Two studies with contradictory results sought to control for productivity by comparing increases from waking hypermnesia techniques with increases from hypnotic hypermnesia techniques. Further research must address the possibility that hypnotic subjects exhibit an increase in accurate memories but an even greater increase in inaccurate memories. Techniques for *removal of amnesia* do not appear reliable because they presuppose a videotape model of memory, which ignores the capacity of memories to be combined with and altered by new information.

Memory research on waking subjects has shown that memory alteration occurs in both retention and retrieval stages of memory processing. Small changes in the wording of questions have been shown to distort a witness' memory for a previously experienced event. The type of question asked can also evoke different responses. Free recall questions are more accurate but less complete, while closed questions are less accurate but more complete. The optimal approach is free recall questions initially, followed by closed, specific questions.

Although results are not entirely consistent, *memory research with hypnotic subjects* has shown that hypnotic subjects are generally more susceptible to inaccurate responses based on leading, suggestive questions than are nonhypnotic subjects. Separating resultant confabulations from original memories is extremely difficult, if not impossible. Regarding *interrogation techniques*, use of a videotape recorder metaphor in interrogation contradicts established memory theory and wrongly implies that memories during hypnosis will be accurate.

Finally, it has been shown that hypnotic subjects not only give more inaccurate responses than waking subjects, they also experience greater conviction in the accuracy of their memory. Ironically, this resulting self-confidence can help an in-court witness testify with greater detail and credibility to the jury while providing inaccurate recollections.

Each of the above dangers shown by memory and hypnosis research is intensified in legal settings because of witnesses' motivation to provide testimony which will aid their cause and avoid acutely undesirable consequences. The aforementioned dangers in the use of hypnosis raise serious questions as to whether hypnosis should ever be used with a witness who must later testify in court.

FORENSIC USE OF HYPNOSIS

Hypnosis first appeared in a forensic context in this country in the late 1800s. The court in *People v. Ewbanks* (1897) held that, "The law of the United States does not recognize hypnosis" (p. 1053). Since then, however, hypnosis has been formally approved by the AMA (1958) and APA (1960, as cited by Hilgard, 1965) and used with increasing frequency and effectiveness as a therapeutic modality (Kroger, 1963). With this acceptance has come renewed interest on the part of law enforcement agencies and attorneys in the introduction of hypnotically derived evidence into the legal process. Most of the literature describing this forensic use of hypnosis consists of anecdotal reports of law enforcement cases in which hypnosis was utilized (Arons, 1967; Kroger and Douce, 1980). Some report great success (Schafer and Rubio, 1978). Others, such as Dorcus (1960), conclude that "recall . . . (is) not greatly improved under hypnosis" but that "when strong emotional elements surround the events to be recalled, some additional information may be secured" (p. 60). Salzberg (1977) states that the subject's motivation and capacity for being hypnotized, the amount of emotional blocking associated with the experience, and the actual knowledge the subject has of the events to be recalled are crucial in forensic cases.

Hypnosis has been used primarily in four types of cases, those in which: (1) no facts are yet known about the perpetrators of the crime, and investigative leads are needed; (2) significant facts are known, a suspect has been identified, and a witness needs to recall details for purposes of court testimony; (3) a witness has given conflicting statements, one of which must be verified as true; and (4) a defendant's mental condition (e.g., lack of memory) impedes his defense or is part of the litigation (e.g., defendant's competency to stand trial or alleged insanity at the time of the crime).

In the first situation, hypnosis has been used successfully to aid victims or witnesses who cannot recall any details or provide leads for police. For example,

Schafer and Rubio (1978) reported a rape case in which the rapist dropped his wallet before leaving the victim's bedroom. The victim quickly took it into her bathroom, locked the door, and looked at its contents. She was only able to glance at his identification card and photograph, however, before he returned a second time. Later, she could not remember his name or photograph. During hypnosis, she could not visualize the identification card name but was able to visualize the photograph and later identify the rapist's mug shot. When the defendant was arrested and fingerprinted, his thumb print matched one found in the victim's room, and he was convicted.

Similarly, Kroger and Douce (1980) reported the Chowchilla kidnapping case in California in which 26 school children and their bus driver were abducted from their bus at gunpoint by masked men and herded into vans. The kidnappers drove the vans to a remote rock quarry, sealed the vans and victims off inside a rectangular-shaped tomb underneath the ground, and fled. After prolonged effort, the bus driver and two older boys dug their way out, and the children were rescued. When the investigation began, the bus driver stated that he had tried unsuccessfully to memorize the license plate on the getaway van. Under hypnosis, however, he called out license plate numbers which led to arrests of suspects who were convicted and sentenced to life imprisonment. Unfortunately, the authors provided no additional details whereby one could reasonably conclude that those convicted were guilty.

In investigative situations such as these, the use of hypnosis poses little danger because no facts or preconceived notions typically exist in investigators' minds regarding the events in question. Any lead obtained from hypnosis can be verified or disconfirmed independently, just like any other lead received by police.

In the second situation, however, hypnosis is used to refresh or buttress the witness' memory about events partially remembered or suspects already identified. In this instance, there is likelihood of conscious or unconscious bias, suggestivity, and leading questions, since authorities already have a factual scenario or suspect in mind. For example, in *State v. White* (1979), a 20-year-old woman named "Sweetie Pie" had been strangled to death several years earlier. Police later received complaints from several women about being beaten and choked by Joe White, who had known "Sweetie Pie." A woman volunteered to be hypnotized and questioned about her past love affair with White. Under hypnosis she was asked leading questions about White's possible role in "Sweetie Pie's" murder. A posthypnotic suggestion was given that she would tell the truth. One week later she told the police that once, while choking her, White screamed, "If you don't behave, I'll do the same thing to you that I did to 'Sweetie Pie'." Whtie was indicted but never convicted of "Sweetie Pie's" murder because the court excluded the woman's hypnotically-induced testimony of White's confession. Because of suggestivity which the court found in the hypnotic procedure, the court ruled that the memory of the witness was more likely created than genuinely remembered. Karlin (1983) reports similar cases in which the reliability of hypnotically-enhanced testimony was questionable.

In the third type of situation, hypnosis is used to ascertain which of an unreliable witness' prior conflicting statements is true. For example, in *In re Milligan* (1978), a multiple murder, the prosecution's key witness was a 14-year-old girl who had given so many conflicting versions that it was speculated that she was involved in the murders herself. The witness' aunt, sister, grandmother, and cousin had been murdered, and the witness could not say whether her memories were of acutal events or dreams. During hypnosis she repeated one version of her story, and it was suggested to her that she would know if this were fact or dream. Thereafter, she became reassured of her version and was consistent and unflappable under cross-examination at trial. In such a case hypnosis can significantly enhance a subject's self-confidence in the particular version of events which she happens to recall during hypnosis.

In another case, *State v. Douglas* (1978), a woman reported that she had been raped and robbed and was receiving threatening notes from the perpetrators. After hypnosis, she identified a perpetrator's mug shot. The prosecutor, originally skeptical about the case, decided to prosecute after the mug shot identification. Later, however, the prosecutor ordered a handwriting analysis of the threatening notes, which were found to have been written by the rape victim. When confronted, the victim admitted concocting the whole story to regain attention from her estranged husband. In this case hypnosis' purported reliability nearly caused irreparable damage.

The fourth situation is that in which a defendant's mental condition either hinders his defense (lack of memory about the alleged crime) or is the focus of the litigation (competency to stand trial or insanity at the time of the crime). An example of the former occurred in *People v. Ritchie* (1977). A man accused of killing a two and half year-old child requested hypnosis to recall forgotten memories about the events in question. In hypnosis he relived events with great affect and remembered seeing his wife commit the murder. A review by experts of a videotape of the session, however, revealed leading questions by the hypnotist and blatant contradictions in the defendant's story. As a result, the court excluded the hypnotic evidence based on its inherent unreliability.

Successful utilization of investigative hypnosis has led to the training of thousands of police officers across the United States in hypnotic techniques for questioning witnesses (Reiser, 1980). The Society for Investigative and Forensic Hypnosis has also been established (Reiser and Neilson, 1980). Some (Orne et al., in press) have questioned who is qualified to administer hypnosis in a forensic setting. Those supporting the use of police officers as hypnotists argue that police officers are trained and experienced in interviewing citizens regarding crimes and that use of police officers would be less expensive than mental health professionals. However, the International Society of Hypnosis (ISH), made up of physicians, psychologists, dentists, and clinical social workers, and its constituent societies in the United States (American Society of Clinical Hypnosis and the Society for Clinical and Experimental Hypnosis) adopted by overwhelming majority a resolution stating that the ISH "is strongly opposed to the training of police officers as hypnotechnicians and the use of hypnosis by the police officer" (ISH, 1979). Primary reasons for this position were the potential for the creation of confabulated memories during hypnosis and the concern that police officers lack training in evaluating psychopathology and handling the significant risk for psychological harm in witnesses or victims of traumatic events. In addition, hypnotists would be unfamiliar with details of the case and free of bias (Orne, 1981b).

In summary, hypnosis has been used with mixed results both before and after criminal suspects have been identified. Risks appear to be least and potential benefits greatest when hypnosis is used to develop investigative leads before any suspects or crucial facts are determined. However, the more hypnosis is used to refresh a witness' existing knowledge of events or strengthen the testimony of an unreliable, wavering witness, the greater the risk for creating confabulated, irreparably altered memories. Moreover, controversy exists over whether police officers are qualified to administer hypnosis or whether it should be done only by mental health professionals. The latter appear more qualified because they are both attuned to psychological dangers inherent in dealing with witnesses to traumatic events and unaware of facts regarding a particular case.

Legal Decisions Regarding Forensic Hypnosis

Recent increased use of hypnosis in the forensic arena has given rise to much legal research and concern (For reviews, see Diamond, 1980; Dilloff, 1977; Murray, 1979; Sarno, 1979; Spector and Foster, 1977; Warner, 1979). Most decisions and reviews have dealt with the use of hypnosis to refresh a witness' memory prior to testimony rather than the use of hypnosis to obtain investigative leads later corroborated by independent evidence. As will be shown, the prevailing trend among courts appears to be to reject the former and accept the latter.

Before reviewing legal decisions, it will be instructive to look at four primary legal issues and objections involved (Worthington, 1979). First, the party contesting the use of hypnosis can argue that hypnosis is not an adequately accepted and reliable scientific technique. The general test for admissibility of a scientific technique was enunciated years ago in *Frye v. United States* (1923), which provided the standard regarding admissibility of such techniques as polygraphs, "truth serums," blood typing, voiceprints, and ballistics tests. The court stated that a scientific principle will be accepted and considered valid when "the thing from which the deduction is made . . . (is) sufficiently established to have gained general acceptance in . . . (its) particular field . . . (p. 1014). Typically, courts require that the reliability of the scientific method be established, that the witness be qualified as an expert in his field, and that correct application of scientific principles in that case be shown before evidence is admissible *(People v. Shirley,* 1982).

Second, the party opposing admission of hypnotically-aided testimony can argue the Sixth Amendment of the United States Constitution, which provides that in any criminal prosecution the accused has the right to be confronted with the witnesses against him. It is argued that hypnosis can cause a subject to confabulate new, inaccurate memories which he will believe are authoritatively true. If this happens, an accused loses the chance to confront the same "witness" who existed at the time of the alleged crime, and the accused's Sixth Amendment rights are violated.

Third, the United States Supreme Court has repeatedly excluded identifications of subjects in impermissibly suggestive circumstances (e.g., when the robber allegedly had a beard and only one person in a group of mug shots shown to the victim has a beard) as violations of the fifth and fourteenth Amendments of the United States Constitution, which provide that no one can be deprived of liberty without due process of law (*Simmons v. United States,* 1968). It is argued that the highly suggestive circumstances involved in hypnotizing a victim who later identifies the defendant are akin to impermissibly suggestive identifications.

Fourth, the prosecution has a legal and ethical duty not to suppress or destory material evidence favorable to the defendant (*Brady v. Maryland,* 1963). Courts can dismiss a case when the prosecution has suppressed or destroyed material evidence, whether intentionally or negligently. It can be argued that hypnotizing a witness before the adverse party gets a chance to cross-examine the witness destroys potentially favorable and material evidence which the adverse party may have obtained, had the witness remained "uncontaminated" by hypnosis.

As far as legal decisions are concerned, courts have generally taken one of three positions: (1) admission, without regard to circumstances under which hypnosis was administered (*Harding v. State,* 1968); (2) exclusion, without regard to circumstances under which hypnosis was administered (*State v. Mack,* 1980); and (3) admission as long as procedural safeguards existed during administration (*State v. Hurd,* 1981).

Regarding the first position, the highest criminal court in Maryland ruled on hypnotically-enhanced testimony in the seminal case of *Harding v. State* (1968).

In that case the prosecuting witness suffered from amnesia after being shot, raped, and abandoned along a deserted road. Under hypnosis she was able to relate the events following the shooting. The court ruled that testimony regarding memories obtained for the first time during hypnosis is admissible and declared that the fact that the witness had achieved her knowledge during hypnosis went only to the question of evidentiary weight to be given to the testimony by the jury, not to admissibility. In other words, instead of not allowing the witness to testify at all, the court allowed her to testify and simply left it up to the jury to decide whether her testimony was credible. The court likened such refreshing of a witness' memory to the commonly accepted procedure of aiding a witness' recollections through review of documentary evidence. However, the court recommended a cautionary instruction urging the jury to weigh hypnotic evidence carefully and not give it greater weight than any other evidence at trial. Other courts thereafter followed *Harding v. State* in admitting hypnotically-aided testimony in criminal cases (*State v. Jorgenson,* 1971; State v. McQueen, 1978; *United States v. Adams,* 1978) and in civil cases (*Kline v. Ford Motor Company, Inc.,* 1975), with reversals of judgments occurring only when the use of hypnosis was not disclosed (*United States v. Miller,* 1969). Further, courts have generally not wavered from a policy of not admitting in-court testimony, tape recording, or written summaries of statements made by the witness while in trance (*State v. Harris,* 1965).

In 1980, the Minnesota State Supreme Court adopted the second of the above three positions. In *State v. Mack* (1980) the court held that a previously hypnotized witness could not testify at trial regarding subject matters adduced during pretrial hypnosis, regardless of whether testimony was offered for the prosecution or defense. The court criticized *Harding v. State* and based its exclusionary decision upon the testimony of expert witnesses regarding the clinical and scientific uses of hypnosis. Those witnesses cited lack of reliability of hypnotically-aided testimony, augmented suggestibility of hypnotic subjects, and unshakeable self-confidence in previously hypnotized witnesses.

Similarly, in a noteworthy recent opinion (*Collins v. State,* 1982) the Maryland court overruled its earlier *Harding v. State* ruling and held that hypnosis did not meet the standard for admission of scientific evidence established in *Frye v. United States.* The court reviewed scientific research regarding hypnosis and concluded that hypnotic refreshing of recollection is not generally accepted as reliable by the relevant scientific community. Other states which have similarly excluded hypnotically-induced recollections of a witness or victim are California (*People v. Shirley,* 1982), Florida (*Shockey v. State,* 1976), Georgia (*Creamer v. State,* 1974), Indiana (*Strong v. State,* 1976), Michigan (*People v. Gonzales,* 1981), Nebraska (*State v. Palmer,* 1981), Pennsylvania (*Commonwealth v. Nazarovitch,* 1981), and Virginia *(Greenfield v. Commonwealth,* 1974). North

Carolina (*State v. Waters,* 1983) and Wyoming (*Chapman v. State,* 1982) have recently admitted hypnotically-enhanced testimony.

The California ruling in *People v. Shirley* is exhaustive and noteworthy. That court concluded that the use of hypnosis to restore the memory of a potential witness was not generally accepted as reliable by the relevant scientific community. Therefore, the court held that since the *Frye v. United States* test had not been met, the testimony of a witness who had undergone hypnosis for the purpose of restoring his memory of the events in issue was not admissible as to any matters relating to those events, from the time of the hypnotic session forward. This ruling, however, allowed a witness to testify regarding topics wholly unrelated to the events that were the subject of the hypnotic session. The ruling also approved the use of hypnosis with a witness for investigative purposes, although the witness is not thereafter allowed to testify regarding the events of the crime.

Two of the most noted legal experts on the law of evidence frown upon admission of hypnotically-aided testimony because of the subject's heightened suggestibility (McCormick, 1972; Wigmore, 1970). McCormick (1972) states:

> Declarations made under hypnosis have been treated judicially in a manner similar to drug-induced statements. The hypnotized person is ultrasuggestible, and this manifestly endangers the reliability of his statements. The courts have recognized to some extent the usefulness of hypnosis, as an investigative technique and in diagnosis and therapy. However, they have rejected confessions induced thereby, statements made under hypnosis when offered by the subject in his own behalf, and opinion as to mental state based on hypnotic examination. (p.510).

Several states have adopted the third position expressed above and ruled that hypnotically induced testimony is admissible but only under limited circumstances. For example, the New Jersey State Supreme Court (*State v. Hurd,* 1981) required that any pretrial hypnosis of a victim or witness be shown by clear and convincing evidence to be minimally reliable. The court also required the party offering the evidence to comply with specific procedural safeguards, which will be enumerated in full below. Finally, the court stated that if these safeguards are present, the trial court can then admit or exclude the testimony based on a determination of whether "the use of hypnosis in the particular case was reasonably likely to result in recall comparable in accuracy to normal human memory" (*State v. Hurd,* 1981, p.111).

Similarly, the Arizona State Supreme Court modified an earlier holding (*State v. Mena,* 1981) which absolutely excluded hypnotically-induced testimony. The court's modification in *Collins v. Superior Court of the State of Arizona* (1982) held that a witness or victim who had been hypnotized could still testify as long as the testimony related to matters which the individual was shown to have remembered before hypnosis. Though such a distinction is logical and attractive, application of this rule could present many difficulties. It would seem imperative, for example, to create an exhaustive record (perhaps by deposition) of all the witness' memories about a matter before hypnosis in order to determine whether a witness' in-court testimony involved a matter which the witness had *not* remembered before hypnosis. Given the complexity of some factual questions, separating one "matter" which the witness recalled before hypnosis from another "matter" which the witness did not recall before hypnosis could be extremely difficult, both for the witness and the court. A final danger from this ruling is that, if hypnosis fails to elicit new details, the witness can still testify and benefit from the significantly enhanced self-confidence of a hypnotic subject.

In summary, opponents of the use of hypnotically-aided testimony argue that hypnotic procedures are unreliable and result in confabulated, irreparably altered memories. Such testimony is opposed on various grounds, such as the failure of hypnosis to comply with legal standards for scientific evidence, violation of the Sixth Amendment requirement that an accused be able to confront witnesses against him, violation of the due process clauses in the form of impermissibly suggestive identifications, and violation of the prosecution's duty not to suppress or destroy material evidence favorable to the defendant. As to hypnotically-enhanced testimony, the current trend among courts appears to be either outright exclusion, or admission when procedural safeguards exist. Courts generally allow the use of hypnosis to develop investigative leads, especially when procedural safeguards are applied.

Procedural Safeguards for Forensic Hypnosis

Orne (1979) proposed the following safeguards, which have been used and cited in virtually every major recent court ruling (e.g., *Collins v. State,* 1982; *People v. Shirley*, 1982; *State v. Hurd,* 1981; *State v. Mack,* 1980):

1. Hypnosis should be carried out by a psychiatrist or psychologist with special training in its use. He should not be informed about the facts of the case verbally; rather, he should receive a written memorandum outlining whatever facts he is to know, carefully avoiding any other communications which might affect his opinion. Thus, his beliefs and possible bias can be evaluated. It is extremely undesirable to have any involvement in the investigation of the case. Further, he should be an independent professional not responsible to the prosecution or the investigators.
2. All contact of the psychiatrist or psychologist with the individual to be hypnotized should be videotaped from the moment they meet until the entire interaction is completed. The casual comments which are passed before or after hypnosis are every bit as important to get on tape as the

hypnotic session itself. (It is possible to give suggestions prior to the induction of hypnosis which will act as posthypnotic suggestions).

Prior to the induction of hypnosis, a brief evaluation of the patient should be carried out and the psychiatrist or psychologist should then elicit a detailed description of the facts as the witness or victim remembers them. This is important because individuals often are able to recall a good deal more while talking to a psychiatrist or psychologist than when they are with an investigator, and it is important to have a record of what the witness' beliefs are before hypnosis. Only after this has been completed should the hypnotic session be initiated. The psychiatrist or psychologist should strive to avoid adding any new elements to the witness' description of his experience, including those which he had discussed in his wake state, lest he inadvertently alter the nature of the witness' memories—or constrain them by reminding him of his waking memories.

3. No one other than the psychiatrist or psychologist and the individual to be hypnotized should be present in the room before and during the hypnotic session. This is important because it is all too easy for observers to inadvertently communicate to the subject what they expect, what they are startled by, or what they are disappointed by. If either the prosecution or the defense wish to observe the hypnotic session, they may do so without jeopardizing the integrity of the session through a one-way screen or on a television monitor.

4. Because the interactions which have preceded the hypnotic session may well have a profound effect on the sessions themselves, tape recordings of prior interrogations are important to document that a witness had not been implicitly or explicitly cued pertaining to certain information which might then be reported for apparently the first time by the witness during hypnosis. (pp. 335–336)

At no time during or after hypnosis should the subject be given posthypnotic suggestions that subsequent memories will be exhaustive and accurate. Further, arrangements should be made for the subject to have a follow-up visit with the hypnotist or another mental health professional to discuss the hypnotic experience or any traumatic memories which may have come to the surface during hypnosis (Orne et al., in press). These aforementioned procedural safeguards promulgated by Orne can preserve the hypnotic subject's emotional well-being, protect the rights of both parties to the litigation, and allow for the possibility that the witness can later testify regarding matters not discussed during hypnosis.

SUGGESTIONS FOR FUTURE RESEARCH

There is a critical need for research in the area of forensic hypnosis. Many investigations are vague case reports which fail to provide enough details for the reader to ascertain whether hypnosis actually assisted in the case. Broad conclusions such as, "Hypnosis helped solve 11 of 17 cases," are not particularly helpful. Reports should include subsequent investigations to ascertain the ultimate truth or falseness of hypnotically-enhanced testimony. One research method might be to analyze (retrospectively) recorded, hypnotic interrogations of persons who witnessed actual crimes. One could then compare the facts as ultimately determined in court, the witness' original statement, and the witness' hypnotically-induced statement to ascertain influences on recovery of memories.

Research on memory and its distortion has been very valuable in evaluating the types of questions which witnesses are asked and establishing base rates of accuracy for various questioning methods. In such memory research, material to be remembered must be contextually meaningful, subjects must experience some level of arousal when observing the events in issue, and events must be viewed unintentionally. Nevertheless, laboratory research on memory and interrogation of eyewitnesses can never completely simulate the witnessing of real crimes. Though difficult, controlled experiments in which "crimes" occur and hypnosis is later used to elicit "unknown" details have been carried out more frequently in recent years (e.g., Timm, 1981). Instead of research on such clinical techniques as hypnotic age regression, more research is needed on hypermnesia for observed "crimes."

Moreover, suggestibility of subjects should be assesed by standardized tests whenever possible. Further studies are needed (e.g., Sheehan and Tilden, 1982) to ascertain whether suggestibility is related to hypnotic effects on memory enhancement and posthypnotic confidence.

Other questions also merit further research. Does hypnosis cause increased productivity of responses due to lowered response criterion? Is the effect of a witness who has been hypnotized greater on a jury than that of an unhypnotized witness? When is the likelihood of confabulation greatest? What effects do specific preconceptions of the hypnotist have on outcome? Does reliving a painful experience without affect produce more accurate memories than doing so with affect? Finally, is hypnosis differentially effective in the recall of information which subjects tried to remember and information which subjects simply noted unintentionally.

In conclusion, hypnosis may be valuable in the practice of psychotherapy, in which the historical accuracy of memories or fantasies obtained during hypnosis is not crucial. However, a different situation prevails in the legal arena, in which truth is of paramount importance. Given the risk of confabulation and memory alteration during hypnosis, the increased suggestibility of hypnotic subjects, and the enhanced confidence and credibility of witnesses and victims who have been hypnotized, the prudent view appears to be to allow the use of hypnosis for purposes of developing investigative leads but to exclude testimony when the witness has undergone pretrial hypnosis for the purpose of refreshing recollection. When hypnosis is utilized to develop investigative leads, previously enumerated procedural safeguards should be present, and the subject should be barred from testifying at trial regarding the events covered during hypnosis.

Laurence and Perry (1983b) have summarized historical precedents in Russia, France, Italy, and Switzerland regarding potential risks in the forensic use of hypnosis. Experts in those countries in the nineteenth century recognized the significant danger of false memories and confabulations when life and liberty were at stake. Today, nearly a century later, in our "modern" era of sophisticated technology and research, we can do no less.

REFERENCES

American Medical Association. (1958). Medical use of hypnosis. *Journal of the American Medical Association, 168,* 186–189.

Arons, H. (1967). *Hypnosis in criminal investigation.* Springfield, IL: Charles C. Thomas.

Augustynek, A. (1978). Remembering under hypnosis. *The Journal for Basic Research in Psychological Sciences, Studia Psychologia, 20,* 256-266.

Augustynek, A. (1979) Hypnotic hypermnesia. *Prace Psychologiczno-Pedagogiczne, 29,* 25-34.

Barber, T. X. (1962). Hypnotic age regression: A critical review. *Psychosomatic Medicine, 24,* 286–299.

Barber, T. X. (1976). *Hypnosis: A scientific approach.* New York: Psychological Dimensions, Inc.

Barber, T. X., & Calverly, D. S. (1966). Effects of recall of hypnotic induction, motivational suggestions, and suggested regression: A methodological and experimental analysis. *Journal of Abnormal Psychology, 71,* 169-180.

Barber, T. X., Spanos, N. P., & Chaves, J. F. (1974). *Hypnosis, imagination, and human potentialities.* New York: Pergamon Press.

Barlett, F. C. (1932). *Remembering.* Cambridge: Cambridge University Press.

Bourne, L. E., Dominowski, R. L., & Loftus, E. F. (1979). *Cognitive processes.* Englewood Cliffs, NJ: Prentice-Hall.

Brady v. Maryland, 373 U.S. 83 (1963).

Breuer, J., & Freud, S. (1955). *Studies on hysteria (The standard edition of the complete psychological works of Sigmund Freud,* Vol. II). London: Hogarth. (Originally published 1895).

Burch, G. W. (1974) *Hypnosis: An aid to police interrogations.* Unpublished master's thesis, California State University Long Beach Calif.

Cady, H. M. (1924). Minor studies from the psychological laboratory of Northwestern University contributed by Robt. H. Gault. On the psychology of testimony. *American Journal of Psychology, 35,* 110-112.

Chapman v. State, 638 P.2d 1280 (1982).

Collins v. State, 52 Md. App. 186, 447 A.2d 1272 (1982).

Collins v. Superior Court of State of Arizona, 132 Ariz. 180, 644 P.2d 1266 (1982).

Commonwealth v. Nazarovitch, 496 Pa. 97, 436 A.2d 170 (Pa. 1981).

Creamer v. State, 232 Ga. 136, 205 S. E. 2d 240 (1974).

Crowder, R. G. (1976). *Principles of learning and memory.* Hillsdale, NJ: Erlbaum.

DePiano, F. A., & Salzberg, H. C. (1981). Hypnosis as an aid to recall of meaningful information presented under three types of arousal. *International Journal of Clinical and Experimental Hypnosis, 29,* 383-400.

Dhanens, T. P., & Lundy, R. M. (1975). Hypnotic and waking suggestions and recall. *International Journal of Clinical and Experimental Hypnosis 23,* 68-79.

Diamond, B. L. (1980). Inherent problems in the use of pretrial hypnosis on a prospective witness. *California Law Review, 68,* 313-349.

Dilloff, J. (1977). The admissibility of hypnotically influenced testimony. *Ohio N. Univ. Law Review, 4,* 18-20.

Dorcus, R. M. (1960). Result under hypnosis of amnesic events. *International Journal of Clinical and Experimental Hypnosis, 7,* 57-61.

Dywan, J. & Bowers, K. (1983). The use of hypnosis to enhance recall. *Science, 222,* 184-185.

Erickson, M. H. (1939). An experimental investigation of the possible anti-social use of hypnosis. *Psychiarty, 2,* 391-414.

Frye v. United States, 293 F. 1013 (D. C. Cir. 1923).

Gidro-Frank, M. G., & Bowers-Buch, M. K. (1948). A study of the plantar response in hypnotic age regression. *Journal of Nervous and Mental Disorders, 107,* 443-458.

Greenfield v. Commonwealth, 214 Va. 710, 204 S E. 2d 414 (1974).

Griffin G. R. (1980). Hypnosis: Towards a logical approach in using hypnosis in law enforcement agencies. *Journal of Police Science and Administration, 8,* 385-389.

Harding v. State, 5 Md. App. 230, 246 A.2d 302, *cert. denied,* 395 U.S. 949 (1968).

Helwig, C. V. (1978). A comparison of the effectiveness of hypnotic-motivational, task-motivational, and relaxation instructions in eliciting the recall of anxiety-inducing material. (Doctoral dissertation, University of Toronto, 1976) *Dissertation Abstracts International, 38,* 6013A.

Hilgard, E. R. (1965). *Hypnotic susceptibility.* New York: Harcourt, Brace and World.

Hilgard, E. R. (1977). *Divided Consciousness: Multiple controls in human thought and action.* New York: Wiley.

Hilgard, E. R., & Loftus, E. F. (1979). Effective interrogation of the eyewitness. *International Journal of Clinical and Experimental Hypnosis, 27,* 342-357.

Hull, C. L. (1933). *Hypnosis and suggestibility.* New York: Appleton-Century-Crofts.

Huse, B. (1930). Does the hypnotic trance favor the recall of faint memories? *Journal of Experimental Psychology, 13,* 519-529.

In re Milligan, No. J-17617 (Superior Court, Monterey County, California, June 29, 1978; unreported).

International Society of Hypnosis. (1979). Resolution. *International Journal of Clinical and Experimental Hypnosis, 27,* 453.

Karlin, R. A. (1983). Forensic hypnosis: Two case reports. *International Journal of Clinical and Experimental Hypnosis, 31,* 227-234.

Kline v. Ford Motor Co., Inc., 523 F. 2d 1067 (9th Cir. 1975).

Kline, M. V., & Guze, H. (1951). The use of a drawing technique in the investigation of hypnotic age regression and progression. *British Journal of Medical Hypnotism, Winter,* 1-12.

Kroger, W. A. (1963). *Clinical and experimental hypnosis.* Springfield, Il: Charles C. Thomas.

Kroger, W. S., & Douce, R. G. (1980). Forensic uses of hypnosis. *American Journal of Clinical Hypnosis, 23,* 86-93.

Laurence, J-R., and Perry, C. (1983). Hypnotically created memory among highly hypnotizable subjects. *Science, 222,* 52?-524. (a)

Laurence, J-R., and Perry, C. (1983). Forensic hypnosis in the late nineteenth century. *International Journal of Clinical and Experimental Hypnosis, 31,* 266-283. (b)

Lindsay, R. C. L., Wells, G. L., & Rumpel, C. M. (1981) Can people detect eyewitness-identification accuracy within and across situations? *Journal of Applied Psychology, 66,* 79-89.

Loftus, E. F. (1975). Leading questions and eyewitness report. *Cognitive Psychology, 7,* 560-572.

Loftus, E. F. (1979). *Eyewitness testimony.* Cambridge, Ma: Harvard University Press.

Loftus, E. F., & Palmer, J. C. (1974). Reconstruction of automobile destruction: An example of the interaction between language and memory. *Journal of Verbal Learning and Verbal Behavior, 13,* 585-589.

Loftus, E. F., & Zanni, G. (1975). Eyewitness testimony: The influence of the wording of a question. *Bulletin of the Psychonomic Society, 5,* 86-88.

Marquis, K. H., Marshall, J., & Oskamp, S. (1972). Testimony validity as a function of the question form, atmosphere, and item difficulty. *Journal of Applied Social Psychology, 2,* 167-186.

McCormick, C. T. *Law of evidence,* sec. 208 (2d ed.). St. Paul: West Pub. Co., 1972.

McGlashan, T. H., Evans, F. J., & Orne, M. T. (1969). The nature of hypnotic analgesia and placebo response to experimental pain. *Psychosomatic Medicine, 31,* 227-246.

Murray, E. K. (1979). Evidence-admissibility of present recollection restored by hypnosis. *Wake Forest Law Review, 15,* 357-374.

O'Connell, D. N., Shor, R. E., & Orne, M. T. (1970). Hypnotic age regression: An empirical and methodological analysis. *Journal of Abnormal Psychology, 76,* (Monograph Supplement No. 3), 1-32.

Orne, M. T. (1951). The mechanisms of hypnotic age regression: An experimental study. *Journal of Abnormal Psychology, 46,* 213-225.

Orne, M. T. (1961). The potential uses of hypnosis in interrogation. In A. D. Biderman and H. Zimmer (Eds.), *The manipulation of human behavior.* New York: Wiley.

Orne, M. T. (1977). The construct of hypnosis: Implications of the definition for research and practice. *Annals of the New York Academy of Sciences 296,* 14-33.

Orne, M. T. (1979). The use and misuse of hypnosis in court. *International Journal of Clinical and Experimental Hypnosis, 27,* 311-341.

Orne, M. T. (1981). The significance of unwitting cues for experimental outcomes: Toward a pragmatic approach. *Annals of the New York Academy of Science, 364,* 152-159. (a)

Orne, M. T. (1981). The use and misuse of hypnosis in court. In M. Tonry and N. Morris (Eds.), *Crime and justice: An annual review of research* (Vol. 3). Chicago: University of Chicago Press. (b)

Ornie, M. T., Soskis, D. A., Dinges, D. F., & Orne, E. C. (in press). Hypnotically induced testimony. In G. L. Wells and E. F. Loftus (Eds.), *Eyewitness testimony: Eyewitness perspectives.* Cambridge: Cambridge University Press.

People v. Ewbanks, 117 Cal. 652, 49 P. 1049 (1897).

People v. Gonzales, 108 Mich. App., 310 N. W. 2d 306 (1981).

People v. Ritchie, No C-36932 (Superior Court, Orange County, California, April 7, 1977; unreported).

People v. Shirley, 31 C. 3d 18, 641 P.2d 775, *cert. denied,* 103 S. Ct. 13 (1982).

Putnam, W. H. (1979) Hypnosis and distortions in eyewitness testimony. *International Journal of Clinical and Experimental Hypnosis, 27,* 437-448.

Reiff, R., & Scheerer, M. (1959). *Memory and hypnotic age regression: Developmental aspects of cognitive function explored through hypnosis.* New York: International Universities Press.

Reiser, M. (1976). Hypnosis as a tool in criminal investigation. *The Police Chief, 43,* 36-40.

Reiser, M. (1980). *Handbook of investigative hypnosis.* Los Angeles, Cal.: Lehi.
Reiser, M., & Nielson, M. (1980). Investigative hypnosis: A developing speciality. *American Journal of Clinical Hypnosis, 23,* 75–84.
Rosenthal, B. G. (1944). Hypnotic recall of material learned under anxiety-and non-anxiety-producing conditions. *Journal of Experimental Psychology, 34,* 369–389.
Salzberg, H. C. (1977). The hypnotic interview in crime detection. *American Journal of Clinical Hypnosis, 19,* 255–258.
Salzberg, H. C., DePiano, F. A. (1980) Hypnotizability and task motivating suggestions: A further look at how they affect performance. *International Journal of Clinical and Experimental Hypnosis, 28,* 261–271.
Sarno, G. G. (1979). Admissibility of hypnotic evidence at criminal trial. *American Law Report, 3d, 92,* 442–468.
Schafer, D. W., & Rubio, R. (1978). Hypnosis to aid the recall of witnesses. *International Journal of Clinical and Experimental Hypnosis, 26,* 81–91.
Shaul, R. D. (1978). Eyewitness testimony and hypnotic hypermnesia. (Doctoral dissertation, Brigham Young University, 1978). *Dissertation Abstracts International, 39,* 2521B. (University Microfilms No. 78-21, 261).
Sheelan, P. W. (1972). *The function and nature of imagery.* New York: Academic Press.
Sheehan, P. W., & Tilden, J. (1983). Effects of suggestibility and hypnosis on accurate and distorted retrieval from memory. *Journal of Experimental Psychology: Learning, Memory, and Cognition, 9,* 283–293.
Shockey v. State, 338 So.2d 33 (Fla. App. 1976).
Shor, R. E., & Orne, E. C. (1962). *The Harvard Group Scale of Hypnotic Susceptibility, Form A.* Palo Alto, C. Consulting Psychologists Press.
Simmons v. United States, 390 U.S. 377 (1968).
Spector, R. S., & Foster, T. E. (1977). Admissibility of hypnotic statements: Is the law of evidence susceptible? *Ohio State Law Journal, 38,* 567–613.
Stager, G. L. (1974). The effect of hypnosis on the learning and recall of visually presented material (Doctoral dissertation, Pennsylvania State University, 1974). *Dissertation Abstracts International, 35,* 3075B. (University Microfilms No. 74–28, 985).
Stager, G. L., & Lundy, R. M. (in press). Hypnosis and the learning and recall of visually presented material. *International Journal of Clincal and Experimental Hypnosis.*
Stalnaker, J. M., & Riddle, E. E. (1932). The effect of hypnosis on long-delayed recall. *Journal of General Psychology, 6,* 429–440.
State v. Douglas, Indictment No. 692-77 (Union County, N. J.), vacated May 23, 1978.
State v. Harris, 241 Or. 224, 405 P. 2d 492 (1965).
State v. Hurd, 86 N. J. 525, 432 A. 2d 86 (1981).
State v. Jorgensen, 8 Or. App. 1, 492 P.2d 312 (1971).
State v. Mack, 292 N. W. 2d 764 (1980).
State v. McQueen, 295 N. C. 96, 244 S. E. 2d 414 (1978).
State v. Mena, 128 Ariz. 226, 624 P.2d 1274 (1981).
State v. Palmer, 210 Neb. 206, 313 N. W. 2d 648 (1981).
State v. Waters, 308 N. C. 348, 302 S. E. 2d 188 (1983).
State v. White, No. J-3665 (Circuit Court, Branch 10, Milwaukee County, Wisconsin, March 27, 1979; unreported).
Strong v. State, 435 N. E. 2d 969 (1982).
Sturm, C. A. (1983). *Eyewitness memory: Effects of guided memory and hypnotic hypermnesia techniques and hypnotic susceptibility.* Unpublished doctoral dissertation, University of Montana, Missoula.

Timm, H. W. (1981). The effects of forensic hypnosis techniques on eyewitness recall and recognition. *Journal of Police Science and Administration, 9,* 188-194.

Timm, H. W. (1982 August). *A theoretical and empirical examination of the effects of forensic hypnosis on eyewitness recall.* Paper presented at the 9th International Congress of Hypnosis and Psychosomatic Medicine, Glasgow, Scotland.

United States v. Adams, 581 F.2d 193, 198-199 (9th Cir.), *cert. denied,* 439 U. S. 1006 (1978).

United States v. Miller, 411 F.2d 825 (2d Cir. 1969).

Wadden, T. A., & Anderton, C. H. (1982). The clinical use of hypnosis. *Psychological Bulletin, 91,* 215-243.

Wagstaff, G. F., Traverse, J., & Milner, S. (1982). Hypnosis and eyewitness memory: Two experimental analogues. *IRCS Medical Science: Psychology and Psychiatry, 10,* 894-895.

Warner, K. E. (1979). The use of hypnosis in the defense of criminal cases. *International Journal of Clinical and Experimental Hypnosis, 27,* 417-436.

Weitzenhoffer, A. M., & Hilgard, E. E. (1959) *Stanford Hypnotic Susceptibility Scales, Forms A and B.* Palo Alto, CA: Consulting Psychologists Press.

Weitzenhoffer, A. M., & Hilgard, E. R. (1962). *Stanford Hypnotic Susceptibility Scale, Form C.* Palo Alto, CA.: Consulting psychologist Press.

Wells, G. L., & Leippe, M. R. (1981). How do triers of fact infer the accuracy of eyewitness identifications? Memory for peripheral detail can be midleading. *Journal of Applied Psychology, 66,* 682-687.

Wells, G. L., Lindsay, R. C. L., & Ferguson, T. J. (1979). Accuracy, confidence, and juror perceptions in eye witness identification. *Journal of Applied Psychology, 64,* 440-448.

White, R. W., Fox, G. F., & Harris, W. W. (1940). Hypnotic hypermnesia for recently learned material. *Journal of Abnormal and Social Psychology, 35,* 88-103.

Wigmore, J. H. (1970). *3A Evidence,* sec. 998 (Chadbourn rev.). Boston: Little Brown and Company.

Worthington, T. S. (1979). The use in court of hypnotically enhanced testimony. *International Journal of Clinical and Experimental Hypnosis, 27,* 402-416.

Yates, A. J. (1961). Hypnotic age regression. *Psychological Bulletin, 58,* 429-440.

Young, P. C. (1926). An experimental study of mental and physical functions in the normal and hypnotic state: Additional results. *American Journal of Psychology, 37,* 345-356.

Zelig, M., & Beidleman, W. B. (1981). The investigative use of hypnosis: A word of caution. *International Journal of Clinical and Experimental Hypnosis, 29,* 401-412.

PART V

Conclusion

Chapter 12

Educational and Ethical Issues in Clinical Hypnosis

Kevin M. McConkey

Macquarie University
North Ryde, NSW, Australia

There has been debate over educational and ethical issues in the area of hypnosis ever since Franz Anton Mesmer formed the *Sociétés de l' Harmonie* over two centuries ago in order to provide training in the theory and application of animal magnetism (see Chapter 1 for a discussion of this era). Although many of the particular concerns about animal magnetism can be understood in terms of the social context of the time and are no longer relevant, many of the underlying educational and ethical issues about hypnosis are a source of continuing controversy.

There is a high level of interest about hypnosis among contemporary health professionals, and this level of interest underscores the need for discussion not only of the type of training that is available for those who wish to employ hypnosis, but also of the type of concerns that arise when hypnosis is used in clinical practice. There are many issues involved in these interrelated areas, and this chapter attempts to coordinate and examine a range of educational and ethical issues in clinical hypnosis.

The approach adopted in this chapter assumes that those interested in clinical hypnosis have received appropriate professional education and certification in the health sciences (e.g., as medical, psychological, or dental practitioners) and that they follow the ethical guidelines of their own professional association (e.g., the American Medical Association, American Psychological Association, or American Dental Association). This assumpton underscores the important point that hypnosis is not an independent science or art, but rather is an adjunctive technique that should be employed only by health science professionals (or professionals-in-training) within their own area of professional competence.

This chapter is designed more for individuals who are new to, rather than experienced in, the area of hypnosis. It is organized around a discussion of five questions that are often asked by those who are new to the area, and just as often debated by those who are experienced in the area. These questions are: (1) What is the nature of hypnosis? (2) What are the current attitudes toward hypnosis? (3) What training is available in hypnosis? (4) What professional concerns are there about hypnosis? (5) What therapeutic concerns are there about hypnosis? Each of these questions incorporates a number of issues, and the chapter attempts to define and clarify these issues, to summarize opinions and research findings about them, and to provide practical recommendations and research suggestions when appropriate. Although the chapter is selective in terms of the issues that are discussed, when it is read together with the chapters in this book, it should provide an informed orientation to the area of hypnosis. The chapter begins with a discussion of the nature of hypnosis.

NATURE OF HYPNOSIS

As can be seen in the other chapters of this book, the area of hypnosis is divergent in terms of the theoretical models employed to understand it, the experimental methods used to investigate it, and the clinical procedures used to apply it. That diversity sometimes overshadows the important point that hypnosis does play a major role as a treatment adjunct in a variety of clinical settings (see Chapter 13 for a summary discussion). Nevertheless, the definition of hypnosis does affect the way in which it is investigated in the laboratory and applied in the clinic (Orne, 1977), and a useful descriptive definition of hypnosis is that it occurs when hypnotic techniques are employed with motivated, hypnotizable individuals and those individuals experience subjective alterations in response to appropriate suggestions from the hypnotist (Orne & Hammer, 1974; Orne & McConkey, 1982).

Hypnotic suggestions can be effective in bringing about desired experiential changes in hypnotizable persons. For example, hypnotizable individuals can experience decreased pain (see Chapter 3), amnesia or hypermnesia (see Chapter 11), and emotional alterations (see Chapter 7) following suggestions from the hypnotist. Such alterations in perception, memory, and mood in response to specific suggestions from the hypnotist, in fact, are the essential defining features of hypnosis (Orne & Hammer, 1974; Orne & McConkey, 1982).

Although hypnosis usually occurs in the context of a dyadic interaction and some type of induction procedure is usually needed (see Chapter 1), it is the level of hypnotizability of the client–and not the "skill" of the hypnotist–that is the major determinant of the experience of hypnosis (Hilgard, 1965; Orne & Hammer, 1974). Individuals vary in their level of hypnotizability; about 15 percent have a very high level, about 5 percent have a very low level, and the remainder vary in between (Hilgard, 1965). The assessment of hypnotizabilty can be an important component of its clinical use because information about a client's level of hypnotizability often allows the therapist to tailor the induction and therapeutic procedures to match the special abilities, as well as the special needs, of that client (Frankel, 1982; Frankel, Apfel, Kelley, Benson, Quinn, Newmark, & Malmaud, 1979; Perry, Gelfand, & Marcovitch, 1979). Further, since therapeutic outcome is dependent on level of hypnotizability in many instances, knowledge of a client's level of hypnotizability often helps the therapist to determine whether hypnosis is the most appropriate technique to employ with that client and, if so, to also determine which hypnotic techniques to employ (Frankel, 1982; Mott, 1979; Perry et al., 1979). In order to provide a scientifically-based assessment of hypnotizability, there are a number of valid and reliable measures of hypnotizability available for use in either the experimental or the clinical setting (see Frankel et al., 1979; Hilgard, 1978/79; Sheehan & McConkey, 1982; for recent reviews).

Hypnotic suggestions that are given to motivated, but low hypnotizable, clients may lead to therapeutic change, but this is because of the substantial nonspecific effects of the hypnotic context rather than to any experiential alterations due to hypnosis. That is, the hypnotic context, rather than the hypnotic experience, can be a very important component of the clinical use of hypnosis (Gruenewald, 1982a; Wadden & Anderton, 1982), and the nature and impact of the hypnotic context needs to be appreciated more widely. McConkey (1984) has outlined the nature and the effects of the contextual shift that occurs when hypnosis is introduced into the therapeutic setting. In general, this shift affects the individual behavior of both the therapist and the client as well as their dyadic interaction.

Therapists who employ hypnosis generally believe in its utility and communicate this to clients both verbally and nonverbally. Further, their behavior often changes when hypnosis is employed because the use of hypnotic techniques tends to legitimize behavior on the part of the therapist (e.g., explicit requests, atypical closeness) that may not be displayed when hypnosis is not involved (McConkey, 1984; Orne, 1965). Clients who accept the use of hypnosis generally believe in its utility irrespective of whether they have a sufficient level of hypnotizability to experience hypnosis. In this sense, hypnotic techniques can be used to legitimize change in individuals who are ready to change by allowing them to (incorrectly) attribute the change to what they perceive as the powerful external means of hypnosis. In terms of the dyadic interaction of therapist and client, the use of hypnosis generally brings about an increased degree of personal involvement on the part of both the therapist and the client. Clients often feel very comfortable with and trusting of the therapist when hypnosis is involved, and these feelings may be reciprocated by the therapist (Sheehan, 1980; Shor, 1959). All of these effects can have a substantial positive impact on therapeutic outcome, but they can also increase transference and countertransference feelings (Fromm, 1968; Gruenewald, 1971). In fact, when hypnosis is used therapists need to be alert to the role that countertransference may play in their behavior (Orne, 1965).

In summary, this section has considered three points about the nature of hypnosis. First, hypnosis is best understood in terms of the experiential alterations that occur in the hypnotized individual. It is these subjective experiences, and not any particular behaviors, that are the essential features of hypnosis (Orne, 1959). Second, it is the hypnotizability of the client and not any special skill of the therapist (apart from the skill of therapy) that is important. Thus, the client brings the necessary hypnotic ability to the setting, and the therapist brings therapeutic techniques (that have been learned through professional training) that are designed to facilitate the client's use of hypnosis for therapeutic purposes. Third, the use of hypnosis leads to a contextual shift that may have both positive and negative effects on the therapeutic interaction. Therapists need to be especially alert to recognize these changes and to employ them in therapeutically positive ways. The effects that occur when hypnosis is used are shaped in part by the attitudes that the therapist and the client hold about hypnosis. Accordingly, the chapter turns now to an overview of current attitudes toward hypnosis.

ATTITUDES TOWARD HYPNOSIS

Laying aside the specialist scientific and professional literature in the area of hypnosis (e.g., *International Journal of Clinical and Experimental Hypnosis* [Editor: Martin T. Orne, 111 North 49th Street, Philadelphia, PA 19139]; *American Journal of Clinical Hypnosis* [Editor: Melvin A. Gravitz, 1325 18th Street, NW, Washington, DC 20036]), attitudes toward hypnosis are shaped by a wide variety of information sources (e.g., newspapers, magazines, books, television). Unfortunately, the accuracy of the information available from these sources varies widely (Sheehan, Dolby, & McDermott, 1975), and is often inconsistent with the scientific and professional literature. For this reason, it is useful to consider what is known about the attitudes of clients and colleagues alike.

There is relatively little information available about public attitudes toward hypnosis (e.g., London, 1961; McIntosh & Hawney, 1983; van der Walde, 1974). London (1961) reported that a survey of students affirmed common stereotypes about hypnosis (e.g., inability to resist hypnotic suggestion, spontaneous posthypnotic amnesia), and van der Walde (1974) reported generally negative attitudes toward hypnosis in an investigation of patient preferences for treatment. More recently, McIntosh and Hawney (1983) reported that one-third of the patients in a general medical practice would accept hypnosis if it was recommended by their physician, and the majority would require further information before making a decision. Further, McIntosh and Hawney (1983) reported meaningful associations between knowledge about and acceptance of hypnosis as well as between information source and attitude toward hypnosis. Specifically, those patients whose knowledge about hypnosis was based on television or stage shows generally considered that hypnosis was not clinically useful and generally held unfavorable attitudes toward it (McIntosh & Hawney, 1983).

Despite the lack of formal data about public attitudes toward hypnosis, therapists typically become familiar with the range of notions held about hypnosis by their clients. For instance, clients typically have misperceptions about hypnosis in terms of its nature (e.g., hypnosis is sleep), its impact (e.g., hypnosis impairs memory), their own role (e.g., hypnotizable individuals are weak-willed), and the role of the hypnotist (e.g., the hypnotist takes total control). Whenever hypnosis is being considered, then, it is important to probe and clarify clients' views for both educational and therapeutic reasons, since therapeutic progress will be impeded if there is not a convergence between the views of the client and the therapist (Sacerdote, 1974). Further, for some clients (e.g., children) the therapist will have to clarify the views of significant others (e.g., parents) as well as the views of the client (Call, 1976). For this reason, Gardner (1974) has described educational, observational, and experiential techniques intended to enhance parents' views about the efficacy of hypnosis with their children. As Clarke and Jackson (1983) have pointed out, a major aspect of contemporary clinical work is not the development of new techniques but rather the development of strategies to enhance clients' expectancies about the techniques that are available. This is especially important in the area of hypnosis because of the large amount of misinformation about hypnosis that is available to the public.

In contrast to the lack of formal surveys of public attitudes toward hypnosis, there has been substantial investigation of the attitudes of various professional groups toward hypnosis (e.g., Gardner, 1976; Kraft & Rodolfa, 1982; Moss, Logan, & Lynch, 1962; Moss, Riggen, Coyne, & Bishop, 1965; Parrish, 1975; Pulver & Pulver, 1975; Rodolfa, Kraft, Reilley, & Blackmore, 1982, 1983; Sheehan & McConkey, 1979; Woody & Herr, 1966; Woody, Houck, & Thompson, 1969). Not surprisingly, these surveys have indicated a strong relationship between knowledge about hypnosis, use of hypnosis, and attitudes toward hypnosis (Sheehan & McConkey, 1979). For example, Kraft and Rodolfa (1982) reported that both general members of the American Psychological Association (APA) and members of the APA Division of Psychological Hypnosis (Division 30) considered that hypnosis was a clinically useful technique and that training and research in hypnosis was worthwhile. In addition, the most positive attitudes toward hypnosis were reported by Division 30 members, and more favorable attitudes were reported by those in the general APA membership who do, rather than do not, use hypnosis in professional practice. Similarly, Rodolfa et al.

(1983) reported that the directors of APA internship sites that offered hypnosis training held more positive attitudes about hypnosis than did those at sites that did not offer hypnosis training; in addition, the directors at sites that did not offer training considered that hypnosis was too controversial and too specialized a clinical technique to be taught.

The surveys have indicated also that professional attitudes toward hypnosis have become more positive in recent years (Sheehan & McConkey, 1979). Although this is due in part to the recognition and official endorsement of hypnosis as a valid treatment adjunct by various professional organizations (e.g., American Medical Association, American Psychological Association), it is probably due more to the substantial increase in research that has occurred in the area of hypnosis. That is, the acceptability of hypnosis has increased in the therapeutic setting largely because the research that has been conducted has provided a more scientific basis for its clinical application. The upsurge in both experimental investigation and clinical application of hypnosis has been most evident among psychologists, who appear to have a substantial investment in the area of hypnosis (Kraft & Rodolfa, 1982). For instance, the *International Journal of Clinical and Experimental Hypnosis* is currently one of the core journals in the field of psychology as a whole (Haynes, 1983).

In summary, this section has considered three points about attitudes toward hypnosis. First, substantial misinformation is available about hypnosis and its clinical application. Thus, the therapist who uses hypnosis needs to appreciate clients' (and colleagues') attitudes toward hypnosis, and the influences that shape those attitudes. Second, despite the official endorsement, the scientific scrutiny, and the indications of clinical utility, hypnosis is misunderstood and regarded with skepticism by many professionals. Third, attitudes toward hypnosis have become more positive in general because of the research that has been conducted into its nature and effects. Further attitudinal change will occur only if there is continued research into hypnosis and increased accountability of its clinical application. Such a situation will be determined in part by the type of training that those who use hypnosis have received, and the chapter turns now to consider current training in hypnosis.

TRAINING IN HYPNOSIS

The basic techniques of hypnosis can be learned by virtually anyone. Its skillful clinical application, however, requires that the therapist is trained not only in therapeutic techniques in general but also in hypnotic techniques in particular. The majority of therapists who employ hypnosis receive their hypnosis training either in university or internship courses or in continuing education or professional society programs. The design, content, implementation, and impact of various hypnosis training programs have been discussed widely in the literature (e.g., American Board of Examiners in Psychological Hypnosis, 1961; Burrows & Dennerstein, 1979; Dorcus, 1958; Fredericks, 1978, 1980; Gardner, 1976; Gubel, 1973; Hartland, 1968; Moss et al., 1962, 1965; Olness, 1977; Parrish, 1975; Pulver & Pulver, 1975; Pulver & Smith, 1961; Rodolfa et al., 1982, 1983; Sheehan & McConkey, 1979; Valett, 1962; Verberne, 1976; Wald & Kline, 1955; Woody et al., 1969).

In terms of university and internship courses, Parrish (1975) reported that training in hypnosis was most available to psychology students and least available to dental students, with medical students occupying a middle position. Further, Moss et al. (1962) reported that whereas the focus of hypnosis training in medical schools was on clinical application, the focus of training in psychology programs was on theoretical and experimental issues as well as on clinical application. Valett (1962) has argued that the integration of hypnosis training into a psychology program usefully leads to hypnosis being employed appropriately as one other psychological technique and to it being incorporated into professional practice and scientific investigation in an optimal way. Consistent with this, Fredericks (1980) and Pulver and Pulver (1975) reported that physicians who had taken hypnosis courses either at medical school or as part of their residency tended to incorporate hypnotic principles into their everyday interactions with patients even if they did not employ hypnosis formally; that is, their training in hypnosis appeared to increase not only their awareness of psychological factors but also their ability to deal with those factors constructively.

In terms of continuing education and society programs in hypnosis, Sheehan and McConkey (1979) reported that the issue of appropriate training in hypnosis has developed as a critical one for professional societies. There is some conflict about the optimal hypnosis training model largely because professionals tend to consider that the type of training that they received themselves is the most appropriate training model; for example, psychologists, more so than physicians or dentists, consider that hypnosis training should emanate from universities rather than from professional societies (Woody et al., 1969). Laying this conflict aside, however, the type of training organized by professional societies currently provides the optimal training opportunity for the health professional interested in the clinical application of hypnosis; that is, training in hypnosis for professionals is best obtained currently in the context of the programs offered by professional societies.

An overlap does occur, of course, between university and society training in hypnosis. For example, Burrows and Dennerstein (1979) reported their experiences in organizing and teaching hypnosis to students in a university setting and to professionals in workshop and seminar settings. They argued that there is a need for a closer association and pooling of university and professional society resources. In addition, they argued that there is a need to provide training to those who teach and supervise in the workshops and seminars offered by professional societies; that is, the quality of the society training programs is only as good as the quality of those who provide those programs. Improved training programs will lead to better trained therapists, improved client management, and a greater understanding of both the benefits and limits of clinical hypnosis (Burrows & Dennerstein, 1979).

There are a number of professional hypnosis societies, and it is important to recognize that they all do not restrict membership to health science professionals nor do they all provide training programs of the same quality. Accordingly, it is useful to consider those societies that provide workshops and courses that are consistent with the aims and orientation of this chapter. These are the Society for Clinical and Experimental Hypnosis [129-A Kings Park Drive, Liverpool, NY 13088], the American Society for Clinical Hypnosis [2250 East Devon Avenue, Suite 336, Des Plaines, IL 60018], and the International Society of Hypnosis [111 North 49th Street, Philadelphia, PA 19139]. In addition, the continuing education courses offered by APA Division 30 [American Psychological Association, Continuing Education Program, 1200 17th Street, Washington, DC 20036] are recommended. These training opportunities are limited to appropriately qualified professionals or professionals-in-training, and the training orientation is that the therapist who employs hypnosis should first be a competent therapist, and the researcher who investigates hypnosis should first be a competent researcher. The programs are conducted by individuals who are experienced in teaching hypnotic techniques and principles at a professional level, and they provide participants with the opportunity to learn hypnotic theory and techniques and to apply these techniques in the context of their own professional activities.

In order to obtain an appreciation of the value of receiving training in hypnosis in the context of such programs, it is useful to consider one of these societies in more detail. The Society for Clinical and Experimental Hypnosis (SCEH) is one of the two major professional hypnosis societies in North America (see Schneck, 1953, for a historical note on its development). This society stimulates and supports research in the area of hypnosis and related areas, encourages cooperation among scientists and practitioners with regard to experimental and clinical hypnosis, supports communication through scientific meetings and publications, maintains standards of adequacy and ethics in the area of hypnosis, and provides formal and standardized training facilities for qualified individuals (Society for Clinical and Experimental Hypnosis, 1981). SCEH limits its membership to physicians, doctoral level psychologists, and dentists who are members or eligible for membership in their respective professional organizations (i.e., American Medical Association, American Psychological Association, and

American Dental Association), and to clinical social workers with masters or doctoral degrees who are listed in the *NASW Register of Clinical Social Workers* or the *National Registry of Health Care Providers in Clinical Social Work.* In addition, interns or residents in medicine and dentistry and advanced graduate students in psychology doctoral programs are eligible for student affiliateship. SCEH is affiliated with the American Association for the Advancement of Science, the World Federation of Mental Health, and the International Society of Hypnosis, and is accredited for continuing education by the American Medical Association and the American Psychological Association.

SCEH has four basic ethical principles to which members are required to subscribe. These are: (1) A member of SCEH shall be a member in good standing of the recognized professional organization in the individual's field. (2) Members of SCEH shall limit their clinical and scientific use of hypnosis to the areas of their competence as defined by the professional standards of their field. (3) The clinical and scientific utilization of hypnosis is an important contribution to human health. It should not be used as a source of entertainment. (4) A member of SCEH shall make clinical and scientific use of hypnosis if it contributes to the welfare of the patient and/or to the advancement of professional knowledge in the member's field. Each of these basic principles has a number of components that are listed in the society's code of ethics (see Society for Clinical and Experimental Hypnosis, 1981).

In summary, this section has considered two major points about training in hypnosis. First, education and training programs in hypnosis tend to be idiosyncratic and a systematic analysis of exactly what constitutes a full training program is lacking. One problem of much of the training that is available is that it is brief and segmented in nature, and it affords little opportunity for supervised integration of hypnosis into clinical practice. Second, optimal training strategies are emerging in the area of hypnosis and the type of training that is offered by the recommended professional hypnosis societies provides the best available training opportunities in hypnosis irrespective of professional discipline or therapeutic orientation. Clearly, active involvement in and membership of these societies provides a training and support network that is aimed toward the optimal integration of hypnosis into professional practice.

PROFESSIONAL CONCERNS ABOUT HYPNOSIS

Hypnosis is employed by a wide variety of individuals for an even wider variety of purposes. Those who use hypnosis range from professionals who employ it in either research or clinical activities to those who employ it as part of a stage show or as part of a criminal investigation. There are many issues involved in the variety of users and uses of hypnosis, and this section focuses on two professional concerns. The first concern is the relationship between professionals who have different emphases in their uses of hypnosis; specifically, the relationship between scientists and practitioners in the area of hypnosis. The second concern is the relationship between professionals and laypersons who use hypnosis in the course of their activities; specifically, the relationship of health professionals with law enforcement personnel who employ hypnosis.

The relationship between experimental and clinical hypnosis has been discussed widely in the literature (e.g., Frankel, 1978; Gruenewald, 1982b, Orne, 1977; Sacerdote, 1982; Sheehan, 1979). Like many other areas, the area of hypnosis suffers in part from a gap between scientific investigation and clinical practice. Udolf (1981) has argued that not only may findings based on experimental hypnosis be inapplicable to clinical hypnosis, but also they may be directly opposite to what would be found in the latter case. Such a view is shortsighted, however, because an analysis of the relationship between clinical and experimental hypnosis in terms of the clinical utility of experimental data, the generality of clinical effects, the relationship between clinical events and the scientific pursuit, and the similarity of scientific and clinical methods, shows that "the competent, intuitive clinician and the systematic researcher have much in common despite the complexities of the different settings in which they work" (Sheehan, 1979, p. 138). From the comparisons that have been conducted of clinical and experimental hypnosis it is clear that good clinicians practice the science, rather than just the art, of therapy in order to be maximally effective, and that good researchers are attuned to therapeutic issues if they want their research to have clinical relevance. As Hilgard and Hilgard (1975) have argued, the cooperation between experimenter and clinician is critical if clinical hypnosis is going to be based on as firm a scientific ground as possible.

One important contribution to narrowing the gap between experimental and clinical hypnosis is clinical research and publication. Increasingly, scientific methodologies that are compatible with the demands of the clinical setting are being developed (see Barlow, Hayes, & Nelson, 1984), and suggestions for communicating clinical research and observation are being provided (e.g., Frankel, 1981; Fromm, 1981; Orne, 1981). Thus, both researchers and clinicians can work to bring experimental and clinical hypnosis toward rapprochement by investigating and communicating the hypnotic processes that they see at work in their particular professional contexts.

In terms of the relationship between professionals and laypersons who use hypnosis, much contemporary debate has focused on the use of hypnosis by law enforcement personnel for investigative purposes (see Carter, 1982; Diamond, 1980; Orne, 1979; Perry & Laurence, 1982; Ruffra, 1983; as well as Chapter 11). A brief examination of this issue helps to sharpen the viewpoint of this chapter, and of the major professional hypnosis societies, that professionals should not support the nonprofessional use of hypnosis.

Some of those involved in the forensic use of hypnosis (e.g., Hibbard & Worring, 1981; Reiser, 1980) consider that forensic hypnosis is a separate specialty, and that only those who are trained in investigative procedures (i.e., law enforcement personnel) should employ hypnosis in the forensic context. Reiser (1980), for instance, has argued that police officers are better qualified than health professionals to employ hypnosis for investigative purposes. This position, however, is inconsistent with the position of the Federal Bureau of Investigation whose policy is to have only health science professionals conduct the hypnotic testing of witnesses or victims of crime (Ault, 1979). Reiser's (1980) position is also inconsistent with the position of major professional societies (e.g., SCEH), which argue that if hypnosis is used in the forensic context, then the hypnotic inquiry should be conducted only by professionals who are trained in the health sciences.

There are a number of reasons for restricting the use of hypnosis to health science professionals. For example, although hypnosis is a relatively safe procedure, only broadly trained professionals are likely to be able to recognize and manage any complications that may arise from its use (see Perry & Laurence, 1982, for a discussion of this and other reasons). One way in which some law enforcement agencies have responded to this objection is to have health professionals act as consultants to the police officer who is conducting the hypnotic session. The tendency of some health professionals to accept such a role has led major hypnosis societies to restate their position that "it is unethical to train lay individuals in the use of hypnosis, to collaborate with laymen in the use of hypnosis, or to serve as a consultant for laymen who are using hypnosis" (Society for Clinical and Experimental Hypnosis, 1979; p. 452).

The professional concern of interacting with laypersons, in general, and law enforcement personnel, in particular, who employ hypnosis has been addressed in a question and answer form by the International Society of Hypnosis (1982). For example, the response to the question of whether professional societies are justified in attempting to restrict the use of hypnosis to their own membership is that hypnosis is simply one clinical tool that should be used in the context of an individual's professional competence and is not something that should be used without the benefit of training in the health sciences. Similarly, the response to the question of whether it might be better to license lay hypnotists in order to have them available for consultation when required is that such licensing and consultation would inappropriately place the emphasis on hypnosis per se, rather than on when and how to use hypnosis in the context of professional practice. The response to the question of whether the ethical constraints against teaching lay individuals can prevent lecturing about hypnosis is that the constraint does not affect the giving of information about hypnosis, but rather the teaching of hypnotic techniques to laypersons. These, and other questions, are answered more fully by the International Society of Hypnosis

(1982). In general, all of these types of questions are clarified if it is remembered that hypnosis is not an independent scientific or therapeutic discipline.

In summary, this section has considered two professional concerns about hypnosis. First, the major data and opinions on the interaction of clinical and experimental hypnosis highlight the similarity that exists in the concerns and findings of practitioners and researchers. The gap that sometimes exists can be narrowed by both of these groups appreciating the benefits of cross-fertilization and by contributing to the scientific and professional literature in the area of hypnosis. Second, support of the use of hypnosis by individuals who lack training in the health sciences is inconsistent with the ethical guidelines of major professional hypnosis societies. It also displays a misunderstanding that hypnosis is a separate discipline or profession, rather than a psychological technique that should be employed only by health professionals.

THERAPEUTIC CONCERNS ABOUT HYPNOSIS

There are many therapeutic concerns about clinical hypnosis that are discussed in the other chapters of this book. Issues such as the types of individuals and types of disorders with which hypnosis can be used in a therapeutically useful way are important concerns. This chapter lays these types of concerns aside, however, and focuses on three other issues relating to potentially negative aspects of hypnosis. These are whether hypnosis has unintentional sequelae, whether it can be used for antisocial purposes, and whether it can negatively affect the therapeutic relationship. These concerns are discussed because there is much misinformation available about the dangers of hypnosis.

In terms of the sequelae of hypnosis, both the clinical and the experimental data indicate clearly that hypnosis is a remarkably safe procedure with virtually no negative sequelae (e.g., Coe & Ryken, 1979; Crawford, Hilgard, & Macdonald, 1982; Faw, Sellers, & Wilcox, 1968; Hilgard, 1974; Hilgard, Hilgard, & Newman, 1961), as long as it is employed by broadly trained professionals in their particular area of competency. That is, there is no evidence that hypnosis itself is dangerous. Problems can arise, however, because of either ignorance about its benefits and limits, overzealous or irresponsible applications, or a lack of understanding of interpersonal relationships in general and the hypnotic relationship in particular (see Kost, 1965; West & Deckert, 1965). Thus, one situation in which problems can occur is when hypnosis is employed by unqualified personnel for trivial purposes, such as stage hypnosis (see Kleinhauz & Beran, 1981; Kleinhauz, Dreyfuss, Beran, Goldberg, & Azikri, 1979). Another situation in which problems can occur is when hypnosis is employed by a therapist who is not well-trained in recognizing and dealing with the problems of resistance, transference, and countertransference, since these problems appear to be intensified when hypnosis is employed (Orne, 1965).

Whether hypnosis can be used to facilitate antisocial behavior has been discussed widely in the literature (e.g., Conn, 1972, 1981; Kline, 1972; Levitt & Baker, 1983; Orne, 1972; Perry, 1979; Sheehan, 1977; Watkins, 1972). Although it is an issue that is difficult to investigate in a scientifically rigorous fashion (Coe, 1977; Orne, 1972), the data provide no support for the popular view that the hypnotist is able to exert a unique form of control over the hypnotized individual. The two main positions on hypnotic coercion are that hypnosis can be a causal factor and that hypnosis cannot be a causal factor (but a close interpersonal relationship can be) in coercion; see Perry (1979) for a stimulating discussion of a legal case that contrasted these two positions. Although the major commentators on the issue of hypnosis and coercion differ in the positions that they adopt and the emphases that they make, they agree that hypnosis can facilitate destructive elements in a disturbed individual and that such an abuse can occur in the context of a close therapist-client relationship. As Orne (1972) has pointed out: "The therapist using hypnosis, like any other therapist, will strive to ally himself with the healthy wishes and aspirations of the patient, but it is of course possible for a disturbed therapist to ally himself with destructive aspects of a patient's personality and facilitate destructive behavior" (pp. 113-114).

Since hypnosis may facilitate a close relationship, then, an individual may become more likely to respond to certain requests just in the same way that he or she may be more likely to respond to requests by someone with whom they have a close personal relationship away from the therapeutic context. There is no evidence, however, that hypnosis directly increases the behavioral control of the hypnotist over that which is already present prior to the introduction of hypnosis. As Orne (1972) has pointed out: "Both the patient and the hypnotherapist are best served by the recognition that both the induction and maintenance of hypnosis involve a cooperative enterprise which may facilitate vivid and meaningful subjective experiences for the patient, but where in an ultimate sense, the patient always remains in control" (p. 115).

The nature of the hypnotic relationship has been discussed widely in the literature in terms of its potentially positive and negative aspects (Fromm, 1968; Gruenewald, 1971; Orne, 1965). Because the use of hypnosis appears to intensify the therapeutic relationship, many therapists consider hypnosis to be contraindicated in the treatment of particular types of clients. For instance, severely depressed individuals have been known to become suicidal following the use of hypnosis (Crasilneck & Hall, 1975). It is important to note, however, that this is not related to the experience of hypnosis, but rather to the shift that occurs in the therapist-client relationship when hypnosis is employed (Burrows, 1980).

Laying aside the problems associated with intensified transference, difficulties can develop also with respect to countertransference. Whereas the potential of such problems accompanies all therapeutic interactions, the possibility of their occurrence is increased when hypnosis is involved (Orne, 1965). Generally, the problems and ethical implications of transference and countertransference can be handled adequately by the trained therapist if he or she recognizes them. In the context of using hypnosis, then, it is very important that the therapist becomes sensitized to recognizing some of the early warning signs of a power struggle or countertransference bind. These signs include such things as whether the therapist uses hypnosis for all clients, derives special gratification from the use of hypnosis, is concerned to have clients experience deep hypnosis, fears that clients may be faking hypnosis, considers that hypnosis is a test of will, or looks forward to hypnotizing attractive clients (Orne, 1965). The therapist who sees such events in his or her behavior should carefully evaluate the motivations underlying the use of clinical hypnosis. As Gardner and Olness (1981) have pointed out, some therapists are attracted to the area of hypnosis because they (mis)perceive that hypnosis can help them to resolve the problems that they are experiencing in dealing with clients.

In summary, this section has considered three therapeutic concerns about hypnosis. First, although hypnosis is a safe procedure in itself, difficulties can arise if it is used either inappropriately or by inexperienced individuals. Second, although hypnosis cannot be employed to coerce individuals, the change that occurs in the interpersonal context when hypnosis is employed may lead to a change in the willingness of individuals to engage in behaviors that they would not engage in if they were in the context of a less close interpersonal relationship; this change is based on the nature of the interpersonal relationship, however, and not on the experience of hypnosis. Third, when difficulties arise during the use of clinical hypnosis, they are likely to be due to transference or countertransference problems. Thus, therapists need to be especially oriented to the subtle changes that may occur in the nature of their interpersonal interactions with clients when hypnosis is introduced.

SUMMARY COMMENTS AND RECOMMENDATIONS

This chapter has considered the nature of hypnosis, attitudes toward hypnosis, training in hypnosis, and professional and therapeutic concerns about hypnosis. For each of these general areas, a number of specific aspects have been discussed. This final section provides a summary comment on these aspects and makes a number of recommendations about educational and ethical issues in clinical hypnosis.

In terms of the nature of hypnosis, much research needs to be conducted to specify more precisely the phenomena and processes involved in hypnosis. Recent research (e.g., Sheehan & McConkey, 1982) has pointed to the value of focusing on the experience of the hypnotized individual, and clinicians would seem to be ideally situated to focus on the nature of hypnosis as it is experienced by their individual clients. Although we know more about the conduct of research in the experimental, than the clinical, setting, methodologies are emerging that allow research to be conducted more easily and more rigorously in the clinical setting (see Chapter 3). Apart from the fact that any clinical application of hypnosis should be tied to a scientific data base, the increased emphasis on accountability in clinical settings suggests that those who employ any clinical technique have an ethical responsibility to investigate that technique (Barlow et al., 1984). Two aspects of clinical hypnosis that need particular investigation are the relevance of hypnotizability and the impact of the hypnotic context. The overemphasis that sometimes occurs on the hypnotic skills of the therapist, rather than the hypnotic abilities of the client, will only be corrected through additional specification of the relevance of hypnotizability to therapeutic process and outcome. Similarly, there is a need to more carefully specify and understand the impact of the hypnotic context on both client and therapist. In particular, research is needed to delineate the specific effects of the experience of hypnosis as opposed to the nonspecific effects of the hypnotic context. Overall, the hypnosis practitioner has a responsibility to understand what aspects of hypnosis lead, or do not lead, to therapeutic gain. Only with such an understanding in hand can the therapist determine how hypnotic techniques are best used to facilitate an individual's physical and psychological well-being.

In terms of attitudes toward hypnosis, there is a need for additional data about public attitudes toward hypnosis, and the influences that shape those attitudes. This type of data would be of value to therapists because it would allow them to determine how to best approach and modify the attitudes that their clients bring into the clinical setting. Given the range of misinformation that is available about hypnosis, therapists should take particular care to discuss the use of hypnosis with clients, should review and clarify clients' views about hypnosis, and should provide a full reply to questions about hypnosis. Because it is often difficult to provide information about hypnosis (or any clinical technique, for that matter) in a way that is both accurate and understandable by clients, therapists could prepare themselves by either reading material that deals directly with this issue (e.g., Hodge, 1974) or by obtaining brochures about hypnosis that have been designed for clients (e.g., Kohn, 1981; Webster, 1982). Although such educational brochures vary in the emphases that they make, they do provide a useful way of orienting clients to hypnosis as well as stimulating them to raise any misgivings about its use. Given that many professionals hold misconceptions and negative attitudes about hypnosis, those who use hypnosis should be prepared to provide accurate information about the benefits and limitations of clinical hypnosis to colleagues. One approach to improving communication about hypnosis was outlined by Olness (1977) who offered an in-service educational program that appeared to improve attitudes toward hypnosis and facilitated the use of hypnosis in a children's hospital. Professional societies are becoming increasingly concerned about the misinformation that is available about hypnosis and are more actively informing both the public and professionals about hypnosis and its appropriate application. For example, APA Division 30 is beginning to disseminate official statements regarding its views of the nature and application of psychological hypnosis (Edmonston, Levitt, & Wick, 1983; for information contact: Eugene E. Levitt, Department of Psychiatry, Institute of Psychiatric Research, Indiana University, 1100 West Michigan Street, Indianapolis, IN 46223). Such communication is important because it not only serves to legitimize the use of hypnosis among professionals, but also highlights the potential relevance of hypnosis as an appropriate treatment technique. Overall, those who employ hypnosis have a responsibility to ensure, through both individual and collective efforts, that accurate information becomes more widely available to members of the public and professional groups alike.

In terms of training in hypnosis, one issue that needs further consideration is the differences in hypnosis training that exist across the various health professionals who employ hypnosis. For instance, psychology programs appear to provide the most complete (i.e., theoretical, experimental, and clinical aspects) and the most integrated (i.e., hypnosis is simply one technique to have available) training in hypnosis, and the implications of this for interdisciplinary interaction and professional relationships in the area of hypnosis need to be considered carefully. Another issue is variability in training approach and quality of training in the area of hypnosis. Clearly, those who are seeking training in hypnosis should examine carefully the credentials and experience of those offering the training. Specifically, the trainers and supervisors not only should be well-trained themselves but also should have the support of university and/or professional society resources; the professional society programs recommended in this chapter meet these criteria. These professional societies also take a clear stand on the unethical use of hypnosis by unqualified personnel, and involvement in these societies can encourage a more active responsibility in alerting the public to the risks involved in the irresponsible use of hypnosis and the protection provided by ethical, professional practice.

In terms of professional concerns about hypnosis, it is clear that a gap sometimes exists between clinical and experimental hypnosis. It is clear also, however, that both the hypnosis practitioner and researcher need to work collaboratively in order to understand the phenomenon of hypnosis fully and to apply the techniques of hypnosis most effectively. Research is a vital part of the activities of any clinician who wishes not only to contribute to individual well-being but also to advance knowledge through scientifc observation, and there are many research strategies that can be integrated into clinical practice (e.g., Barlow et al., 1984). One area in which scientists and practitioners converge is in their general viewpoint that support should not be given to the use of hypnosis by laypersons. The forensic use of hypnosis was discussed in this respect, and it is important to recognize the general opposition that is emerging to the use of hypnosis by law enforcement personnel, and the professional risks that are involved in supporting such uses.

In terms of therapeutic concerns about hypnosis, it is clear that hypnosis is not a dangerous procedure and cannot be used for antisocial purposes, although negative events (both intentional and unintentional) can occur because of the nature of the therapeutic relationship when hypnosis is involved. Further specification is needed of the exact nature of the hypnotic relationship and of the limits of interpersonal interactions in the hypnotic situation. In addition, specification is needed of the personal involvement of the hypnotist in the hypnotic interaction, since much clinical data point to the need for therapists who use hypnosis to be attuned to their own motivations and behaviors during the use of hypnosis. Overall, research and clinical observation could usefully focus on the contextual shift associated with the introduction of hypnosis.

Finally, education and ethical issues in the area of hypnosis will continue to evolve over time. Many of the issues discussed here are complex ones, and the position adopted in this chapter reflects current findings and informed opinion. New information becomes available and changes in opinion occur, of course. Those new to hypnosis need to become informed about the concerns of the area. As importantly, however, they have the opportunity to contribute to and guide the future course of clinical hypnosis.

REFERENCES

American Board of Examiners in Psychological Hypnosis. (1961). Report. *American Psychologist, 16,* 203-205.

Ault, R. L., Jr. (1979). FBI guidelines for use of hypnosis. *International Journal of Clinical and Experimental Hypnosis, 27,* 449-451.

Barlow, D. H., Hayes, S. C., & Nelson, R. O. (1984). *The scientist-practitioner: Research and accountability in clinical and educational settings.* New York: Pergamon Press.

Burrows, G. D. (1980). Affective disorders and hypnosis. In G. D. Burrows & L. Dennerstein (Eds.), *Handbook of hypnosis and psychosomatic medicine.* Amsterdam: Elsevier/North-Holland.

Burrows, G. D., & Dennerstein, L. (1979). Teaching hypnosis in Victoria. *Australian Journal of Clinical and Experimental Hypnosis, 7,* 207-213.

Call, J. D. (1976). Children, parents, and hypnosis: A discussion. *International Journal of Clinical and Experimental Hypnosis, 24,* 149-155.

Carter, D. J. (1982). The use of hypnosis to refresh memory: Invaluable tool or dangerous device? *Washington University Law Quarterly, 60,* 1059-1085.

Clarke, J. C., & Jackson, J. A. (1983). *Hypnosis and behavior therapy: The treatment of anxiety and phobias.* New York: Springer.

Coe, W. C. (1977). The problem of relevance versus ethics in researching hypnosis and antisocial conduct. *Annals of the New York Academy of Sciences, 296,* 90–104.

Coe, W. C., & Ryken, K. (1979). Hypnosis and risks to human subjects. *American Psychologist, 34,* 673–681.

Conn, J. H. (1972). Is hypnosis really dangerous? *International Journal of Clinical and Experimental Hypnosis, 20,* 61–79.

Conn, J. H. (1981). The myth of coercion through hypnosis: A brief communication. *International Journal of Clinical and Experimental Hypnosis, 29,* 95–100.

Crasilneck, H. B., & Hall, J. A. (1975). *Clinical hypnosis: Principles and applications.* New York: Grune & Stratton.

Crawford, H. J., Hilgard, J. R., & Macdonald, H. (1982). Transient experiences following hypnotic testing and special termination procedures. *International Journal of Clinical and Experimental Hypnosis, 30,* 117–126.

Diamond, B. L. (1980). Inherent problems in the use of pretrial hypnosis on a prospective witness. *California Law Review, 68,* 313–349.

Dorcus, R. M. (1958). Editorial. Training in hypnosis for therapy. *Journal of Clinical and Experimental Hypnosis, 6,* i–iv.

Edmonston, W. E., Jr., Levitt, E. E., & Wick, E. E. (1983, December). Project enlightenment. *Division 30 Newsletter,* p. 3.

Faw, V., Sellers, D. J., & Wilcox, W. W. (1968). Psychopathological effects of hypnosis. *International Journal of Clinical and Experimental Hypnosis, 16,* 26–37.

Frankel, F. H. (1978). The relationship between research and clinical practice: Bridging the gap. *Australian Journal of Clinical and Experimental Hypnosis, 6,* 7–15.

Frankel, F. H. (1981). Reporting hypnosis in the medical context: A brief communication. *International Journal of Clinical and Experimental Hypnosis, 29,* 10–14.

Frankel, F. H. (1982). Hypnosis and hypnotizability scales: A reply. *International Journal of Clinical and Experimental Hypnosis, 30,* 377–392.

Frankel, F. H., Apfel, R. J., Kelley, S. F., Benson, H., Quinn, T., Newmark, J., & Malmaud, R. (1979). The use of hynotizability scales in the clinic: A review after six years. *International Journal of Clinical and Experimental Hypnosis, 27,* 63–73.

Fredericks, L. E. (1978). Teaching hypnosis in the overall approach to the surgical patient. *American Journal of Clinical Hypnosis, 20,* 175–183.

Fredericks, L. E. (1980). The value of teaching hypnosis in the practice of anesthesiology. *International Journal of Clinical and Experimental Hypnosis, 28,* 6–15.

Fromm, E. (1968). Transference and countertransferences in hypnoanalysis. *International Journal of Clinical and Experimental Hypnosis, 16,* 77–84.

Fromm, E. (1981). How to write a clinical paper: A brief communication. *International Journal of Clinical and Experimental Hypnosis, 29,* 5–9.

Gardner, G. G. (1974). Parents: Obstacles or allies in child hypnotherapy. *American Journal of Clinical Hypnosis, 17,* 44–49.

Gardner, G. G. (1976). Attitudes of child health professionals toward hypnosis: Implications for training. *International Journal of Clinical and Experimental Hypnosis, 24,* 63–73.

Gardner, G. G., & Olness, K. (1981). *Hypnosis and hypnotherapy with children.* New York: Grune & Stratton.

Gruenewald, D. (1971). Transference and countertransference in hypnosis. *International Journal of Clinical and Experimental Hypnosis, 19,* 71–82.

Gruenewald, D. (1982a). Some thoughts on the distinction between the hypnotic situation and the hypnotic condition. *American Journal of Clinical Hypnosis, 25,* 46–51.

Gruenewald, D. (1982b). Problems of relevance in the application of laboratory data to clinical situations. *International Journal of Clinical and Experimental Hypnosis, 30,* 345-353.

Gubel, I. (1973). From hypnosis to sophrology: Eleven years of teaching. *American Journal of Clinical Hypnosis, 15,* 258-262.

Hartland, J. (1968). Education in hypnosis. *American Journal of Clinical Hypnosis, 11,* 119-124.

Haynes, J. P. (1983). An empirical method for determining core psychology journals. *American Psychologist, 38,* 959-962.

Hibbard, W. S., & Worring, R. W. (1981). *Forensic hypnosis: The practical application of hypnosis in criminal investigations.* Springfield, IL: Charles C. Thomas.

Hilgard, E. R. (1965). *Hypnotic susceptbility.* New York: Harcourt, Brace, & World.

Hilgard, E. R. (1978/79). The Stanford hypnotic susceptibility scales as related to other measures of hypnotic responsiveness. *American Journal of Clinical Hypnosis, 21,* 68-83.

Hilgard, E. R., & Hilgard, J. R. (1975). *Hypnosis in the relief of pain.* Los Altos, CA: William Kaufman.

Hilgard, J. R. (1974). Sequelae to hypnosis. *International Journal of Clinical and Experimental Hypnosis, 22,* 291-298.

Hilgard, J. R., Hilgard, E. R., & Newman, M. (1961). Sequelae to hypnosis with special reference to earlier chemical anesthesia. *Journal of Nervous and Mental Disease, 133,* 461-478.

Hodge, J. R. (1974). What patients may ask about hypnosis. *Medical Times, 102,* 123-133.

International Society of Hypnosis. (1982). *Membership Directory.* Philadelphia: Author.

Kleinhauz, M., & Beran, B. (1981). Misuses of hypnosis: A medical emergency and its treatment. *International Journal of Clinical and Experimental Hypnosis, 29,* 148-161.

Kleinhauz, M., Dreyfuss, D. A., Beran, B., Goldberg, T., & Azikri, D. (1979). Some aftereffects of stage hypnosis: A case study of psychopathological manifestations. *International Journal of Clinical and Experimental Hypnosis, 27,* 219-226.

Kline, M. V. (1972). The production of antisocial behavior through hypnosis: New clinical data. *International Journal of Clinical and Experimental Hypnosis, 20,* 80-94.

Kohn, H. (1981). *Modern clinical hypnosis: An educational brochure.* San Jose, CA: California Society of Clinical Hypnosis.

Kost, P. F. (1965). Dangers of hypnosis. *International Journal of Clinical and Experimental Hypnosis, 13,* 220-225.

Kraft, W. A., & Rodolfa, E. R. (1982). The use of hypnosis among psychologists. *American Journal of Clinical Hypnosis, 24,* 249-257.

Levitt, E. E., & Baker, E. L. (1983). The hypnotic relationship—Another look at coercion, compliance and resistance: A brief communication. *International Journal of Clinical and Experimental Hypnosis, 31,* 125-131.

London, P. (1961). Subject characteristics in hypnosis research: Part I. A survey of experience, interest, and opinion. *International Journal of Clinical and Experimental Hypnosis, 9,* 151-161.

McConkey, K. M. (1984). Clinical hypnosis: Differential impact on volitional and nonvolitional disorders. *Canadian Psychology, 25,* 79-83.

McIntosh, I. B., & Hawney, M. (1983). Patient attitudes to hypnotherapy in a general medical practice: A brief communication. *International Journal of Clinical and Experimental Hypnosis, 31,* 219-223.

Moss, C. S., Logan, J. C., & Lynch, D. (1962). Present status of psychological research and training in hypnosis: A developing professional problem. *American Psychologist, 17,* 542-549.

Moss, C. S., Riggen, G., Coyne, L., & Bishop, W. (1965). Some correlates of the use (or disuse) of hypnosis by experienced psychologist-therapists. *International Journal of Clinical and Experimental Hypnosis, 13,* 39-50.

Mott, T. (1979). The clinical importance of hypnotizability. *American Journal of Clinical Hypnosis, 21,* 263-269.

Olness, K. (1977). In-service hypnosis education in a children's hospital. *American Journal of Clinical Hypnosis, 20,* 80-83.

Orne, M. T. (1959). The nature of hypnosis: Artifact and essence. *Journal of Abnormal and Social Psychology, 58,* 277-299.

Orne, M. T. (1965). Undesirable effects of hypnosis: The determinants and management. *International Journal of Clinical and Experimental Hypnosis, 13,* 226-237.

Orne, M. T. (1972). Can a hypnotized subject be compelled to carry out otherwise unacceptable behavior? A discussion. *International Journal of Clinical and Experimental Hypnosis, 20,* 101-117.

Orne, M. T. (1977). The construct of hypnosis: Implications of the definition for research and practice. *Annals of the New York Academy of Sciences, 296,* 14-33.

Orne, M. T. (1979). The use and misuse of hypnosis in courts. *International Journal of Clinical and Experimental Hypnosis, 27,* 311-341.

Orne, M. T. (1981). The why and how of a contribution to the literature: A brief communication. *International Journal of Clinical and Experimental Hypnosis, 29,* 1-4.

Orne, M. T., & Hammer, A. G. (1974). Hypnosis. *Encyclopaedia Britannica* (Vol. 15). Chicago, IL: Benton.

Orne, M. T., & McConkey, K. M. (1982). Hypnosis and self-hypnosis. In L. Kristal (Ed.), *The ABC of psychology.* New York: Penguin Books.

Parrish, M. J. (1975). Predoctoral training in clinical hypnosis: A national survey of availability and educator attitudes in schools of medicine, dentistry, and graduate clinical psychology. *International Journal of Clinical and Experimental Hypnosis, 23,* 249-265.

Perry, C. (1979). Hypnotic coercion and compliance to it: A review of evidence presented in a legal case. *International Journal of Clinical and Experimental Hypnosis, 27,* 187-218.

Perry, C., Gelfand, R., & Marcovitch, P. (1979). The relevance of hypnotic susceptibility in the clinical context. *Journal of Abnormal Psychology, 88,* 592-603.

Perry, C., & Laurence, J. -R. (1982) [Review of *Handbook of investigative hypnosis*]. *International Journal of Clinical and Experimental Hypnosis, 30,* 443-448.

Pulver, S. E., & Pulver, M. P. (1975). Hypnosis in medical and dental practice: A survey. *International Journal of Clinical and Experimental Hypnosis, 23,* 28-47.

Pulver, S. E., & Smith, L. H. (1961). Teaching medical hypnosis: A pilot course at a university medical school. *Comprehensive Psychiatry, 2,* 157-162.

Reiser, M. (1980). *Handbook of investigative hypnosis.* Los Angeles: LEHI.

Rodolfa, E. R., Kraft, W. A., Reilley, R. R., & Blackmore, S. H. (1982). Hypnosis training in APA and non-APA approved clinical/counseling doctoral programs. *Professional Psychology, 13,* 670-673.

Rodolfa, E. R., Kraft, W. A., Reilley, R. R., & Blackmore, S. H. (1983). The status of research and training in hypnosis at APA accredited clinical/counseling psychology internship sites: A national survey. *International Journal of Clinical and Experimental Hypnosis, 31,* 284-292.

Ruffra, P. S. (1983). Hynotically induced testimony: Should it be admitted? *Criminal Law Bulletin, 19,* 293-324.

Sacerdote, P. (1974). Convergence of expectations: An essential component for successful hypnotherapy. *International Journal of Clinical and Experimental Hypnosis, 22,* 95–111.

Sacerdote, P. (1982). A non-statistical dissertation about hynotizability scales and clinical goals: Comparisons with individualized induction and deepening procedures. *International Journal of Clinical and Experimental Hypnosis, 30,* 354–376.

Schneck, J. M. (1953). An outline of the development of the Society for Clinical and Experimental Hypnosis. *Journal of Clinical and Experimental Hypnosis, 1,* 2.

Sheehan, P. W. (1977). Antisocial behavior in hypnosis: Some theoretical and professional issues. *Australian Journal of Clinical Hypnosis, 5,* 79–85.

Sheehan, P. W. (1979). Clinical and research hypnosis: Toward rapprochement. *Australian Journal of Clinical and Experimental Hypnosis, 7,* 135–146.

Sheehan, P. W. (1980). Factors influencing rapport in hypnosis. *Journal of Abnormal Psychology, 89,* 263–281.

Sheehan, P. W., Dolby, R. M., & McDermott, D. (1975). Report on hypnotherapy clinics and their function. *Australian Psychologist, 10,* 213–224.

Sheehan, P. W., & McConkey, K. M. (1979). Hypnosis in Australia: A survey of the membership of the Australian Society for Clinical and Experimental Hypnosis. [Monograph]. *Australian Journal of Clinical and Experimental Hypnosis, 7,* 43–101.

Sheehan, P. W., & McConkey, K. M. (1982). *Hypnosis and experience: The exploration of phenomena and process.* Hillsdale, NJ: Erlbaum.

Shor, R. E. (1959). Hypnosis and the concept of the generalized reality-orientation. *American Journal of Psychotherapy, 13,* 582–602.

Society for Clinical and Experimental Hypnosis. (1979). Resolution. *International Journal of Clinical and Experimental Hypnosis, 27,* 452.

Society for Clinical and Experimental Hypnosis (1981). *SCEH Directory.* Liverpool, NY: Author.

Udolf, R. (1981). *Handbook of hypnosis for professionals.* New York: Van Nostrand Reinhold.

Valett, R. E. (1962). Psychological training in hypnosis in New Zealand. *International Journal of Clinical and Experimental Hypnosis, 10,* 119–121.

van der Walde, P. H. (1974). Patient's preference for treatment: Attitudes toward hypnosis. *International Journal of Clinical and Experimental Hypnosis, 22,* 46–53.

Verberne, T. (1976). Clinical hypnosis in Australia: The 1974/75 survey of full members of the Australian Society for Clinical and Experimental Hypnosis. *Australian Journal of Clinical Hypnosis, 4,* 4–8.

Wadden, T. A., & Anderton, C. H. (1982). The clinical use of hypnosis. *Psychological Bulletin, 91,* 215–243.

Wald, A., & Kline, M. V. (1955). A university training program in clinical hypnosis. *Journal of Clinical and Experimental Hypnosis, 3,* 183–187.

Watkins, J. G. (1972). Antisocial behavior under hypnosis. Possible or impossible? *International Journal of Clinical and Experimental Hypnosis, 20,* 95–100.

Webster, W. C. (1982). *Questions and answers about clinical hypnosis.* Columbus, OH: Ohio Psychology Publishing.

West, L. J., & Deckert, G. H. (1965). Dangers of hypnosis. *Journal of the American Medical Association, 192,* 9–12.

Woody, R. H., & Herr, E. L. (1966). Psychologists and hypnosis: Part II. Use in educational settings. *American Journal of Clinical Hypnosis, 9,* 254–256.

Woody, R. H., Houck, J. E., & Thompson, K. F. (1969). Proposals for education and training in clinical hypnosis. *American Journal of Clinical Hypnosis, 12,* 95–99.

Chapter 13

Future Directions of Hypnosis

Frank A. De Piano
Nova University

Herman C. Salzberg
University of South Carolina

Review of the chapters contained in this text gives an indication of the widely varying set of disorders with which hypnosis has been successfully (and in some cases unsuccessfully) employed. Certainly as one reviews each of these areas both obvious and more subtle recommendations for future research and better presented clinical application come into focus. These issues have been discussed in each of the individual chapters and need not be rediscussed here. If one is to view the various content areas as a group, it is clear that some areas have been more active, both in terms of research and clinical practice (although there does not always appear to be a strong correspondence between activity in research and acitivity in clinical practice). For example, hypnosis in pain management, due largely to the work of E. Hilgard, P. Sacerdote and their associates, appears to have been especially active. In recent years innovative and parsimonious theories have been developed in order to explain the interaction between hypnosis and pain management. One might predict that, due to this rich theorizing, the area of hypnosis in pain management will continue to develop.

Other areas, such as those associated with smoking, weight management, and cognitive performance, appear ripe for theory development. In each of these areas, substantial amounts of laboratory and clinical data have been compiled. Much of these data, however, appear to be fragmented and unrelated. These growing bodies of literature are much in need of solid theorizing which attempts to account for all facets of the data as opposed to individual aspects of them. With these areas, the authors are reminded of other areas within the behavioral sciences which have accumulated large amounts of seemingly contradictory data, but which when pulled together by creative theorizing have suddenly appeared to "make sense." For example, within social psychology, the area of social facilitation has had a long history of seemingly inconsistent findings. Not until Zajonc (1965) reviewed multiple aspects of these data, and tied the findings together, did one obtain a sense of comprehension of this field.

Still other areas discussed in this text are in need of extended information gathering, both in the laboratory and in the field, before any intelligent theorizing can begin. For example, few data have been accumulated in the areas of treatment of phobias, enhanced physical performance, and forensic applications of hypnosis. Theorizing in these areas would be premature and misleading in that not enough has yet been observed. Theorizing might well prove misleading in that many "facts" are yet to be identified.

Finally, other areas such as those associated with catharsis and uncovering therapies and, to a less extent, those involving psychosomatic disorders have not been operationalized to the point where intelligent data gathering can proceed. For example, the researcher interested in examining aspects of catharsis does not have a generally acceptable operationalized definition readily available. Thus, only anecdotal data have been accumulated to date. Due to this deficit in operationalizing these areas, there appears to be little likelihood of growth and expansion in the near future. As a result, it is likely that the clinical utilization of hypnosis in these areas will be restricted to those who are committed to the efficacy of hypnosis a priori.

To summarize, it appears that to make predictions and recommendations about hypnosis as a field is as sensible as making recommendations about medicine or psychology as fields. Only when statements are made with specific reference to well-defined areas within each of these more general conceptual areas can we begin to make sense.

Another approach in attempting to anticipate the future direction of hypnosis is to understand it in respect to other areas within the behavioral sciences in general, and psychology and behavior change in particular.

First, that hypnosis has undergone criticism, disfavor, discredit, and general periods of decline in popularity (both in lay and professional circles) and yet has maintained enough professional interest to be regularly taught as part of the curriculum for clinical psychologists, physicians, dentist, and other areas is a testimony to the perceived potential efficacy of this mode of behavior change. In part, this "longevity" of hypnosis can be attributed to the rather profound behavior effects manifested in a relatively brief period of time by those hypnotized. For example, the hypnotized individual, asked to talk about aspects of his or her life, or utilize imagery to an extensive degree, will be able to do so quite readily. While it is true that a nonhypnotized individual will be capable of much the same behavior, the *willingness* to engage in such behavior can only be attained after much relationship building has occurred.

After a rather brief hypnotic induction, the hypnotized individual engages in rather profound behavior change, that is, body posture changes, speed of verbalization changes, emotional changes occur, and so on. These changes, while possible under a variety of conditions, simply do not occur as readily under many of the other conditions. It is perhaps this aspect of hypnosis—the fact that behavior changes rapidly and profoundly—which continues to draw those who are interested in behavior change.

As one continues to compare hypnosis to other areas, it is difficult not to be impressed with the level of sophistication which has developed in this field. This sophistication is due largely to the rigorous and constructively critical approaches taken by those involved in the area, such as E. Hilgard, M. Orne, and T. X. Barber. Orne's contribution of the notion of demand characteristics has greatly enhanced to research methodology in general and hypnosis in particular. Few published studies in hypnosis fail to address this concept. Likewise, the control for motivational factors advocated by Barber has driven the researcher to determine to what extent ***beyond motivation*** hypnosis enhances performance, reduces pain, and so on.

When one compares these developments to other areas involved with behavior change one can only be struck with the relative sophistication in the area of hypnosis research. For example, the behavioral orientation within psychotherapy is generally regarded as one of the most rigorous areas within the field of behavior change. Few behavior modification studies, however, meaningfully attempt to ferret out differences between demand characteristics of setting the "true effects" due to the behavior modification per se. Many hypnosis studies, however, do precisely this.

This is not to say that there are not numerous studies within the field which continue to be plagued by methodological shortcomings. The variability among hypnosis methodologists is great; however, the methodological refinements continue to grow and the proportion of sound studies is on the rise.

Hypnosis will continue to be an area of both intrigue and professional curiosity. Perhaps as systematic research progresses some of those individuals drawn by the more sensationalistic aspects of the phenomena will lose interest. However, those scientifically curious, who had heretofore been turned off by the exaggerated claims and lack of methodological vigor, will be drawn into the field.

REFERENCE

Zajonc, R. B. (1965). Social facilitation. *Science, 149,* 269-274.

Author Index

Subject Index